T0319376

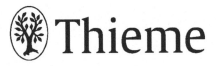

Cervical Spondylotic Myelopathy and Ossification of Posterior Longitudinal Ligament

WFNS Spine Committee Book

Mehmet Zileli, MD
Professor of Neurosurgery
Department of Neurosurgery
Ege University
Izmir, Turkey

Jutty Parthiban, MD, FNS
Head of Department of Neurosurgery;
Course Director for National Board of Examination
Kovai Medical Center and Hospital
Coimbatore, Tamil Nadu, India

Thieme
Delhi • Stuttgart • New York • Rio de Janeiro

Publishing Director: Ritu Sharma
Development Editor: Dr Gurvinder Kaur
Director- Editorial Services: Rachna Sinha
Project Managers: Snehil Sharma and Arindam Banerjee
Vice President, Sales and Marketing: Arun Kumar Majji
Managing Director & CEO: Ajit Kohli

Thieme Medical and Scientific Publishers Private
Limited.
A - 12, Second Floor, Sector - 2, Noida - 201 301,
Uttar Pradesh, India, +911204556600
Email: customerservice@thieme.in
www.thieme.in

Cover design: Thieme Publishing Group
Typesetting by RECTO Graphics, India

Printed in India

5 4 3 2

ISBN 978-93-90553-20-4
Also available as e-book:
eISBN 978-93-90553-28-0

Important note: Medicine is an ever-changing science undergoing continual development. Research and clinical experience are continually expanding our knowledge, in particular, our knowledge of proper treatment and drug therapy. Insofar as this book mentions any dosage or application, readers may rest assured that the authors, editors, and publishers have made every effort to ensure that such references are in accordance with **the state of knowledge at the time of production of the book.**

Nevertheless, this does not involve, imply, or express any guarantee or responsibility on the part of the publishers in respect to any dosage instructions and forms of applications stated in the book. **Every user is requested to examine carefully** the manufacturers' leaflets accompanying each drug and to check, if necessary, in consultation with a physician or specialist, whether the dosage schedules mentioned therein or the contraindications stated by the manufacturers differ from the statements made in the present book. Such examination is particularly important with drugs that are either rarely used or have been newly released in the market. Every dosage schedule or every form of application used is entirely at the user's own risk and responsibility. The authors and publishers request every user to report to the publishers any discrepancies or inaccuracies noticed. If errors in this work are found after publication, errata will be posted at www.thieme. com on the product description page.

Some of the product names, patents, and registered designs referred to in this book are in fact registered trademarks or proprietary names even though specific reference to this fact is not always made in the text. Therefore, the appearance of a name without designation as proprietary is not to be construed as a representation by the publisher that it is in the public domain.

Contents

Foreword

Spinal surgery is a large section of neurosurgery. It is evolving fast and new diagnostic and surgical techniques are emerging. It has also a conjunction with orthopaedics and creates a competence for many years.

Cervical spondylotic myelopathy and ossification of posterior longitudinal ligament (OPLL) is one of the most challenging subjects of spinal surgery. I congratulate Dr. Mehmet Zileli and Dr. Jutty Parthiban for preparing a comprehensive book with 28 chapters discussing all aspects of the topic.

The WFNS Spine Committee has done a tremendous work during the last 4 years. It undertakes many educational activities, including live courses, webinars, virtual symposia, and consensus meetings. The committee also published recommendations for some common spinal disorders. This book is an addition to the multiple productions of the committee.

Franco Servadei, MD
President
World Federation of Neurosurgical Societies
Milan, Italy

Foreword

I feel privileged and honored to write the foreword to the book titled *Cervical Spondylotic Myelopathy and Ossification of Posterior Longitudinal Ligament*, edited by Dr. Mehmet Zileli and Dr. Jutty Parthiban. As Founder and President of Neuro Spinal Surgeons Association of India, and former Chairman of WFNS Spine Committee, it is my privilege to write this foreword.

This monograph will prove to be very valuable as it contains comprehensive knowledge on the subject. The question that arises is the necessity for such a publication in the era of the digital world. I am convinced that even today books have a tremendous role to play as these are comprehensive resources, backed by expertise and experience, such as this one, as compared to the information easily available on the internet which is widespread, yet unverified most times.

Once this book is available on the internet, the interested students, undergraduate and postgraduate, can download it on their tablets and read it at leisure anywhere and at any time.

I have gone through the manuscript and I am really happy that the monograph contains all that teachers and postgraduate students need. Chapter 1 compiled by Dr. George Dohrmann, et al is informative and gripping, particularly for the doctors who are interested in the history of CSM and OPLL. The section on the operative treatment of this ailment, compiled elaborately by Dr. Salman Sharif et al, is knowledgeable. It is indeed a difficult proposition, even for the experts, to select the right patient for the right type of surgical decompression and stabilization, in order to achieve fusion. Overwhelming advances in technology and the enormous choice of implants call for astute judgment by the surgeon, if one has to achieve success.

CSM tends to be diffused with myelomalacia and in many cases, it is associated with diffuse idiopathic skeletal hyperostosis (DISH). In addition to this, Dr. Kiyoshi Hirabayashi also felt that the anterior approach created several complications in patients, thus, he started posterior laminoplasty. OPLL is no more restricted to Far East countries and is seen commonly in most countries these days; however, Dr. Mehmet Zileli has rightly pointed out in Chapter 3 that it is still more common in Asian countries. K-line is often involved in diffuse OPLL when sagittal alignment of the cervical spine is disturbed. Biomechanics, environmental, genetic, and biochemical factors play an important role in its production.

A surgical approach is important, but it is my perception that conservative management with physiotherapy is much more significant. Such patients are elderly and have a compromised breathing power along with weak muscles and weakened mental capacity. Physiotherapy specialists have an important role to play to compose the minds, improve breathing power, stabilize gait, and strengthen muscles along with mobilization of joints. Home therapy has been advocated in many countries. There should be a special team to improve the morale of these patients and rehabilitate them in the society.

Minimally invasive spinal surgery and endoscopic spinal surgery are making life more comfortable for the patients. These techniques are replacing traditional surgical approaches that we practiced. Dr. Enrique Osorio-Fonseca, an expert in this field, has illustratively outlined in Chapter 23 the benefits of this surgical procedure.

It is much easier to write a monograph single-handedly than with multiple contributions coming from 59 authors for 28 chapters, as mentioned by Dr. Zileli and Dr. Parthiban in the preface. To assemble such a monograph appears to be a herculean task but with patience, modesty, perseverance, and tenacity, both have succeeded. I congratulate them and admire their patience.

The monograph is indeed thought-provoking and has the power to motivate surgeons to rise and act, and make a difference in patients' lives. I find the monograph anecdotal and aphoristic for doctors, as well as for researchers interested in this aspect of medicine.

I wish the monograph a big success and once again congratulate Dr. Mehmet Zileli and Dr. Jutty Parthiban for their patience and tenacity.

P. S. Ramani, MD
Professor and Head
Department of Neuro-spinal surgery
Lilavati Hospital and Research Centre;
Retd. Professor and Head
Department of Neuro-spinal surgery
University of Mumbai
Mumbai, Maharashtra, India

Foreword

Cervical Spondylotic Myelopathy and OPLL: WFNS Spine Committee Book is a remarkable contribution to the spine literature. It is edited by two surgeons, Dr. Mehmet Zileli and Dr. Jutty Parthiban, with impeccable track records, both as clinicians and as academicians. The preface of this book clearly outlines the content and rationale of the book. There is no need to repeat them here, as it has been well-captured by the editors in the preface.

The book is both well-written and well-illustrated. It is a comprehensive resource laid out to provide information in a logical and sequential manner. In this vein, the book could be used as both a reference source and a textbook to be read from cover to cover. The editors have done a remarkable job of crafting a creative infrastructure that facilitates the transmission of information in an efficient and pleasing manner.

The book contains 28 chapters written by 59 authors. The list of authors is a veritable international who's who of spine surgeons. Each one of them has done an incredible job of presenting the material at hand in an easy-to-digest manner.

Once they have read the book, all its readers will understand what I meant above about the book being comprehensive and laid out logically and in a sequential manner. I recommend this book to all young and experienced spine surgeons alike. Please read and enjoy.

Edward C. Benzel, MD
Professor of Neurosurgery
Cleveland Clinic
Cleveland, Ohio, USA

Preface

Treatment of neurologic deficits due to cervical spinal stenosis either by degenerative changes or ossification of the posterior longitudinal ligament (OPLL) has been an essential part of spine surgery. Cervical spondylotic myelopathy (CSM) and OPLL are the most common spinal cord diseases in adults following cervical disk disease. The discussion on diagnostic techniques, indications, type of surgeries, and prediction of outcomes continues to be a topic of interest.

The book has 28 chapters written by 59 authors. It starts with the history of CSM and OPLL, followed by pathophysiology, biomechanics, balance measurements, incidence and natural course, clinical tests, differential diagnosis, diagnostic imaging, electrophysiology, treatment options, surgical techniques, minimally invasive approaches, and outcome analysis. Both classical knowledge and recent information are summarized with evidence-based data.

The book contains contemporary information, such as new imaging tools and descriptions of not widely used surgical techniques, such as oblique corpectomy, anterior controllable anterior displacement and fusion (ACAF) surgery for multisegmented OPLL, and anterior and posterior minimally invasive decompression techniques. It also covers the current recommendations of the WFNS Spine Committee, prepared at recent consensus meetings.

Most chapters contain color illustrations and images to facilitate understanding. We believe this book will help understand this challenging subject. Spinal neurosurgeons, orthopaedic spine surgeons, neurologists, physical therapists, current residents in training, and fellows will benefit from it.

This book is not the first of the WFNS Spine Committee books. It was started by our senior chairman Professor P.S. Ramani with his publications *Surgical Management of Cervical Disc Herniation* (2012) and *Textbook on Thoracic Spine* (2016).

The current book is a continuation of multiple productions of the WFNS Spine Committee since 2017. The WFNS Spine Committee is the most active and academic-oriented group of eminent neurosurgeons from around the world, dedicating time and efforts in continuously organizing consensus meetings, publishing articles, and bringing out quality books on spinal disorders and neurospinal surgery. We hope that this collaboration will continue in the future and help propagate the knowledge of neurospinal surgery that helps in understanding and solving spinal disorders all over the world. We are extremely thankful to all the authors for their contribution to this book. We look forward to continuing support in our next endeavors.

We thank Professor Franco Servadei, President, World Federation of Neurosurgical Societies (WFNS), Professor Edward Benzel, Editor-in-Chief, *World Neurosurgery*, and Professor P.S. Ramani, former Chairman, WFNS Spine Committee, for providing forewords.

We are thankful to the staff at Thieme Publishers, Delhi, for their commitment and hard work in bringing out this book.

It is a great feat accomplished during the worldwide pandemic by the contributors and the publisher.

We sincerely thank everyone.

Mehmet Zileli, MD
Jutty Parthiban, MD, FNS

Acknowledgments

Dedicated to WFNS Spine Committee members who spent their precious time and collaborated extensively to achieve many goals.

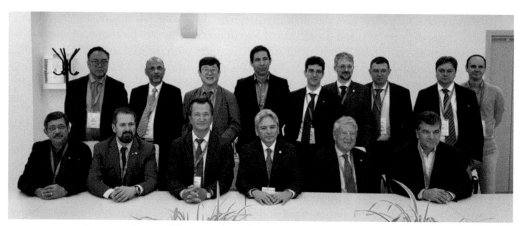

A group photo with some members of the WFNS Spine Committee.

Contributors

Abdul Hafid Bajamal, MD, PhD
Professor
Department of Neurosurgery
Faculty of Medicine
Airlangga University
Dr. Soetomo Academic General Hospital
Surabaya, Indonesia

Achal Gupta, MD
Senior Resident
Department of Neurosurgery
Lilavati Hospital and Research Centre
Mumbai, Maharashtra, India

Anand Kaul, MD
Resident
Department of Neurosurgery
Lewis Katz School of Medicine
Temple University
Philadelphia, Pennsylvania, USA

Anna Prajsnar-Borak, MD
Fellow
Department of Neurosurgery
University Hospital of Saarland and Faculty of
Medicine
University of Saarland
Homburg, Germany

Ben Roitberg, MD
Professor and Chair
Department of Neurological Surgery
Case Western Reserve University
Cleveland, Ohio, USA

Bong-Soo Kim, MD, FAANS
Professor of Neurosurgery
Director, Spine Surgery
Director, Minimally Invasive and Complex Spine
Fellowship Program
Department of Neurosurgery
Lewis Katz School of Medicine
Temple University
Philadelphia, Pennsylvania, USA

Carla D Anania, MD
Associate Professor
Department of Neurosurgery
Humanitas Clinical and Research Center
Rozzano, Italy

Carolina Ramírez-Martínez, MD
Orthopedic Surgeon
Jesús Uson Minimally Invasive Surgery Center
Bogotá, Colombia

D'jamel Kitumba, MD
Department of Neurosurgery
Hospital Lusíadas Porto
Porto, Portugal

Eko Agus Subagio, MD, PhD
Chief of Surabaya Neuroscience Institute
Department of Neurosurgery
Faculty of Medicine
Airlangga University
Dr. Soetomo Academic General Hospital
Surabaya, Indonesia

Enrique Osorio-Fonseca, MD
Neurosurgeon
Chief of Neurosurgery
Loscobos Medical Center;
Associate Professor
Spine Surgery Program
Universidad El Bosque
Bogotá, Colombia

Fabio Galbusera, PhD
Laboratory Head
IRCCS Istituto Ortopedico Galeazzi
Milan, Italy

Fengzeng Jian, MD, PhD
Department of Neurosurgery
Division of Spine
Xuanwu Hospital
Capital Medical University,
Beijing, China

Francesco Costa, MD
Head of the Surgical Spine Oncology Section
Neurosurgery Department
Humanitas Clinical and Research Center
Rozzano, Italy

Gabriel Oswaldo Alonso-Cuéllar, DVM, MSc
Director
Education and Research of the Minimally Invasive
    Spine Center
Bogotá, DC, Colombia

George J. Dohrmann, MD, PhD
Professor
Department of Neurological Surgery
University of Chicago
Chicago, Illinois, USA

Ibet Marie Y. Sih, MD, FAFN, FPCS
Program Director for Neurosurgery
Institute for the Neurosciences
St. Luke's Medical Center
Metro Manila, Philippines

Jesus Lafuente, PhD, MD, FRCS Ed.
Neurosurgeon & Spine Surgeon
Director of Spinal Center
Hospital Universitario del Mar
Barcelona, Spain

Joachim M.K. Oertel, MD
Professor and Head
Department of Neurosurgery
University Hospital of Saarland and Faculty of
Medicine
University of Saarland
Homburg, Germany

João Flávio G. Madureira, MD
School of Medicine UNICEPLAC
Department of Neurosurgery
Hospital Lago Sul
Clínica Quéops Millennium
Brasília, Brazil

Joel Passer, MD
Chief Resident
Department of Neurosurgery
Lewis Katz School of Medicine
Temple University
Philadelphia, Pennsylvania, USA

Jorge Felipe Ramírez-León, MD
Orthopedic surgeon
Minimally Invasive Spine Center;
Reina Sofía Clinic;
Fundación Universitaria Sanitas
Bogotá, DC, Colombia

José Alberto Israel Romero Rangel, MD
Neurosurgeon
Member of the Spine Clinic of the Neurological
    Center
The American-British Cowdray Medical Center IAP
Campus Santa Fe
Mexico City, Mexico

José Antonio Soriano Sánchez, MD
Professor and Head
Spine Clinic of the Neurological Center
The American-British Cowdray Medical Center IAP
Campus Santa Fe
Mexico City, Mexico

José Gabriel Rugeles-Ortíz, MD
Orthopedic surgeon
Minimally Invasive Spine Center;
Reina Sofía Clinic;
Fundación Universitaria Sanitas
Bogotá, DC, Colombia

Jutty Parthiban, MD, FNS
Head of Department of Neurosurgery;
Course Director for National Board of Education
    Neurosurgery
Kovai Medical Center and Hospital
Coimbatore, Tamil Nadu, India

Karlo M. Pedro, MD
Resident
Section of Neurosurgery
Department of Neurosciences
University of the Philippines-Manila
Philippine General Hospital
Metro Manila, Philippines

Khrisna Rangga Permana, MD, PhD
Resident
Department of Neurosurgery
Faculty of Medicine
Airlangga University
Dr. Soetomo Academic General Hospital
Surabaya, Indonesia

Krešimir Rotim, MD, PhD
Professor and Head
Neurosurgery Clinic
UHC Sisters of Mercy
Vinogradska, Zagreb, Croatia

Krishna Sharma, DNB
Associate Professor
Nepal Medical College
Kathmandu University
Kathmandu, Nepal

Marcos Masini, MD, PhD
Professor
School of Medicine UNICEPLAC
Department of Neurosurgery
Hospital Lago Sul
Clínica Quéops Millennium
Brasília, DF, Brazil

Marina Zmajević Schönwald, MD PhD
Head
Unit for Clinical Neurophysiology Monitoring
Neurosurgery Clinic
UHC Sisters of Mercy
Vinogradska, Zagreb, Croatia

Maurizio Fornari, MD
Professor and Director
Department of Neurosurgery
Humanitas University
Milan, Italy

Mehmet Zileli, MD
Professor of Neurosurgery
Department of Neurosurgery
Ege University
Izmir, Turkey

Muhammad Faris, MD, PhD
Head of Spine Division
Department of Neurosurgery
Faculty of Medicine
Airlangga University
Dr. Soetomo Academic General Hospital
Surabaya, Indonesia

Nevhis Akıntürk, MD
Consultant Neurosurgeon
Department of Neurosurgery
Ege University
Bornova, Izmir, Turkey

Nicholas Ahye, MD
Chief Resident
Department of Neurosurgery
Lewis Katz School of Medicine
Temple University
Philadelphia, Pennsylvania, USA

Nicolás Prada-Ramírez, MD
Orthopedic Surgeon
Pontificia Universidad Javeriana
Bogotá, DC, Colombia

Nikolay Konovalov, MD, PhD
Professor and Chairman
Spinal Neurosurgery Department
Burdenko Neurosurgical Center
Moscow, Russia

Nobuyuki Shimokawa, MD
Head
Department of Neurosurgery
Tsykazaki Hospital,
Himeji, Hyogo, Japan

Onur Yaman, MD
Associate Professor
Department of Neurosurgery
Memorial Hospital
Istanbul, Turkey

Oscar L. Alves, MD
Head
Department of Neurosurgery
Hospital Lusíadas Porto
Porto, Portugal

P. S. Ramani, MD
Professor and Head
Department of Neuro-spinal Surgery
Lilavati Hospital and Research Centre;
Retd. Professor and Head
Department of Neuro-spinal surgery
University of Mumbai
Mumbai, Maharashtra, India

R. David Fessler, MD, PhD
Department of Neurosurgery
Rush University Medical Center
Chicago, Illinois, USA

Richard G. Fessler, MD, PhD
Professor
Department of Neurosurgery
Rush University Medical Center
Chicago, Illinois, USA

Rui Reinas, MD
Resident
Department of Neurosurgery
Centro Hospitalar de Vila Nova de Gaia/Espinho
Portugal

Salman Sharif, MD, FRCS(SN), IFAANS
Co-Chair, WFNS Spine Committee
Professor & Chief
Department of Neurosurgery
Liaquat National Hospital & Medical College
Karachi, Pakistan

Sandeep Vaishya, MCh (Neurosurgery)
Executive Director
Department of Neurosurgery
Fortis Memorial Research institute
Gurgaon, Haryana, India

Scott C. Robertson, MD, FACS, FAANS
Adjunct Clinical Professor
University of the Incarnate Word School of
    Osteopathic Medicine;
Director of Neurosurgery
Laredo Medical Center
Laredo Spine &Neurosurgical Associates
Laredo, Texas, USA

Se-Hoon Kim, MD, PhD
Professor and Director of Spinal Neurosurgery
Department of Neurosurgery
Ansan Hospital
Korea University Medical Center
Ansan, Gyeonggi-do, Korea

Stanislav Kaprovoy, MD
Resident
Burdenko Neurosurgical Center
Moscow, Russia

Sumeet Sasane, MD
Junior Consultant
Department of Neurosurgery
Lilavati Hospital and Research Centre
Mumbai, Maharashtra, India

Syed Maroof Ali, MD
Resident
Department of Neurosurgery
Liaquat National Hospital & Medical College
Karachi, Pakistan

Toshihiro Takami, MD
Associate Professor
Chief of Neurospine
Department of Neurosurgery,
Osaka Medical and Pharmaceutical University
Takatsuki, Osaka, Japan

Umesh Srikantha, MD, FMISS
Consultant Neurosurgeon
Head of Spine services
Aster CMI Hospital
Bengaluru, Karnataka, India

Vasiliy Korolishin, MD
Neurosurgeon
Axis Special Hospital
Moscow, Russia

Yousuf Shaikh, MD
Resident
Department of Neurosurgery
Liaquat National Hospital & Medical College
Karachi, Pakistan

Zan Chen, MD, PhD
Professor
Department of Neurosurgery
Division of Spine
Xuanwu Hospital
Capital Medical University,
Beijing, China

Zhenlei Liu, MD
Department of Neurosurgery
Division of Spine
Xuanwu Hospital
Capital Medical University
Beijing, China

01 Cervical Spondylotic Myelopathy: A Historical Review

George J. Dohrmann and Jutty Parthiban

Introduction

The history of operating on the cervical spine is a long one. The first recorded cervical laminectomy was done as part of the mummification process to remove the brain of Tutankhamun, the 18th dynasty pharaoh[1] (**Fig. 1.1**). The first therapeutic laminectomy was attributed to Paul of Aeginia in 600 AD[2] (**Fig. 1.2**).

19th Century

In 1803, Portal described spinal cord compromise related to a degenerative small spinal canal and, therefore, recorded the first description of what is now termed "cervical spondylotic myelopathy"[3] (**Fig. 1.3**). The British surgeon, H.J. Cline, in 1814, performed

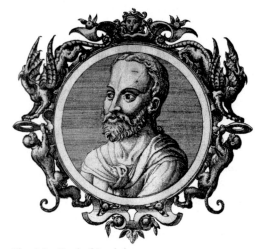

Fig. 1.2 Paul of Aeginia.

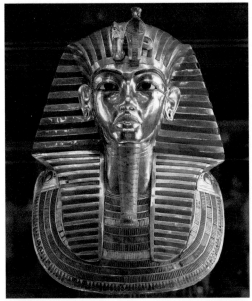

Fig. 1.1 Tutankhamun, 18th dynasty pharaoh.

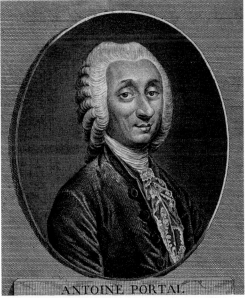

Fig. 1.3 The first description of what is now termed "cervical spondylotic myelopathy" was by A. Portal in 1803.

a multilevel laminectomy to decompress the spinal cord in a patient with a spine fracture, and he reported it in the New England Journal of Medicine in 1815.[4] Two years later in the journal, Lancet, Tyrell reported 100% mortality in patients with spinal dislocation/neurological injury treated surgically.[5] The first laminectomy performed in North America was done in 1828 for relief of paralysis from spinal fracture, and it resulted in what was described as "partial success." The operation was done by Alben Smith, a surgeon in Danville, Kentucky, and he credited the operation a success as the paraplegia "improved."[6]

Another report published in the American Journal of Medical Science in 1835 noted that surgical decompression for paraplegia was discouraging.[7] A bony bar, now known as a "spondylotic bar," causing paraplegia was reported by Key in 1838[8]. "Vertebral exostosis," causing spinal cord compression, was described by Gowers in 1892.[9] The following year William Lane described spondylolisthesis with spinal cord compression causing progressive paralysis, and the paralysis improved after decompressive laminectomy.[10] The discovery of X-rays by Conrad Roentgen in

1895 greatly aided spinal diagnosis and treatment.[11] Makins and Abbott in 1896 reported a successful laminectomy procedure for vertebral osteomyelitis with neural compression.[12]

20th Century

In 1901, British neurosurgeon Victor Horsley decompressed the cervical spinal cord in a patient with progressive neurological decline due to compression, "cervical spondylotic myelopathy"[13] (**Fig. 1.4**). The hemilaminectomy procedure was done by Taylor in 1910.[14] Neurosurgeon Charles Elsberg (**Fig. 1.5**), in 1916, published a book in which he noted "a spinal operation may finally be required in some cases of arthritis or spondylitis on account of compression of the nerve roots or the cord by new-formed bone."[15]. How arthritis in the cervical spine was responsible for spinal cord compression was noted by Elliott in 1926.[16]

Compression of the spinal cord was divided into three regions by Stookey in 1928: (1) comprising half of the posterior region; (2) comprising both halves of the spinal cord; (3) comprising the nerve roots laterally.[17] Between 1929 and 1932, Schmorl,

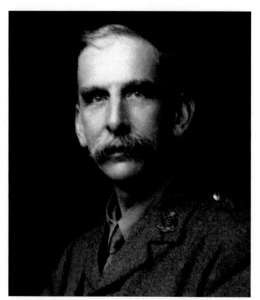

Fig. 1.4 Neurosurgeon, Victor Horsley.

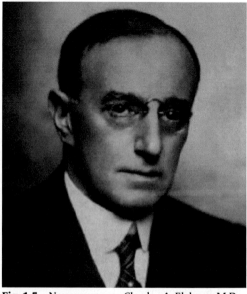

Fig. 1.5 Neurosurgeon, Charles A. Elsberg, M.D.

Junghans, and Andrae described the anatomical and pathologic aspects of intervertebral disc protrusion from the spine. Semmes and Murphy in 1943 described cervical disc rupture and neural compromise.[18] Posterolateral decompression was advocated by Spurling and Scoville in 1944,[19] and by Frykholm[20] in 1947, with long-term follow-up published about laminoforaminotomy ("keyhole facetectomy") by Scoville, Dohrmann and Corkill[21] and long-term follow-up of posterior cervical spine operations by Dohrmann (**Fig. 1.6**) and Hsieh.[22] Brain in 1948 defined spondylosis as a chronic osteophytic process that was more apt to produce myelopathic symptoms.[23] In 1952, Brain, Northfield, and Wilkinson summarized the neurological manifestations of cervical spondylosis.[24]

Anterior Approach

For years, decompression of the spinal cord/nerve roots was done posteriorly; then, in 1955, Robinson and Smith,[25] and in 1958, Smith and Robinson,[26] published their anterior decompression and fusion procedure. In 1958, Cloward (**Fig. 1.7**) published a variation on the anterior cervical decompression/fusion procedure.[27] In 1960, Bailey and Badgley recommended onlay strut grafting to stabilize the cervical spine and decrease cervical spinal cord compression and cervical spinal cord injury from abnormal movement.[28] The natural history of cervical spondylotic myelopathy (no treatment) was published by Lees and Alden-Turner[29] in the British Medical Journal in 1963. Spinal cord and nerve root lesions that develop in association with cervical spondylosis were delineated by Hughes and Wilkinson.[30,31] Verbiest, in 1968, described anterolateral decompression of the cervical spine.[32] Multilevel cervical corpectomies and grafting have been recommended for multilevel cervical spondylosis with considerable anterior compression.[33] Boni et al, in 1984, published the technique called "multiple subtotal somatectomy."[34] Later, this technique was modified and simplified to decrease the rate of possible complications at multiple levels. The lateral walls of the vertebral body were preserved and the central part of the vertebral body was fully removed. The original technique, as described by Boni et al, required modified Cloward instrumentation at multiple levels, widening of the holes at the multiple levels, and

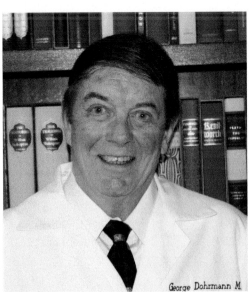

Fig. 1.6 Neurosurgeon, George J. Dohrmann, M.D., Ph.D.

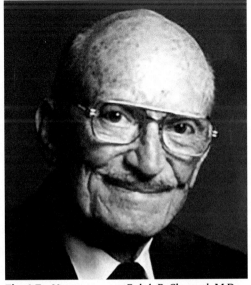

Fig. 1.7 Neurosurgeon, Ralph B. Cloward, M.D.

deepening of the bony trench, with removal of the posterior walls of the vertebral bodies up to the posterior longitudinal ligament and removal of any element compressing the spinal cord.[35]

Laminoplasty

Cervical laminoplasty has been advocated as an alternative to laminectomy to overcome some limitations of laminectomy, in order to treat degenerative cervical spinal stenosis at multiple levels. It all started with Kirita in 1968 who devised a technique to drill out laminae and split them at midline to remove them, in order to achieve total decompression of the spinal cord.[36] It was technically demanding but with fewer complications. In 1973 in Japan, Oyama and Hattori first introduced laminoplasty to prevent post-laminectomy invasion of the laminectomy membrane.[37] This procedure has not been widely accepted because of the technical difficulties of the operation, which are related to the need to thin the entire lamina, in order to perform a Z-plasty at each level. This created long operative times.

To avoid these problems and prevent postlaminectomy instability with consequent malalignment and rigidity, subsequent to fusion, a new surgical technique called "expansive open-door laminoplasty" was devised by Hirabayashi in 1977 (published in 1978) to replace ordinary laminectomy of the cervical spine. This idea came from Hirabayashi's serendipitous observation of the pulsation of the dura mater at the open-door stage of the laminectomy before removing the laminae "en bloc" and while performing a modified Kirita technique[38] (**Figs. 1.8 and 1.9**).[39] It has become the treatment of choice for patients affected by multilevel ossification of the posterior longitudinal ligament. Since then, several laminoplasty techniques have been described and currently used as one of the surgeon's options for posterior decompression operations.

To decrease the incidence of postlaminectomy kyphosis, Ducker and Ziedman[40] summarized the voluminous literature and made recommendations. For severe spondylotic compression of the spinal cord/nerve roots, both anteriorly and posteriorly, the use of postdecompression instrumentation has been summarized by Jackson and Gokaslan.[33]

Further details of spinal surgery technique development, relative to decompression/cervical spondylotic myelopathy/spinal instrumentation, over the years, have been summarized by Alberstone and Benzel[41] (**Fig. 1.10**).

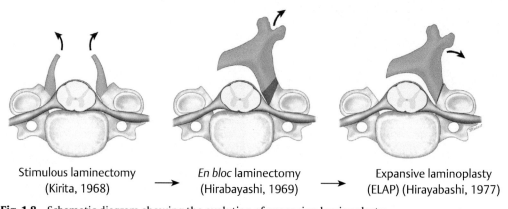

Stimulous laminectomy (Kirita, 1968)	*En bloc* laminectomy (Hirabayashi, 1969)	Expansive laminoplasty (ELAP) (Hirayabashi, 1977)

Fig. 1.8 Schematic diagram showing the evolution of expansion laminoplasty.

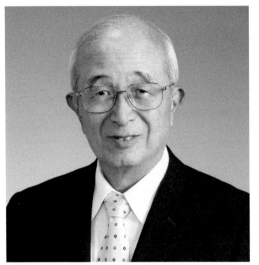

Fig. 1.9 Orthopaedic surgeon, Kiyoshi Hirabayashi, M.D.

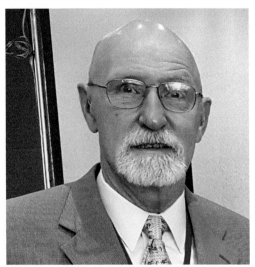

Fig. 1.10 Neurosurgeon, Edward C. Benzel, M.D.

References

1. Fielding JW. Introduction: Cervical spine surgery - past, present, and future potential. In: Camins MB, O'Leary PF, eds. Disorders of the Cervical Spine. Baltimore, MD: Williams and Wilkins; 1992:xxxiii–xxvii
2. Adams F. Paulus Aeginata. Vol. 2. London: Sydenham Society; 1816
3. Portal A. Coursd'AnatomicMedicale on Elements de l'Anatomic de Homme. Vol. 1. Paris: Baudouin; 1803
4. Cline HJ Jr. (cited by Hayward G): An account of a case of fracture and dislocation of the spine. N Engl J Med 1815;4:13
5. Tyrell F. Compression of the spinal marrow from displacement of the vertebrae consequent upon injury. Operation of removing the arch and spinous processes of the vertebrae. Lancet 1827;11:685–688
6. Smith AG. Account of a case in which portions of three dorsal vertebrae were removed for the relief of paralysis from fracture, with partial success. North Am Med Surg J. 1829;8:94–97
7. Rogers DL. A case of fractured spine with decompression of the spinous processes, and the operation for its removal. Am J Med Sci 1835;16:91–94
8. Key C. Guys Hosp Rep 1838;3:17
9. Gowers W. Diseases of the Nervous System. Vol. 1. 2nd ed. London: Churchill; 1892:260
10. Lane WA. Case of spondylolisthesis associated with progressive paraplegia;laminectomy. Lancet 1893;1:991
11. Röentgen WC. Übercine Neve Art Von Strahlen: Sitzungsberichte der Physik Wurzburg. Med Ges 1895;•••:132
12. Makins GH, Abbott FC. On primary osteomyelitis of the vertebrae. Ann Surg 1896; 23(5):510–539
13. Hoff JT. Cervical disc disease and cervical spondylosis. In: Wilkins RH, Rengachary SS, eds. Neurosurgery. New York, NY: McGraw-Hill; 1985:ch286:2230
14. Taylor AS. Unilateral laminectomy. Ann Surg 1910;51(4):529–533
15. Elsberg CA. Diseases of the Spinal Cord and Its Membranes. Philadelphia, PA: WB Saunders; 1916
16. Elliott GR. A contribution to spinal osteoarthritis involving the cervical region. J Bone Joint Surg Am 1926;8:42–52
17. Stookey B. Compression of the spinal cord due to ventral extradural cervical chondromas: Diagnosis and surgical treatment. Arch Neurol Psychiatry 1928;20:275–291
18. Semmes RE, Murphey F. The syndrome of unilateral rupture of the sixth cervical intervertebral disk. JAMA 1943;121:1209–1214
19. Spurling RG, Scoville WB. Lateral rupture of the cervical intervertebral discs. Surg Gynecol Obstet 1944;78:350–358

20. Frykholm R. Deformities of dural pouches and strictures of dural sheaths in the cervical region producing nerve-root compression; a contribution to the etiology and operative treatment of brachial neuralgia. J Neurosurg 1947;4(5):403–413

21. Scoville WB, Dohrmann GJ, Corkill G. Late results of cervical disc surgery. J Neurosurg 1976;45(2):203–210

22. Dohrmann GJ, Hsieh JC. Long-term results of anterior versus posterior operations for herniated cervical discs: analysis of 6,000 patients. Med Princ Pract 2014;23(1):70–73

23. Brain WR, Knight GC, Bull JW. Discussion of rupture of the intervertebral disc in the cervical region. Proc R Soc Med 1948; 41(8):509–516

24. Brain WR, Northfield D, Wilkinson M. The neurological manifestations of cervical spondylosis. Brain 1952;75(2):187–225

25. Robinson RA, Smith GW. Anterolateral cervical disc removal and interbody fusion for cervical disc syndrome. Bull Johns Hopkins Hosp 1955;96:223–224

26. Smith GW, Robinson RA. The treatment of certain cervical-spine disorders by anterior removal of the intervertebral disc and interbody fusion. J Bone Joint Surg Am 1958;40-A(3):607–624

27. Cloward RB. The anterior approach for removal of ruptured cervical disks. J Neurosurg 1958;15(6):602–617

28. Bailey RW, Badgley CE. Stabilization of the cervical spine by anterior fusion. J Bone Joint Surg Am 1960;42-A:565–594

29. Lees F, Turner JW. Natural history and prognosis of cervical spondylosis. BMJ 1963; 2(5373):1607–1610

30. Hughes JT. Pathology of the Spinal Cord. London: Lloyd-Luke Med Books; 1966

31. Wilkinson M. Cervical Spondylosis: Its Early Diagnosis and Treatment. 2nd ed. Philadelphia, PA: Saunders; 1971

32. Verbiest H. A lateral approach to the cervical spine: technique and indications. J Neurosurg 1968;28(3):191–203

33. Jackson RJ, Gokaslan ZL. Treatment of disk and ligamentous diseases of the cervical spine. In: Winn HR, ed. Youmans Neurological Surgery. 5th ed. Philadelphia, PA: Saunders; 2004:4395–4407

34. Boni M, Cherubino P, Denaro V, Benazzo F. Multiple subtotal somatectomy. Technique and evaluation of a series of 39 cases. Spine 1984;9(4):358–362

35. Boni M, Di Guglielmo L, Denaro V. CT evaluation of the multiple subtotal somatectomy results. In: Kehr P, Weidner A, eds. Cervical Spine. Vienna, Austria: Springer-Verlag; 1987:124–130

36. Kirita Y. En bloc laminectomy using a burr. Chubu Seisai 1968;13:241–242

37. Oyama M, Hattori S. A new method of cervical laminectomy. Chubu Seisaishi. 1973; 16:792–794

38. Hirabayashi K. Expansive open-door laminoplasty for cervical spondylotic myelopathy. Operation (Japan) 1978;32:1159–1163

39. Hirabayashi K, Watanabe K. A review of my invention of expansive laminoplasty. Neurospine 2019;16(3):379–382

40. Ducker T, Ziedman S. Cervical radiculopathies and myelopathies: posterior approaches. In: Frymoyer J, ed. The Adult Spine: Principles and Practice. 2nd ed. Philadelphia, PA: Lippincott; 1997:1381–1400

41. Alberstone CD, Benzel EC. History. In: Benzel EC, ed, Spine Surgery: Techniques, Complication Avoidance, and Management. New York, NY: Churchill Livingstone; 1999:1–40

P. S. Ramani, Sumeet Sasane, and Achal Gupta

Cervical Spondylotic Myelopathy (CSM)

Introduction

Cervical spondylosis is a systemic disease affecting connective tissue. It is one of the many manifestations of degenerative spine disease. It was presumed to be an age-related process. But, recent studies have shown that there are several other factors contributing to the degeneration. It involves multiple disc degeneration, osteophytes formation in vertebral bodies, and instability is usually seen (**Fig. 2.1**). A basic understanding of its pathophysiology is necessary before establishing a diagnosis, considering any surgical intervention for this very common degenerative condition.

Background

Cervical spondylotic myelopathy (CSM) is the most common cause of disability in the elderly.[1,2] The exact incidence and prevalence of CSM is unknown.[3] By authors' knowledge, there is high incidence of spondylosis in young children suffering from athetoid or dystonic movements.[4,5] CSM is a neurological condition that develops insidiously over time as degenerative changes of the spine result in overgrowth of bone and thickening of ligaments, resulting in compression of the cord and nerve roots (**Fig. 2.2**).[6] The natural history of CSM depends on the severity of the condition. It is generally accepted that patients with severe symptoms will not improve and will undergo a steady progression of disability along with pain.[7] The key clinical features of CSM include decreased dexterity of upper limbs and gait instability in the lower limbs. Motor dysfunction is frequently observed besides hypertonia. Sensory loss is observed less frequently, although there is a significant complaint of numbness and paresthesia. Early diagnosis and prompt management, preferably with surgical decompression of the spinal

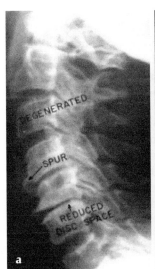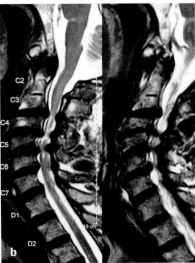

Fig. 2.1 (a, b) X-ray and MRI cervical spine (sagittal view) showing degenerative cervical spondylosis.

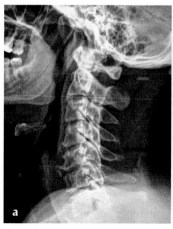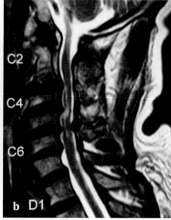

Fig. 2.2 (a, b) X-ray and MRI cervical spine (sagittal view) showing cervical spondylotic myelopathy (CSM).

cord and nerve roots with added stabilization of spine when necessary, is required.

Pathophysiology

The main factors responsible in producing myelopathy and hypertonia, followed by stiffness in the limbs and the trunk in spondylosis, are as follows:[8]

- The cervical canal is narrow: as developmental primary anomaly or secondary in origin due to degeneration in the spine.[1]
- Multiple spondylotic hypertrophy of bone causes a cumulative effect of narrowing the bony canal and causing spinal cord compression.
- Dynamic and static factors can exacerbate stenosis (shortening of neck from multiple disc degeneration; neck extension; thick and incurled ligamentum flavum; thickened other ligaments, etc.) and cause damage to the spinal cord, particularly in watershed areas.
- Disruption of arterial blood supply causes ischemia in the spinal cord in the presence of mechanical compression.

Other Factors Responsible for Myelopathy

In healthy adults, the intervertebral discs in the cervical spine have a similar structure to

that of the lumbar spine, consisting of the annulus fibrosus and nucleus pulposus.[9]

With advancing age, the intervertebral discs loses water content and elasticity due to loss of proteoglycan matrix, which predisposes the disc space to collapse and cause biomechanical incompetence.[10,11] Management involves not only decompression of neural tissue but also an attempt to stabilize the spine to halt progression of degenerative process.

Therefore, with degenerative progression, the movements of the cervical spine are restricted. Any further extension of neck may cause further damage to the cord due to compression. During normal flexion, the spinal cord lengthens, but in CSM patients, it can result in stretching of spinal cord causing damage.[2] The dynamic changes are presumed to cause CSM through increasing tension in the spinal cord, but Breig proved it by examining the effects of spondylotic bars and positioning of the cervical spine on the spinal cord geometry and blood flow.[12] Other workers showed that the dynamic shortening of the posterior cord and dorsal columns in extension may account for the difficulties with balance in CSM patients.[13]

Goel proposed that the primary nodal point of pathogenesis is instability of the spine, which is first manifested at the facets in the cervical spine.[14] The instability is of "vertical" type, wherein the superior facets slip over the inferior facets, resulting in their listhesis or telescoping.[15] Although retrolisthesis of facets has been identified in spinal degeneration, it has been considered as a secondary phenomenon to the effect of disc space reduction and degeneration. Instability of the spine is related to standing human posture, muscle weakness due to intervention (surgical) or injury or disuse from lack of exercise and toning. The profile of cervical and dorsal spinal facets is oblique, and identification of listhesis or instability at this level is difficult, even with modern imaging techniques.

Pathogenesis

Narrow cervical canal, diffuse degenerative, dynamic, and ischemic changes together produce myelopathy. The changes in the spinal cord, studied macro and microscopically, have helped to grade the damage in three grades, depending on the severity:[8]

- Incidental and repeated minor trauma add to the destruction of neuronal tissue and lead to irreversible clinical signs and symptoms.
- Extensive destruction of anterior horn cells is required before the clinical symptoms of motor loss can appear.
- Irreversible changes in the spinal cord is a long-standing proposition, taking about 20 years to develop.

Conclusion

CSM is a common cause of severe disability in elderly population. The incidence of the disease is likely to increase as the life span increases. An understanding of the pathogenesis, thorough clinical examination, and appropriate radiological investigation are crucial for diagnosis and management of the ailment.

Ossification of the Posterior Longitudinal Ligament

Introduction

Ossification is a misnomer, as it is not a reactive calcification which has ossified. Ossification of the posterior longitudinal ligament (OPLL) is an entity by itself, but its etiology and pathogenesis are not clearly understood. OPLL can be defined as an ectopic ossification in the tissues of spinal ligament, showing a hyperostotic condition. The pathophysiology of OPLL remains unknown. OPLL is most commonly found in elderly men and among Asian patients. The disease can start with mild or no symptoms and progress slowly to develop symptoms of myelopathy. An accurate diagnosis with plain radiographs, CT scan and MR imaging is very important to make diagnosis and decisions regarding a treatment plan.

Background

OPLL as an anatomical entity was first described by Key in 1838.[16,17] Oppenheimer in 1942 described calcification to be present in the vertebral ligaments, particularly the posterior longitudinal ligament.[18,19] Tsukimoto introduced it as a disease that caused myelopathy from compression on spinal cord.[20] Many clinical studies conducted in Japan have strongly suggested that OPLL is a multifactorial disease in which complex genetic and environmental factors interact. Development in molecular biology and genetics have enabled us to further understand this complex disease process.

Pathophysiology

Ossification of spinal ligaments is a part of the natural aging process of the musculoskeletal system. OPLL is clinically important because it causes myelopathy. There is no inflammatory reaction. There is increase in osteoblastic cell population. The bone is formed within the matrix. The blood vessels then penetrate the mass. The bone is reformed and trabeculated, resulting in ossification (**Figs. 2.3–2.6**).[21]

The most common classification of cervical OPLL is from the Investigation Committee on OPLL of the Japanese Ministry of Health and Welfare.[22] A lateral radiograph is used to classify OPLL into four subtypes: (1) continuous, (2) segmental, (3) mixed and (4) localized (**Fig. 2.7**).

The continuous type is an ossified mass that spans several vertebral bodies and the intervening disc spaces. The segmental type involves ossification behind each vertebral body. The mixed type is a mixture of both continuous and segmental types. The localized type has been described as a variant pattern in that the ossification is localized to the intervertebral disc space without involvement of the vertebral body. The mixed and continuous types are most frequently associated with myelopathy.[23]

Genetics

Matsunaga et al found that the prevalence of OPLL is higher in the siblings sharing identical human leukocyte antigen (HLA) haplotypes from families of 24 OPLL patients.[24] In 1991, Sakou et al studied 33 families of patients with OPLL and examined the HLA haplotypes of these families. They found that there were 6 HLA haplotypes that were observed frequently in that population and 3 of these haplotypes were found to be exceedingly rare in the general Japanese population, suggesting an association of OPLL and these rare haplotypes.

The conclusion was that the gene responsible for OPLL would likely to fall on the same chromosome that coded HLA (chromosome 6).[25,26] Several studies have found the associated genetic loci linked to OPLL and some of these will be discussed further.

Collagen-related genes: Collagen helps to form bone and cartilage and mediates the interaction between extracellular matrix components and cell surface proteins. Mutations and/or aberrant expressions of

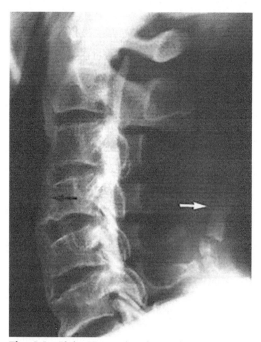

Fig. 2.3 Plain X-ray showing spinal ligaments clearly (bright).

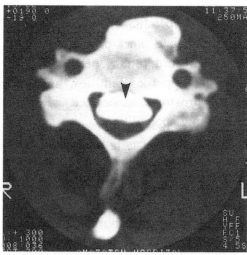

Fig. 2.4 CT showing gross ossification causing compression of the spinal cord (axial view).

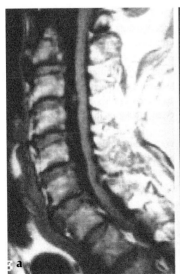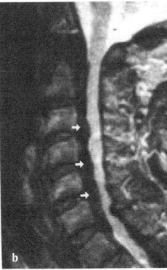

Fig. 2.5 (a, b) MRI pictures showing gross and continuous ossification of the posterior longitudinal ligament (OPLL) (sagittal).

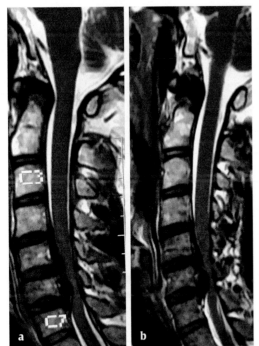

Fig. 2.6 (a, b) MRI pictures showing mixed ossification of the posterior longitudinal ligament (OPLL) (sagittal).

collagen genes may induce various pathological phenotypes in connective tissues. Many collagen genes are shown to be associated with OPLL, including COL11A2, COL6A1 and collagen 17A1.[27–35] The specific roles of these single-nucleotide polymorphisms (SNPs) of collagen genes in the pathogenesis of OPLL remains unclear, although their contributions to the formation of extracellular matrix scaffold facilitates endochondral ossification.

Nucleotide pyrophosphatase (NPPS): The "tiptoe walking (TTW)" mouse is an excellent model for OPLL, because it exhibits ossification of the spinal ligaments similar to OPLL, with almost complete mass formation as in humans.[36–37] The mice has natural potency to create enlargement of the nucleus pulposus, regenerative proliferation of annulus fibrosus cartilaginous tissues, and neovascularization with metaplasia of primitive mesenchymal cells to osteoblasts in the spinal ligaments.[38] It is now confirmed that a mutation within the NPPS gene is the cause of the "TTW" condition. The mutation results

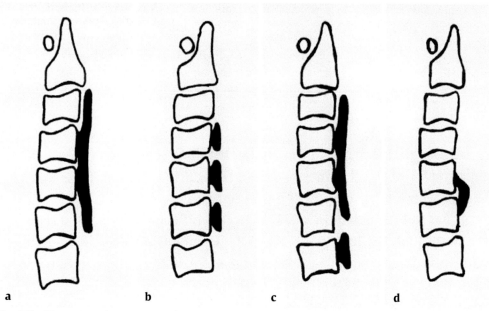

Fig. 2.7 Diagrammatic representation of different types of ossification of the posterior longitudinal ligament (OPLL): **(a)** continuous; **(b)** segmental; **(c)** mixed; **(d)** localized or other.

in truncation of the gene product and probably causes dysfunction of NPPS.[39] The human counterpart of this gene, NPPS also known as ectonucleotide pyrophosphatase (ENPP1), has been cloned.[40,41] NPPS has been shown to be expressed in a variety of tissues, including bone and cartilage and in cells of the osteoblastic cell lineage and chondrocytes.[42] Nakamura et al[42] suggested that NPPS plays an important role in the etiology of OPLL as it does in mice.

TGF-β: Transforming growth factor (TGF)– β induces the differentiation of mesenchymal cells into a chondrocytes phenotype and stimulates bone formation.[43–45] TGF-β is enriched in bone and cartilage to contain a large number of target cells for TGF-β. TGF-β is critical to maintain and expand mesenchymal stem cells (MCS)/progenitor cells and progenitors of osteoblasts via autocrine and paracrine stimulations.[15,46,47] TGF-β is present in the ossified matrix and chondrocytes of adjacent cartilaginous areas of OPLL, but not in multipotent stem cells (MSCs)

and nonossified ligament, suggesting it may stimulate bone formation at a later stage of ectopic ossification.[48] Polymorphisms of TGF-b1 and TGF-b3 are significantly associated with OPLL.[51–54] Three polymorphisms of TGF-β receptor 2 (TGFBR2) gene have been associated with OPLL.[53]

BMP: Bone morphogenetic proteins (BMPs) are multifunctional transcriptional factors that are members of the TGF-β superfamily of proteins and are involved in regulating cartilage and bone formation.[27,54,55] BMP-2 is produced in certain clusters of mesenchymal cells within the posterior longitudinal ligament at levels close to the intervertebral disc and endplate. Abnormal proliferation of chondrocytes (mostly fibrocartilage cells) contributes to the development of the early stages of ossification.[33] Many studies have shown association between BMP SNPs and OPLL, the significant being BMP-2, BMP-4, and BMP-9.[56–64]

Genetics of OPLL is an ever evolving subject. Authors have given a brief summary of major genes involved. The detailed evaluation of genetics of OPLL is beyond the scope of this chapter.

Nongenetic Factors

Multiple investigations have revealed that various exogenous and modifiable risk factors may be responsible for the development of OPLL. The prevalence of ossification of the posterior longitudinal ligament is high in patients with noninsulin-dependent diabetes mellitus and obesity with diabetes mellitus.

Such patients often exhibit increased secretion and impaired action of insulin. It is possible that changes in the secretion or action of insulin may play a role in the progression of the disease.[65,66] It is interesting to note that increased production of insulin may act on osteoprogenitor cells in the spinal ligament to induce ossification.[67]

Other factors which may induce ossification in PLL are:

- Hyperleptinemia.[68]
- Hyperinsulenimia.[69]
- Lumbago.[70]
- Family history of myocardial infarction.
- Limited intake of vegetables and salads.
- Long working hours.[26,71]
- Skeletal fluorosis.[72]

Associated Endocrine Disorder

Patients with OPLL may have deranged metabolism, hypoparathyroidism, vitamin D-resistant rickets/osteomalacia, alteration in sex hormones, and alteration in growth hormone secretion.[73-77]

Mechanical Stress

Mechanical stress can produce OPLL, as stress elevates prostacyclin synthesis in ligament cells derived from OPLL patients and induces osteogenic differentiation.[78-79] Vimentin, a type III intermediate filament protein, is also involved in responding to mechanical stretch in OPLL cells. Vimentin plays an important role in the progression of OPLL through the induction of osteogenic differentiation in OPLL.[80,81]

Multipotent Stem Cells (MSCs)

MSCs are multipotent progenitor cells that can differentiate into a variety of cell types, including osteoblasts and chondrocytes. MSCs plays a role in pathogenic development of several ossification processes. Harada et al[82] suggested that osteogenic differentiation potential of OPLL-derived MSCs could be a cause to produce ossification in spinal ligaments.

OPLL and Forestier's Disease

Forestier and Rotés-Querol published a landmark paper in 1950 on, what they termed as, senile ankylosing hyperostosis of the spine.[83] This pathological entity is known as diffuse idiopathic skeletal hyperostosis (DISH) or Forestier's disease today, and is characterized by exuberant osteophytes formation along the vertebral body. The commonly accepted Resnick and Niwayama classification criteria require "flowing osteophytes over at least four vertebral bodies."[84-85] The most prominent features of DISH appear on the spine as flowing appositions of newly formed ectopic bone along the anterolateral aspect of the spine, with preservation of intervertebral body heights.[86] DISH and OPLL can coexist.[87] The association of this gene with DISH is not found in Czech patients (**Fig. 2.8**).[86,88]

OPLL Progression

Takatsu et al found that growth of the OPLL occurred more rapidly in the surgical group.[89,90] Iwasaki et al found that OPLL progresses more with younger patients than older patients and that load of increased motion helps to proliferate OPLL.[91-92] Growth of OPLL continues in the first 2 to 5 years after laminoplasty followed by gradual termination.[93,94]

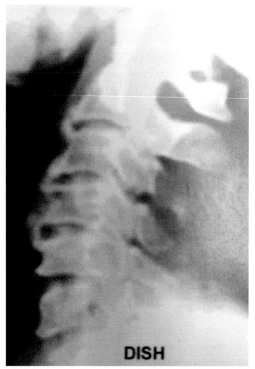

DISH

Fig. 2.8 X-ray cervical spine of diffuse skeletal hyperostosis (DISH)/Forestier disease.

Conclusion

Irrespective of the cause, OPLL is an abnormal growth of bone, and it interferes with normal functioning of spine.

Surgical procedures to excise OPLL are not always easy and has the potential to produce neurological damage. Experience and expertise helps in timely diagnosis and management.

Take-home Points

- CSM occurs as a result of static and dynamic factors of degeneration.
- OPLL tends to be diffuse.
- OPLL is associated with degenerative disorder, such as DISH.
- Myelomalacia is common in OPLL.

References

1. Young WF. Cervical spondylotic myelopathy: a common cause of spinal cord dysfunction in older persons. Am Fam Physician 2000;62(5):1064–1070, 1073
2. Baron EM, Young WF. Cervical spondylotic myelopathy: a brief review of its pathophysiology, clinical course, and diagnosis. Neurosurgery 2007; 60(1, Suppl 1):S35–S41
3. Kalsi-Ryan S, Karadimas SK, Fehlings MG. Cervical spondylotic myelopathy: the clinical phenomenon and the current pathobiology of an increasingly prevalent and devastating disorder. Neuroscientist 2013;19(4):409–421
4. Jameson R, Rech C, Garreau de Loubresse C. Cervical myelopathy in athetoid and dystonic cerebral palsy: retrospective study and literature review. Eur Spine J 2010; 19(5):706–712
5. Duruflé A, Pétrilli S, Le Guiet JL, et al. Cervical spondylotic myelopathy in athetoid cerebral palsy patients: about five cases. Joint Bone Spine 2005;72(3):270–274
6. McCormick JR, Sama AJ, Schiller NC, Butler AJ, Donnally CJ III. Cervical spondylotic myelopathy: a guide to diagnosis and management. J Am Board Fam Med 2020; 33(2):303–313
7. Shiban E, Meyer B. Treatment considerations of cervical spondylotic myelopathy. Neurol Clin Pract 2014;4(4):296–303
8. Ramani PS. Textbook of Cervical Spondylosis. Pathology of Cervical Spondylosis. 1st ed. Daryaganj, New Delhi: Jaypee Brother Medical Publisher; 2004
9. Mercer S, Bogduk N. The ligaments and annulus fibrosus of human adult cervical intervertebral discs. Spine 1999;24(7): 619–626, discussion 627–628
10. Clark C, Frymoyer JW. The Adult Spine: Principles and Practice. 2nd ed. Philadelphia, USA: Lippincott-Raven publications; 1997: 1323–1348
11. Virdi G. Cervical Myelopathy: Pathophysiology, Diagnosis, and Management. Spine Research. 2017 (e-pub ahead of print). doi:10.21767/2471-8173.100032
12. Breig A, Turnbull I, Hassler O. Effects of mechanical stresses on the spinal cord in

cervical spondylosis. A study on fresh cadaver material. J Neurosurg 1966;25(1):45–56

13. Lebl DR, Hughes A, Cammisa FP Jr, O'Leary PF. Cervical spondylotic myelopathy: pathophysiology, clinical presentation, and treatment. HSS J 2011;7(2):170–178

14. Goel A. Is instability the nodal point of pathogenesis for both cervical spondylotic myelopathy and ossified posterior longitudinal ligament? Neurol India 2016;64(4):837–838

15. Goel A. Vertical facetal instability: Is it the point of genesis of spinal spondylotic disease? J Craniovertebr Junction Spine 2015;6(2):47–48

16. Key CA. On paraplegia depending on disease of the ligaments of the spine. Guys Hosp Rep 1838;3:17–34

17. Yan L, Gao R, Liu Y, He B, Lv S, Hao D. The pathogenesis of ossification of the posterior longitudinal ligament. Aging Dis 2017;8(5):570–582

18. Oppenheimer A. Calcification and ossification of vertebral ligaments (spondylitis ossificans ligamentosa): roentgen study of pathogenesis and clinical significance. Radiology 1942;38:160–173

19. Sakou T, Matsunaga S. History of research on ossification of the posterior longitudinal ligament. In: Yonenobu K, Sakou T, Ono K, eds. OPLL. Tokyo: Springer; 1997

20. Tsukimoto H. A case report: autopsy of syndrome of compression of spinal cord owing to ossification within spinal canal of cervical spines. Nippon Geka Hokan 1960;29:1003–1007

21. Ramani PS. Textbook of Cervical Spondylosis. 1st ed. Daryaganj, New Delhi: Jaypee Brother Medical Publisher; 2004

22. Tsuyama N. Ossification of the posterior longitudinal ligament of the spine. Clin Orthop Relat Res 1984; (184):71–84

23. Abiola R, Rubery P, Mesfin A. Ossification of the posterior longitudinal ligament: etiology, diagnosis, and outcomes of nonoperative and operative management. Global Spine J 2016;6(2):195–204

24. Matsunaga S, Yamaguchi M, Hayashi K, Sakou T. Genetic analysis of ossification of the posterior longitudinal ligament. Spine 1999;24(10):937–938, discussion 939

25. Sakou T, Taketomi E, Matsunaga S, Yamaguchi M, Sonoda S, Yashiki S. Genetic study of ossification of the posterior longitudinal ligament in the cervical spine with human leukocyte antigen haplotype. Spine 1991;16(11):1249–1252

26. Stetler WR, La Marca F, Park P. The genetics of ossification of the posterior longitudinal ligament. Neurosurg Focus 2011;30(3):E7

27. Koga H, Sakou T, Taketomi E, et al. Genetic mapping of ossification of the posterior longitudinal ligament of the spine. Am J Hum Genet 1998;62(6):1460–1467

28. Maeda S, Ishidou Y, Koga H, et al. Functional impact of human collagen alpha2(XI) gene polymorphism in pathogenesis of ossification of the posterior longitudinal ligament of the spine. J Bone Miner Res 2001;16(5):948–957

29. Maeda S, Koga H, Matsunaga S, et al. Gender-specific haplotype association of collagen alpha2 (XI) gene in ossification of the posterior longitudinal ligament of the spine. J Hum Genet 2001;46(1):1–4

30. Sakou T, Matsunaga S, Koga H. Recent progress in the study of pathogenesis of ossification of the posterior longitudinal ligament. J Orthop Sci 2000;5(3):310–315

31. Tanaka T, Ikari K, Furushima K, et al. Genomewide linkage and linkage disequilibrium analyses identify COL6A1, on chromosome 21, as the locus for ossification of the posterior longitudinal ligament of the spine. Am J Hum Genet 2003;73(4):812–822

32. Kim KH, Kuh SU, Park JY, et al. Association between BMP-2 and COL6A1 gene polymorphisms with susceptibility to ossification of the posterior longitudinal ligament of the cervical spine in Korean patients and family members. Genet Mol Res 2014;13(1):2240–2247

33. Kong Q, Ma X, Li F, et al. COL6A1 polymorphisms associated with ossification of the ligamentum flavum and ossification of the posterior longitudinal ligament. Spine 2007;32(25):2834–2838

34. Tsukahara S, Miyazawa N, Akagawa H, et al. COL6A1, the candidate gene for ossification of the posterior longitudinal ligament, is associated with diffuse idiopathic skeletal hyperostosis in Japanese. Spine 2005;30(20):2321–2324

35. Wei W, He HL, Chen CY, et al. Whole exome sequencing implicates PTCH1 and COL17A1 genes in ossification of the posterior longitudinal ligament of the cervical spine in Chinese patients. Genet Mol Res 2014; 13(1):1794–1804

36. Hosoda Y, Yoshimura Y, Higaki S. A new breed of mouse showing multiple osteochondral lesions--twy mouse. Ryumachi 1981;21(Suppl):157–164

37. Goto S, Yamazaki M. Pathogenesis of ossification of the spinal ligaments. In: Yonenobu K, Sakou T, Ono K, eds. Ossification of the Posterior Longitudinal Ligament. Tokyo Berlin Heidelberg New York: Springer; 1997:29–37

38. Uchida K, Yayama T, Sugita D, et al. Initiation and progression of ossification of the posterior longitudinal ligament of the cervical spine in the hereditary spinal hyperostotic mouse (twy/twy). Eur Spine J 2012;21(1):149–155

39. Okawa A, Nakamura I, Goto S, Moriya H, Nakamura Y, Ikegawa S. Mutation in Npps in a mouse model of ossification of the posterior longitudinal ligament of the spine. Nat Genet 1998;19(3):271–273

40. Buckley MF, Loveland KA, McKinstry WJ, Garson OM, Goding JW. Plasma cell membrane glycoprotein PC-1. cDNA cloning of the human molecule, amino acid sequence, and chromosomal location. J Biol Chem 1990;265(29):17506–17511

41. Funakoshi I, Kato H, Horie K, et al. Molecular cloning of cDNAs for human fibroblast nucleotide pyrophosphatase. Arch Biochem Biophys 1992;295(1):180–187

42. Nakamura I, Ikegawa S, Okawa A, et al. Association of the human NPPS gene with ossification of the posterior longitudinal ligament of the spine (OPLL). Hum Genet 1999;104(6):492–497

43. Carrington JL, Roberts AB, Flanders KC, Roche NS, Reddi AH. Accumulation, localization, and compartmentation of transforming growth factor beta during endochondral bone development. J Cell Biol 1988;107(5): 1969–1975

44. Joyce ME, Roberts AB, Sporn MB, Bolander ME. Transforming growth factor-beta and the initiation of chondrogenesis and osteogenesis in the rat femur. J Cell Biol 1990;110(6):2195–2207

45. Noda M, Camilliere JJ. In vivo stimulation of bone formation by transforming growth factor-beta. Endocrinology 1989;124(6): 2991–2994

46. Chen G, Deng C, Li YP. TGF-β and BMP signaling in osteoblast differentiation and bone formation. Int J Biol Sci 2012;8(2):272–288

47. Bonewald LF, Mundy GR. Role of transforming growth factor-beta in bone remodeling. Clin Orthop Relat Res 1990; (250):261–276

48. Kawaguchi H, Kurokawa T, Hoshino Y, Kawahara H, Ogata E, Matsumoto T. Immunohistochemical demonstration of bone morphogenetic protein-2 and transforming growth factor-beta in the ossification of the posterior longitudinal ligament of the cervical spine. Spine 1992; 17(3, Suppl): S33–S36

49. Bonewald LF, Dallas SL. Role of active and latent transforming growth factor beta in bone formation. J Cell Biochem 1994; 55(3):350–357

50. Kamiya M, Harada A, Mizuno M, Iwata H, Yamada Y. Association between a polymorphism of the transforming growth factor-beta1 gene and genetic susceptibility to ossification of the posterior longitudinal ligament in Japanese patients. Spine 2001; 26(11):1264–1266, discussion 1266–1267

51. Kawaguchi Y, Furushima K, Sugimori K, Inoue I, Kimura T. Association between polymorphism of the transforming growth factor-beta1 gene with the radiologic characteristic and ossification of the posterior longitudinal ligament. Spine 2003; 28(13):1424–1426

52. Horikoshi T, Maeda K, Kawaguchi Y, et al. A large-scale genetic association study of ossification of the posterior longitudinal ligament of the spine. Hum Genet 2006; 119(6):611–616

53. Jekarl DW, Paek CM, An YJ, et al. TGFBR2 gene polymorphism is associated with ossification of the posterior longitudinal ligament. J Clin Neurosci 2013;20(3):453–456

54. Yonemori K, Imamura T, Ishidou Y, et al. Bone morphogenetic protein receptors and activin receptors are highly expressed in ossified ligament tissues of patients with ossification

of the posterior longitudinal ligament. Am J Pathol 1997;150(4):1335–1347

55. Stapleton CJ, Pham MH, Attenello FJ, Hsieh PC. Ossification of the posterior longitudinal ligament: genetics and pathophysiology. Neurosurg Focus 2011;30(3):E6

56. Li JM, Zhang Y, Ren Y, et al. Uniaxial cyclic stretch promotes osteogenic differentiation and synthesis of BMP2 in the C3H10T1/2 cells with BMP2 gene variant of rs2273073 (T/G). PLoS One 2014;9(9):e106598

57. Wang H, Liu D, Yang Z, et al. Association of bone morphogenetic protein-2 gene polymorphisms with susceptibility to ossification of the posterior longitudinal ligament of the spine and its severity in Chinese patients. Eur Spine J 2008;17(7):956–964

58. Wang H, Yang ZH, Liu DM, Wang L, Meng XL, Tian BP. Association between two polymorphisms of the bone morpho-genetic protein-2 gene with genetic susceptibility to ossification of the posterior longitudinal ligament of the cervical spine and its severity. Chin Med J (Engl) 2008;121(18):1806–1810

59. Yan L, Chang Z, Liu Y, Li YB, He BR, Hao DJ. A single nucleotide polymorphism in the human bone morphogenetic protein-2 gene (109T > G) affects the Smad signaling pathway and the predisposition to ossification of the posterior longitudinal ligament of the spine. Chin Med J (Engl) 2013;126(6):1112–1118

60. Meng XL, Wang H, Yang H, Hai Y, Tian BP, Lin X. T allele at site 6007 of bone morphogenetic protein-4 gene increases genetic susceptibility to ossification of the posterior longitudinal ligament in male Chinese Han population. Chin Med J (Engl) 2010;123(18):2537–2542

61. Furushima K, Shimo-Onoda K, Maeda S, et al. Large-scale screening for candidate genes of ossification of the posterior longitudinal ligament of the spine. J Bone Miner Res 2002;17(1):128–137

62. Ren Y, Feng J, Liu ZZ, Wan H, Li JH, Lin X. A new haplotype in BMP4 implicated in ossification of the posterior longitudinal ligament (OPLL) in a Chinese population. J Orthop Res 2012;30(5):748–756

63. Chen R, Kong D, Xi Y, et al. Association between bone morphogenetic protein and ossification of posterior longitudinal

ligament: a meta-analysis. Int J Clin Exp Med 2017;10(1):79–87

64. Ren Y, Liu ZZ, Feng J, et al. Association of a BMP9 haplotype with ossification of the posterior longitudinal ligament (OPLL) in a Chinese population. PLoS One 2012; 7(7):e40587

65. Kawagishi T, Harata M. Studies of the prevalence of the ossification of the posterior longitudinal ligaments of the cervical spine in diabetic patients. Rinsho Seikei Geka 1979;14:718–722 Japanese

66. Takeuchi Y, Matsumoto T, Takuwa Y, et al. High incidence of obesity and elevated serum immunoreactive insulin level in patients with paravertebral ligamentous ossification: a relationship to the development of ectopic ossification. J Bone Miner Metab 1989; 7:17–21

67. Akune T, Ogata N, Seichi A, Ohnishi I, Nakamura K, Kawaguchi H. Insulin secretory response is positively associated with the extent of ossification of the posterior longitudinal ligament of the spine. J Bone Joint Surg Am 2001;83(10):1537–1544

68. Shirakura Y, Sugiyama T, Tanaka H, Taguchi T, Kawai S. Hyperleptinemia in female patients with ossification of spinal ligaments. Biochem Biophys Res Commun 2000;267(3):752–755

69. Li H, Liu D, Zhao CQ, Jiang LS, Dai LY. Insulin potentiates the proliferation and bone morphogenetic protein-2-induced osteogenic differentiation of rat spinal ligament cells via extracellular signal-regulated kinase and phosphatidylinositol 3-kinase. Spine 2008;33(22):2394–2402

70. Kobashi G, Washio M, Okamoto K, et al; Japan Collaborative Epidemiological Study Group for Evaluation of Ossification of the Posterior Longitudinal Ligament of the Spine Risk. High body mass index after age 20 and diabetes mellitus are independent risk factors for ossification of the posterior longitudinal ligament of the spine in Japanese subjects: a case-control study in multiple hospitals. Spine 2004;29(9):1006–1010

71. Kobashi G, Ohta K, Washio M, et al; Japan Collaborative Epidemiological Study Group for Evaluation of Ossification of the Posterior Longitudinal Ligament of the Spine Risk. FokI variant of vitamin D receptor gene and

factors related to atherosclerosis associated with ossification of the posterior longitudinal ligament of the spine: a multi-hospital case-control study. Spine 2008;33(16):E553–E558

72. Reddy DR. Neurology of endemic skeletal fluorosis. Neurol India 2009;57(1):7–12

73. Adams JE, Davies M. Paravertebral and peripheral ligamentous ossification: an unusual association of hypoparathyroidism. Postgrad Med J 1977;53(617):167–172

74. Okazaki T, Takuwa Y, Yamamoto M, et al. Ossification of the paravertebral ligaments: a frequent complication of hypoparathyroidism. Metabolism 1984;33(8):710–713

75. Rasmussen H, Anast C. Familiar hypophosphatemic rickets and vitamin D-dependent rickets. In: Stanbury JB, Wyngaarden JB, Fredrickson DS, et al., eds. The Metabolic Basis of Inherited Diseases. New York: McGraw-Hill; 1983:1743–1773

76. Ikegawa S, Kurokawa T, Hizuka N, Hoshino Y, Ohnishi I, Shizume K. Increase of serum growth hormone-binding protein in patients with ossification of the posterior longitudinal ligament of the spine. Spine 1993;18(13):1757–1760

77. Motegi M, Musha Y, Morisu M, Wada A, Furufu T. Etiological study on spinal ligament ossification with special reference to dietary habits and serum sex hormones. (in Japanese). Seikei Geka 1993;44:1017–1026

78. Furukawa K. Current topics in pharmacological research on bone metabolism: molecular basis of ectopic bone formation induced by mechanical stress. J Pharmacol Sci 2006;100(3):201–204

79. Ohishi H, Furukawa K, Iwasaki K, et al. Role of prostaglandin I2 in the gene expression induced by mechanical stress in spinal ligament cells derived from patients with ossification of the posterior longitudinal ligament. J Pharmacol Exp Ther 2003;305(3):818–824

80. Shapiro F, Cahill C, Malatantis G, Nayak RC. Transmission electron microscopic demonstration of vimentin in rat osteoblast and osteocyte cell bodies and processes using the immunogold technique. Anat Rec 1995;241(1):39–48

81. Zhang W, Wei P, Chen Y, et al. Down-regulated expression of vimentin induced by mechanical stress in fibroblasts derived from patients with ossification of the posterior longitudinal ligament. Eur Spine J 2014;23(11):2410–2415

82. Harada Y, Furukawa K, Asari T, et al. Osteogenic lineage commitment of mesenchymal stem cells from patients with ossification of the posterior longitudinal ligament. Biochem Biophys Res Commun 2014;443(3):1014–1020

83. Forestier J, Rotés-Querol J. Senile ankylosing hyperostosis of the spine. Ann Rheum Dis 1950;9(4):321–330

84. Resnick D, Niwayama G. DiVuse idiopathic skeletal hyperostosis (DISH): ankylosing hyperostosis of Forestier and Rotés-Querol. In: Resnick D, ed. Diagnosis of Bone and Joint Disorders. 3rd ed. Philadelphia, London, Toronto, Montreal, Sydney, Tokyo: Saunders; 1995:1463–95

85. Resnick D, Niwayama G. Radiographic and pathologic features of spinal involvement in diffuse idiopathic skeletal hyperostosis (DISH). Radiology 1976;119(3):559–568

86. Havelka S, Veselá M, Pavelková A, et al. Are DISH and OPLL genetically related? Ann Rheum Dis 2001;60(9):902–903

87. Mader R, Verlaan JJ, Eshed I, et al. Diffuse idiopathic skeletal hyperostosis (DISH): where we are now and where to go next. RMD Open 2017;3(1):e000472

88. Tsukahara S, Miyazawa N, Akagawa H, et al. COL6A1, the candidate gene for ossification of the posterior longitudinal ligament, is associated with diffuse idiopathic skeletal hyperostosis in Japanese. Spine 2005;30(20):2321–2324

89. Takatsu T, Ishida Y, Suzuki K, Inoue H. Radiological study of cervical ossification of the posterior longitudinal ligament. J Spinal Disord 1999;12(3):271–273

90. Vaziri S, Lockney DT, Dru AB, Polifka AJ, Fox WC, Hoh DJ. Does ossification of the posterior longitudinal ligament progress after fusion? Neurospine 2019;16(3):483–491

91. Iwasaki M, Kawaguchi Y, Kimura T, Yonenobu K. Long-term results of expansive laminoplasty for ossification of the posterior longitudinal ligament of the cervical spine: more than 10 years follow up. J Neurosurg 2002; 96(2, Suppl):180–189

92. Chen Y, Guo Y, Chen D, Wang X, Lu X, Yuan W. Long-term outcome of laminectomy and

instrumented fusion for cervical ossification of the posterior longitudinal ligament. Int Orthop 2009;33(4):1075–1080

93. Chiba K, Yamamoto I, Hirabayashi H, et al. Multicenter study investigating the post-operative progression of ossification of the posterior longitudinal ligament in the cervical spine: a new computer-assisted measurement. J Neurosurg Spine 2005;3(1): 17–23

94. Hirabayashi K, Miyakawa J, Satomi K, Maruyama T, Wakano K. Operative results and postoperative progression of ossification among patients with ossification of cervical posterior longitudinal ligament. Spine 1981; 6(4):354–364

03 Incidence and Natural Course of Cervical Spondylotic Myelopathy and OPLL

Mehmet Zileli and Nevhis Akıntürk

Introduction

Cervical spondylotic myelopathy (CSM) is a common disease among the elderly population. The following two factors are mainly responsible for it: static factor involves spinal stenosis and cord compression, and dynamic factor involves micromovements and movement-related compression of the spinal cord.[1]

Incidence of CSM

The epidemiology of CSM is still not well studied. The incidence is more common in Asian countries.[2-4] In North America, the incidence is more than 4.1 per 100,000, respectively.[5] In the Netherlands, the incidence is 1.6/100,000 inhabitants,[6] and in Taiwan, it is 4.04/100,000 person-years for hospitalizations.[7]

It is more frequent in males. The frequency increases with age. In an MRI study, incidental cord compression was found in 31% at the age range of 40 to 50 years, and it increased to 67% between the age range of 70 to 80 years.[8]

As much as 8% of people who have incidental canal stenosis and no symptoms are estimated to develop myelopathy at 1 year and 23% at the median of a 44-month follow-up.[9]

Incidence of Ossified Posterior Longitudinal Ligament

Ossified Posterior Longitudinal Ligament (OPLL) differs from CSM. Its prevalence is higher in the Asian population.[10] Many factors have been claimed to be responsible of OPLL, especially environmental, genetic, and biochemical factors.[1-4,11] It may also have a familial distribution.[12] It is quite common in patients with diffuse idiopathic skeletal hyperostosis (DISH).[3]

For epidemiological studies, it is difficult to place trust in earlier series which used direct radiograms for detection of OPLL. The prevalence of cervical OPLL in Asian countries has been found to be between 1.9 and 6.3%; however, it is between 0.7 and 1.3% among the White population of the USA.[13]

In a US-based study, the incidence of OPLL in normal population was searched among 2917 patients on CT scans; 74 had OPLL (2.5%).[14] OPLL prevalence in asymptomatic patients is about 2.5%. The incidence was more common among patients with diabetes. Segmental OPLL was found to be more common than the other types. Caudal extension of the OPLL mostly involved C6-7 level.

In another study from 2015[15] using CT scans, the incidence of OPLL was as follows: White population 1.3%, Asian population 4.8%, Hispanic population 1.9%, Afro-American population 2.1%. In another Japanese study examining 1500 persons, the prevalence was 6.3%.[16] In a recent Chinese study that used CT scans on 2000 patients,[13] the OPLL prevalence was 4.1%.

Kawaguchi et al[17] have defined an ossification index (OS index) to describe the extension of the ossification. OS index is the sum of the vertebral body and intervertebral disc levels involved in ossification of the spinal ligaments. Hirai et al[18] classified OPLL according to the cervical OP index in the following manner:

- Grade 1 OPLL: patients with a cervical OP index ≤ 5.
- Grade 2 OPLL: patients with a cervical OP index 6 to 9.
- Grade 3 OPLL: patients with a cervical OP index ≥ 10.

They termed the grade 3 cases as severe cases (OP index of whole spine ≥ 20). In a recent multicenter study by Mori et al,[19] the authors compared the severe group (cervical OP index ≥ 10) with the nonsevere group (cervical OP index ≤ 9).

A total of 234 patients with symptomatic cervical OPLL (57 females and 177 males) with a mean age of 65 years underwent whole spine CT to determine the epidemiological features of this condition.[19]

Cervical laminoplasty was developed in Japan. According to Hirabayashi et al, there are two reasons for this: a narrower spinal canal and a high prevalence rate of OPLL in the Japanese population.[20]

Dural Ossification with OPLL

Dural ossification of OPLL is an important feature, since an anterior surgery of these cases may cause dura laceration and cerebrospinal fluid (CSF) fistula. Mizuno et al[21] examined 111 OPLL patients who had anterior surgeries and found 17 (15.3%) patients with ossification of the dura mater. They described three dural ossification patterns: isolated, double-layer, and en-bloc types. Bone-window CT scanning was found to be very useful for identification of dural ossification as well as OPLL.

Cervical Curvature and OPLL

The recent trend is to measure sagittal balance of cervical spine and whole spine by erect standing radiograms. The K-line is a straight line connecting the midpoints of the spinal canal at C2 and C7 on a neutral cervical lateral radiograph. The maximum occupying ratio of OPLL is calculated from a sagittal CT image of the cervical spine. K-line (+) means OPLL does not exceed the K line. K-line (-) means OPLL exceeds the K line.[22]

Natural Course of CSM

There are still many unknown points for the natural course of CSM. A combination of three symptoms makes the clinic: neck pain, radiculopathy, and myelopathy. Although we commonly use the term "cervical spondylotic myelopathy", it may not be appropriate if there is no myelopathy.

The most common form of the disease involves a long and constant period of ailment with a series of new episodes, symptoms, and signs.[23,24] Continuous symptom progression is not common.

The natural course of CSM in moderate-to-severe CSM patients (modified Japanese Orthopaedic Association [mJOA] scores less than 13) have reported progressions. For this reason, most authors recommend a surgical treatment.[23,25,26] If conservative treatment is chosen, almost 75% of patients can undergo progression of the disease.[23]

A very old paper from the 1960s reported that among 28 patients managed conservatively, 17 patients have improved.[24]

The management of mild CSM patients (mJOA scores between 13–17) is more controversial. Conservative therapy or simple follow-up may be a more viable option in mild CSM patients.[27] However, systematic reviews have reported that a worsening of myelopathy should be expected in 20 to 62% of patients if managed conservatively.[25,28-31] In a series of mild CSM cases reported by Matsumoto et al, symptom progression during conservative management was about 35%.[29] In general 1/5th of patients who did not undergo surgery initially would need surgery during follow-up.

There are some cases in which significant cord compression present on MRI, but there are no symptoms. They comprise approximately 5% of patients.[32] Some authors call them premyelopathic patients; however, Kovalova termed them "nonmyelopathic spondylotic cervical cord compression" (NMSCCC).[8]

It is important to predict the cases which will deteriorate. The incidence of myelopathy development has been estimated at 8% at 1-year follow-up and 23% at 4-year follow-up.[9] The main concern in these premyelopathic patients is minor trauma, which may cause worsening of such patients. The rate of progression to myelopathy in patients with significant canal stenosis and having no symptoms have been well observed in two studies.[33,34] The risk of developing myelopathy has been estimated to be approximately 3% per year.[35]

The same is true for OPLL patients. In a report comprising 323 OPLL patients with significant cervical stenosis but having no symptoms, with a mean 17.6-year follow-up time, only 17% developed myelopathy.[34]

Since radiologic investigations are being ordered more commonly, incidental diagnosis of cervical canal stenosis has also increased. This has led to more common usage of surgery for CSM patients. Number of CSM surgeries is rising.[36,37] If the surgical treatment of CSM continues to increase that much, the costs and its global burden will be more apparent.[38]

Natural Course of OPLL

OPLL is a progressive calcification of the posterior longitudinal ligament, which then creates spinal canal stenosis.[1] In OPLL development, genetic, environmental, biomechanical, and biochemical factors can be responsible.[2-4,11] It has also a relation with DISH.[3,4] Half of the patients with DISH have also OPLL. OPLL is also common among CSM patients, with its incidence observed in about 10% of patients.[10]

OPLL Progression

In general, OPLL is a slow progressive disease. Although laminoplasty has been a traditional surgery for multilevel OPLL cases, its popularity has decreased after reports showing the arrest of OPLL growth only with fusion surgery.[39] There must be a potential relationship between OPLL growth and biomechanical factors. In a study done by Kawaguchi et al, radiographic progression of OPLL after laminoplasty has been reported in 73% of patients and more with longitudinal progression than axial progression.[40,41]

In a systematic review, the incidence of postoperative OPLL progression was reported to be between 3.3 and 74.5%.[41] Progression should be expected more in multiple-level OPLL cases and younger cases. Radiologic progression is more common after laminoplasty than laminectomy and fusion.[41] On the other hand, radiologic progression does not correlate well with neurologic worsening.

Risk factors for cervical OPLL have been studied in a large cohort in Korea.[42] They aimed to predict OPLL risk factors and found hypertension, ischemic stroke, diabetes mellitus, hypothyroidism, and osteoporosis as risk factors for the development of OPLL.

In conclusion, the natural course of patients with cervical stenosis and signs of myelopathy is quite variable. Prediction for which patients will have disease progression and neurologic worsening is not well known. Risk of worsening of patients with no symptoms but having significant stenosis (premyelopathic) is approximately 3% per year.

In a recent review, the WFNS Spine Committee announced their recommendations for natural course of CSM.[43] The statements of that review are as follows: (1) Natural course of patients with cervical stenosis and signs of myelopathy greatly vary. (2) Progression of the disease is possible, but prediction of those patients is not well known. Some patients may remain static for lengthy periods, and some patients with severe disability can improve without treatment. (3) For patients with no symptoms but having significant stenosis (premyelopathic), risk of developing myelopathy with cervical stenosis is approximately 3% per year.[43]

Take-home Points

- The incidence of CSM is more than 4 per 100,000 population. It is more common in males and elderly.

- OPLL is more common in Asian countries. The prevalence of cervical OPLL in Asian countries is between 1.9 to 6.3%, while it is between 0.7 to 1.3% among White populations. Additional dural ossification in OPLL cases is around 15%.

- Moderate-to-severe CSM cases tend to worsen neurologically (approximately 75%), and many authors recommend a surgical decompression to deal with them. In mild CSM patients, neurological worsening with follow-up is less common (20–62%); therefore, a conservative therapy is a viable option.

- The so-called premyelopathic patients (significant cord compression on MRI, but no symptoms), who comprise approximately 5%, can be followed-up. However, a minor trauma can cause neurologic symptoms, and the patients must be informed about this possibility. The risk of developing myelopathy in these premyelopathic patients has been estimated as approximately 3% per year.

- Progression of OPLL can continue if laminoplasty is chosen as technique of decompression. Progression is less likely if a fusion is performed.

References

1. Aljuboori Z, Boakye M. The natural history of cervical spondylotic myelopathy and ossification of the posterior longitudinal ligament: a review article. Cureus 2019; 11(7):e5074

2. Inamasu J, Guiot BH, Sachs DC. Ossification of the posterior longitudinal ligament: an update on its biology, epidemiology, and natural history. Neurosurgery 2006;58(6): 1027–1039, discussion 1027–1039

3. Matsunaga S, Yamaguchi M, Hayashi K, Sakou T. Genetic analysis of ossification of the posterior longitudinal ligament. Spine 1999;24(10):937–938, discussion 939

4. Sugrue PA, McClendon J Jr, Halpin RJ, Liu JC, Koski TR, Ganju A. Surgical management of cervical ossification of the posterior longitudinal ligament: natural history and the role of surgical decompression and stabilization. Neurosurg Focus 2011;30(3):E3

5. Nouri A, Tetreault L, Singh A, Karadimas SK, Fehlings MG. Degenerative cervical myelopathy: epidemiology, genetics, and pathogenesis. Spine 2015;40(12):E675–E693

6. Boogaarts HD, Bartels RH. Prevalence of cervical spondylotic myelopathy. Eur Spine J 2015;24(Suppl 2):139–141

7. Wu JC, Ko CC, Yen YS, et al. Epidemiology of cervical spondylotic myelopathy and its risk of causing spinal cord injury: a national cohort study. Neurosurg Focus 2013;35(1):E10

8. Kovalova I, Kerkovsky M, Kadanka Z, et al. Prevalence and imaging characteristics of nonmyelopathic and myelopathic spondylotic cervical cord compression. Spine 2016; 41(24):1908–1916

9. Wilson JR, Barry S, Fischer DJ, et al. Frequency, timing, and predictors of neurological dysfunction in the nonmyelopathic patient with cervical spinal cord compression, canal stenosis, and/or ossification of the posterior longitudinal ligament. Spine 2013; 38(22, Suppl 1)S37–S54

10. Nouri A, Martin AR, Tetreault L, et al. MRI Analysis of the Combined Prospectively Collected AOS pine North America and International Data: the prevalence and spectrum of pathologies in a global cohort of patients with degenerative cervical myelopathy. Spine 2017;42(14):1058–1067

11. Nam DC, Lee HJ, Lee CJ, Hwang SC. Molecular pathophysiology of ossification of the posterior longitudinal ligament (OPLL). Biomol Ther (Seoul) 2019;27(4):342–348

12. Terayama K. Genetic studies on ossification of the posterior longitudinal ligament of the spine. Spine 1989;14(11):1184–1191

13. Liang H, Liu G, Lu S, et al. Epidemiology of ossification of the spinal ligaments and associated factors in the Chinese population: a cross-sectional study of 2000 consecutive individuals. BMC Musculoskelet Disord 2019;20(1):253

14. Bakhsh W, Saleh A, Yokogawa N, Gruber J, Rubery PT, Mesfin A. Cervical ossification of the posterior longitudinal

ligament: a computed tomography-based epidemiological study of 2917 patients. Global Spine J 2019;9(8):820–825

15. Fujimori T, Le H, Hu SS, et al. Ossification of the posterior longitudinal ligament of the cervical spine in 3161 patients: a CT-based study. Spine 2015;40(7):E394–E403

16. Fujimori T, Watabe T, Iwamoto Y, Hamada S, Iwasaki M, Oda T. Prevalence, concomitance, and distribution of ossification of the spinal ligaments: results of whole spine CT scans in 1500 Japanese patients. Spine 2016;41(21):1668–1676

17. Kawaguchi Y, Nakano M, Yasuda T, Seki S, Hori T, Kimura T. Ossification of the posterior longitudinal ligament in not only the cervical spine, but also other spinal regions: analysis using multidetector computed tomography of the whole spine. Spine 2013;38(23):E1477–E1482

18. Hirai T, Yoshii T, Iwanami A, et al. Prevalence and distribution of ossified lesions in the whole spine of patients with cervical ossification of the posterior longitudinal ligament a multicenter study (JOSL CT study). PLoS One 2016;11(8):e0160117

19. Mori K, Yoshii T, Hirai T, et al. The characteristics of the patients with radiologically severe cervical ossification of the posterior longitudinal ligament of the spine: A CT-based multicenter cross-sectional study. J Orthop Sci 2019 (e-pub ahead of print). doi:10.1016/j.jos.2019.09.018

20. Hirabayashi S, Kitagawa T, Yamamoto I, Yamada K, Kawano H. Development and achievement of cervical laminoplasty and related studies on cervical myelopathy. Spine Surg Relat Res 2019;4(1):8–17

21. Mizuno J, Nakagawa H, Matsuo N, Song J. Dural ossification associated with cervical ossification of the posterior longitudinal ligament: frequency of dural ossification and comparison of neuroimaging modalities in ability to identify the disease. J Neurosurg Spine 2005;2(4):425–430

22. Shimokawa N, Sato H, Matsumoto H, Takami T. Review of radiological parameters, imaging characteristics, and their effect on optimal treatment approaches and surgical outcomes for cervical ossification of the posterior longitudinal ligament. Neurospine 2019;16(3):506–516

23. Clarke E, Robinson PK. Cervical myelopathy: a complication of cervical spondylosis. Brain 1956;79(3):483–510

24. Lees F, Turner JW. Natural history and prognosis of cervical spondylosis. BMJ 1963; 2(5373):1607–1610

25. Tetreault LA, Karadimas S, Wilson JR, et al. The natural history of degenerative cervical myelopathy and the rate of hospitalization following spinal cord injury: an updated systematic review. Global Spine J 2017; 7(3, Suppl)28S–34S

26. Yarbrough CK, Murphy RKJ, Ray WZ, Stewart TJ. The natural history and clinical presentation of cervical spondylotic myelopathy. Adv Orthop 2012;2012:480643

27. Sumi M, Miyamoto H, Suzuki T, Kaneyama S, Kanatani T, Uno K. Prospective cohort study of mild cervical spondylotic myelopathy without surgical treatment. J Neurosurg Spine 2012;16(1):8–14

28. Karadimas SK, Erwin WM, Ely CG, Dettori JR, Fehlings MG. Pathophysiology and natural history of cervical spondylotic myelopathy. Spine 2013; 38(22, Suppl 1)S21–S36

29. Matsumoto M, Chiba K, Ishikawa M, Maruiwa H, Fujimura Y, Toyama Y. Relationships between outcomes of conservative treatment and magnetic resonance imaging findings in patients with mild cervical myelopathy caused by soft disc herniations. Spine 2001;26(14):1592–1598

30. Kadanka Z, Mares M, Bednarík J, et al. Predictive factors for mild forms of spondylotic cervical myelopathy treated conservatively or surgically. Eur J Neurol 2005;12(1):16–24

31. Shimomura T, Sumi M, Nishida K, et al. Prognostic factors for deterioration of patients with cervical spondylotic myelopathy after nonsurgical treatment. Spine 2007;32(22):2474–2479

32. Kato F, Yukawa Y, Suda K, Yamagata M, Ueta T. Normal morphology, age-related changes and abnormal findings of the cervical spine. Part II: Magnetic resonance imaging of over 1,200 asymptomatic subjects. Eur Spine J 2012;21(8):1499–1507

33. Bednarik J, Kadanka Z, Dusek L, et al. Presymptomatic spondylotic cervical cord compression. Spine 2004;29(20):2260–2269

34. Matsunaga S, Sakou T, Taketomi E, Komiya S. Clinical course of patients with ossification of the posterior longitudinal ligament: a minimum 10-year cohort study. J Neurosurg 2004; 100(3, Suppl Spine):245–248

35. Fassett DR, Jeyamohan S, Harrop J. Asymptomatic cervical stenosis: to operate or not? Semin Spine Surg 2007;19:47–50

36. Marquez-Lara A, Nandyala SV, Fineberg SJ, Singh K. Current trends in demographics, practice, and in-hospital outcomes in cervical spine surgery: a national database analysis between 2002 and 2011. Spine 2014;39(6):476–481

37. Nouri A, Cheng JS, Davies B, Kotter M, Schaller K, Tessitore E. Degenerative cervical myelopathy: a brief review of past perspectives, present developments, and future directions. J Clin Med 2020;9(2):535

38. Dieleman JL, Squires E, Bui AL, et al. Factors associated with increases in US health care spending, 1996–2013. JAMA 2017;318(17):1668–1678

39. Vaziri S, Lockney DT, Dru AB, Polifka AJ, Fox WC, Hoh DJ. Does ossification of the posterior longitudinal ligament progress after fusion? Neurospine 2019;16(3):483–491

40. Kawaguchi Y, Kanamori M, Ishihara H, et al. Progression of ossification of the posterior longitudinal ligament following en bloc cervical laminoplasty. J Bone Joint Surg Am 2001;83(12):1798–1802

41. Wang L, Jiang Y, Li M, Qi L. Postoperative progression of cervical ossification of posterior longitudinal ligament: a systematic review. World Neurosurg 2019;126:593–600

42. Shin J, Choi JY, Kim YW, Chang JS, Yoon SY. Quantification of risk factors for cervical ossification of the posterior longitudinal ligament in Korean populations: a nationwide population-based case-control study. Spine 2019;44(16):E957–E964

43. Zileli M, Borkar SA, Sinha S, et al. Cervical spondylotic myelopathy: natural course and the value of diagnostic techniques -WFNS Spine Committee Recommendations. Neurospine 2019;16(3):386–402

04 Biomechanics of the Healthy and the Degenerative Cervical Spine

Francesco Costa and Fabio Galbusera

Introduction

Biomechanics applies physical laws to investigate the mechanics of biological structures such as muscles, ligaments, joints, etc. Because of the complex architecture of the human spine, alterations to its structures due to degeneration or trauma may affect its alignment and biomechanical response; for example, changes in the position of the skull (occiput or C0) on top of the cervical spine may affect the biomechanical capability of the cervical spine to hold the head vertical, therefore also impacting the normal mobility. Indeed, the functional program of the cervical spine ensures maximal mobility of the head for the visual and auditory exploration of the space, as well as protects the spinal cord and vertebral arteries. In order to achieve these functions, the cervical spine has peculiar anatomical and biomechanical properties that are described further in this chapter.

Spine Biomechanics

The spinal column consists of various complex anatomical structures; therefore, it is essential to fully understand the biomechanically relevant anatomy and its mechanical properties. From a biomechanical point of view, the cervical spine can be classified into two main regions: the anterior and the posterior columns. The vertebral bodies, intervertebral discs, and related ligaments (anterior and posterior longitudinal ligaments) comprise the anterior vertebral column and provide for the majority of the axial load-bearing of the spine. The pedicles, lamina, spinous process and facet joints, with the ligament complex, define the posterior column and restrict spinal motion. The facet joints assume the axial load-bearing capacity primarily when the spine is in a lordotic posture, which is considered normal in the standing posture.[1] For descriptive purposes, the cervical spine can be divided into two main regions, with proper characteristics, both anatomical and functional: the upper cervical spine comprising the occiput (also named C0), C1, and C2 and the subaxial cervical spine from C3 to C7.[2]

The motion of the cervical spine, similarly to the other regions of the spine, is commonly described by means of a conventional naming scheme, adopted by the Scoliosis Research Society and consistent with the standard ISO 2631 (VDI 2057) (**Fig. 4.1**).[3] Three main axes of motion are defined; rotation around those axes are named flexion-extension, lateral bending, and axial rotation. In *in vitro* tests conducted on cadaveric specimens as well as in numerical simulations with finite element models, pure moments around those axes of motion are applied by means of material testing systems or purposely designed apparatuses. The specimen is constrained at its lower end, most typically the lower endplate of its most caudal vertebra; the pure moments are applied to the upper vertebra by means of appropriate actuators. Apart from the constrained area, the specimen should be left free to move in all six degrees of freedom. The resulting three-dimensional motion can then be measured with motion capture systems; the rotation measured in correspondence with the maximal applied moment is conventionally named as the range of motion (ROM).

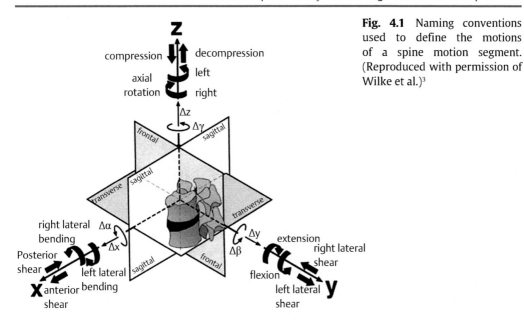

Fig. 4.1 Naming conventions used to define the motions of a spine motion segment. (Reproduced with permission of Wilke et al.)[3]

Flexibility and Motion of the Healthy Cervical Spine

Panjabi et al measured the flexibility of 16 human cervical spine specimens by applying pure moments of 1 Nm in flexion-extension, lateral bending, and axial rotation (**Fig. 4.2**).[4] The results highlighted strong differences among the various levels, especially between the upper and the subaxial cervical spines. Due to the peculiar anatomy of the C0–C1 and C1–C2 motion segments, higher ROMs in flexion-extension and axial rotation with respect to the subaxial cervical spine have been found.[5] In the latter region, a trend toward an increase of flexibility from C2–C3 to C4–C5 followed by a decrease proceeding caudally was observed in all three motion planes. In general, C4–C5 and C5–C6 were found to be the most flexible segments in the subaxial region.

The subaxial cervical spine exhibits specific motion patterns that are not observed or are less evident in the other spinal regions. If a pure moment is applied around the lateral bending axis, due to the peculiar orientation of the facet joints and the saddlelike shape of the vertebral bodies, the resulting rotation would not be around the same axis but would

have a component in axial rotation; lateral bending and axial rotation are therefore coupled.[4,6] Indeed, previous studies proposed the definition of the two main axes of cervical motion[2,7]; the first axis is orthogonal to the sagittal plane and passes through a point slightly caudal to the center of the intervertebral disc, whereas the second axis is orthogonal to the plane defined by the facet joints. Motion around the third hypothetical axis, which is orthogonal to the other two axes, is prevented by the facet joints (**Fig. 4.3**).

A powerful tool for investigating the motion patterns of the cervical spine, in both *in vivo* and *in vitro* tests, is the calculation of the helical axes of motion, that is, the line which is the axis of rotation and simultaneously the direction of translation of a body in motion. Studies determined that the helical axes are an effective method to describe the quality of the motion of the spine, in addition to the quantity which is well described by the ROM.[8] The direction of the helical axes during flexion–extension, lateral bending, and axial rotation of the neck has been measured *in vivo* by means of biplanar fluoroscopy.[9] Indeed, results showed that, in the subaxial spine, the helical axes in lateral bending and axial rotation are very similar

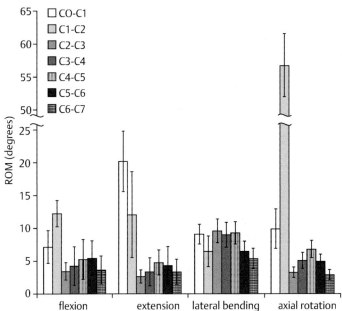

Fig. 4.2 Ranges of motion (ROM) of the cervical motion segments in flexion, extension, lateral bending, and axial rotation, measured in *in vitro* tests on cadaver specimens.[4]

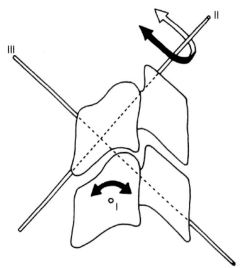

Fig. 4.3 The main motion axes of a cervical motion segment; motion around the axis "III" is prevented by the action of the facet joints. (Reproduced with permission of Bogduk and Mercer.)[2]

and in both cases oriented orthogonally to the facet joints, consistently with the hypothesis of the two main axes of cervical motion[2] (**Fig. 4.4**).

Biomechanics of the Degenerative Cervical Spine

Similar to their lumbar counterparts, cervical motion segments undergo degeneration with aging. Degenerative changes include the reduction of the height and water content of the intervertebral disc, modifications to its mechanical properties due to changes in the tissue composition, development of osteophytes,[10] alterations of the vertebral bone and endplates such as sclerosis and Modic changes (i.e., edema and inflammation of the bone marrow or replacement of bone with fatty marrow visible on magnetic resonance images),[11] as well as osteoarthritis of the facet joints.[12]

As the disc changes are at the basis of the degenerative process, the subaxial cervical spine, in correlation with its functional aim to guarantee the flexion-extension movements, is mainly involved. In fact, the spondylosis, often preceded by mild segmental instability, is defined as "vertebral osteophytosis secondary to degenerative disc disease" and is associated with the arthritic inflammatory process involving the facet joints and

Extension Movement | Flexion Movement

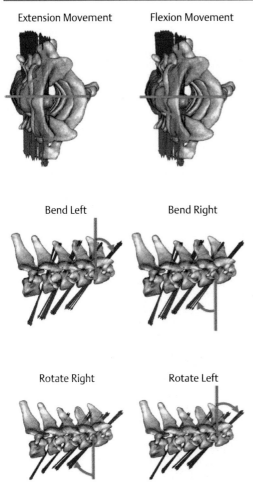

Bend Left | Bend Right

Rotate Right | Rotate Left

Fig. 4.4 The helical axes of motion in flexion-extension (*upper*), lateral bending (*middle*), and axial rotation (*lower*) measured *in vivo*. (Reproduced with permission of Anderst et al.)[9]

osteophyte formation. Due to the degenerative changes, the disc desiccates, resulting in disc height loss: considering the continuous application of motions, which then alters the load transmission across and along the cervical spine, there is a progressive alteration of the endplates, facet joints, finally leading to the formation of osteophytes. As the flexion-extension is the main motion, osteophytes are mainly located anteriorly and posteriorly. Cervical spondylotic myelopathy (CSM) is the direct consequence of repetitive trauma to the spinal cord, thus resulting in abnormal motor and sensory findings, and ultimately

cervical spondylosis can lead to chronic kyphotic deformation. These changes are frequently associated with neck pain and low quality of life.[13] Several classification schemes aimed at grading the degree of cervical degeneration have been introduced and are frequently employed in clinical practice.[14-18] Based on most schemes, a score ranging from "no degeneration" to "severe degeneration" with some in-between grades is used to describe the overall degree of degeneration of the motion segment, which takes into account the various features describing the degenerative phenotypes such as osteophytes, disc height reduction, etc. (**Fig. 4.5**).

The biomechanical impact of the single degenerative feature has been investigated and described in a relatively low number of studies, whereas a larger number of papers addressed the biomechanics of surgeries such as fixation and fusion as well as cervical disc replacement. Most papers investigating cervical degeneration were based on numerical simulations, whereas the response of degenerated cadaveric specimens subjected to *in vitro* testing remains relatively unexplored.

The importance of osteophytes was demonstrated by Kumaresan et al,[19] who built a finite element model of the C4–C6 spine region and used it to quantitatively determine the impact of disc degeneration at the C5–C6 level on the resulting segmental biomechanics. The authors modeled mild and moderate disc degeneration by altering the material properties of the disc and severe degeneration by additionally reducing the height of the intervertebral space. In general, disc degeneration was associated with an increase of both stiffness of the motion segment and stress in the bone tissue adjacent to the disc itself, especially in the anterior region. The paper concluded that such a stress increase may trigger bone remodeling, inducing the formation of the osteophytes that are commonly present in degenerated segments.

A research group in Chesterfield, Missouri published several papers about the impact of cervical degeneration on the adjacent segments, using a finite element model of the

Grade 0 (no degeneration) (C2-3, male 59 years):

lateral radiograph   *midsagittal frozen cut*

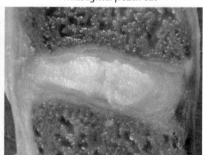

Fig. 4.5 Classification scheme for cervical disc degeneration based on disc height loss, osteophytosis, and diffuse sclerosis. (Reproduced with permission of Kettler et al.)[15]

Grade 1 (mild degeneration) (C5-6, female, 72 years):

lateral radiograph   *midsagittal frozen cut*

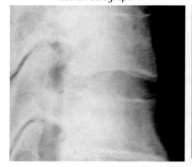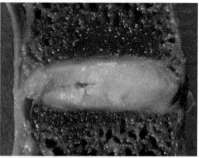

Grade 2 (moderate degeneration) (C4-5, female, 81 years):

lateral radiograph   *midsagittal frozen cut*

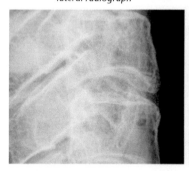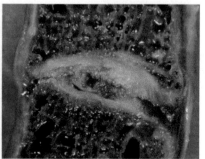

Grade 3 (severe degeneration) (C3-4, female, 92 years):

lateral radiograph   *midsagittal frozen cut*

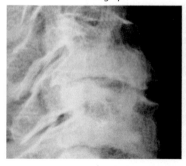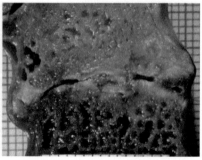

C3–T1 region and modeling degeneration at the C5–C6 level (**Fig. 4.6**).[20-24] The porous-elastic nature of the model allowed for investigation of the flow of water content in the discs, thereby assessing the time-dependent response of the spine under the application of loads with varying speeds. The study confirmed that disc degeneration is associated with a decrease of flexibility at the index level; at the adjacent segments, higher mobility was observed, more evidently at C6–C7 than at C4–C5, especially in flexion-extension.[20] Interestingly, another research group found contrasting results by using a model of the C3–C7 region in which degeneration was implemented at C5–C6 by altering disc height and shape of the endplates as well as by adding osteophytes (**Fig. 4.7**).[25] Indeed, the model confirmed the decreased ROM at the degenerative level, but a moderate flexibility decrease was also observed in the adjacent segments. It should be noted that the analysis of flexion-extension radiographs seems to confirm that the *in vivo* motion at the segments adjacent to a degenerated disc indeed increases, on an average by 0.8° for each degree of degeneration, whereas a ROM decrease is strongly associated with degeneration at the index level.[26]

Increases in the loads transmitted through the facet joints were also observed, at both the adjacent segments and degenerated level itself,[22,25] whereas intradiscal pressures at the adjacent segments were modestly affected.[23] The caudal adjacent segment was more strongly affected than the cranial one also in terms of facet loads. Finally, the authors demonstrated that the patterns of disc height reduction in the anterior and posterior zones also have an influence on the segmental biomechanics, with the posterior height loss being more critical.[21]

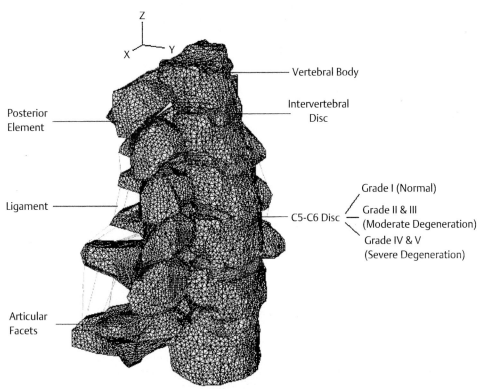

Fig. 4.6 A finite element model of the C3–T1 region, integrating degenerative features at the C5–C6 level. (Reproduced with permission of Hussain et al.)[21]

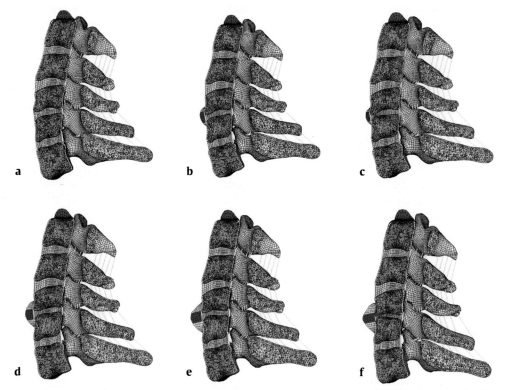

Fig. 4.7 Six finite element models of the subaxial cervical spine integrating progressive degeneration at the C5–C6 level. (**a**) Mild changes of material properties and disc height. (**b**) Mild changes of material properties and disc height, small anterior osteophyte, and mild endplate sclerosis. (**c**) Moderate changes of material properties and disc height, small anterior osteophyte, and mild endplate sclerosis. (**d**) Moderate changes of material properties and disc height, moderate anterior osteophyte, and moderate endplate sclerosis. (**e**) Severe changes of material properties, moderate disc height loss, large anterior osteophyte, and moderate endplate sclerosis. (**f**) Severe changes of material properties and disc height, large anterior osteophyte, and severe endplate. (Reproduced with permission of Cai et al.)[25]

The relevance of the composition of the intervertebral disc in terms of content of proteoglycans and tissue permeability was investigated by the Chesterfield research group by using a finite element model of the C5–C6 motion segment, in which disc swelling behavior was modeled by simulating a fixed charge density.[24] The model revealed that implementing a strain-dependent permeability had a larger effect on the biomechanical response than the fixed charge density. Due to the preliminary nature of the work and the lack of an experimental validation, the authors concluded that further studies would be necessary to corroborate the findings.

Biomechanics of Injury and Defects

In comparison with the relatively poorly investigated field of the biomechanics of cervical degeneration, a larger number of studies have been conducted to assess the biomechanical impact of defects and lesions, such as those resulting from injury or due to invasive surgical treatments, for example, the decompression of a stenotic spinal canal or the resection of a tumor.

The impact on spinal flexibility and stability of injuries due to hyperextension was investigated by Richter et al by using six cadaver specimens of the C4–C7 region. Incremental lesion conditions were implemented at C5-C6 by resecting the anterior longitudinal ligament–the intertransverse ligament, by an incision in the anterior annulus fibrosus, by resecting the flaval, interspinous, and supraspinous ligaments, and finally by capsulotomy.[27] Increasing instability in flexion-extension was observed in all simulated conditions, whereas capsulotomy also determined a destabilization in torsion. Hartwig et al simulated car accidents by means of a purposely designed apparatus[28] (**Fig. 4.8**) and demonstrated that the resulting injuries to facet joint capsules and intervertebral discs determined a ROM increase in lateral bending and, less pronouncedly, in axial rotation.[29]

An interesting *in vitro* study conducted on seven cadaver specimens of the C2–T1 region investigated the changes in cervical stability after simulated decompression surgery for the treatment of spinal stenosis,[30] which was modeled by suturing wooden hemispherical beads inside the spinal canal between C4 and C7 in order to achieve approximately 50% occlusion. The flexibility of the specimens was then measured after simulating stenosis, laminoplasty, and finally laminectomy. Results showed that ROMs were largely unaffected by simulated stenosis and laminoplasty, but laminectomy significantly decreased the stability by 12% in flexion and 17% in extension.

Biomechanics of the Spinal Cord and Cervical Myelopathy

The spinal cord, especially when the cervical spine is in a degenerative condition, is subjected to mechanical strain during neck motion and, possibly, in the standing

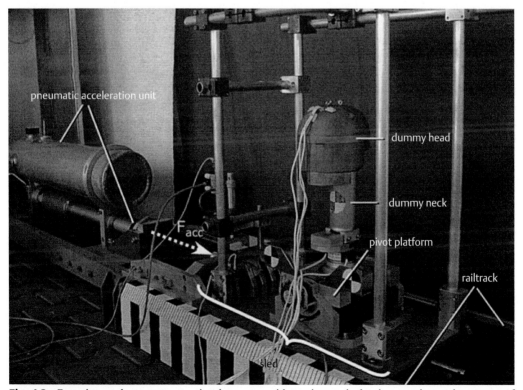

Fig. 4.8 Experimental apparatus to simulate car accidents in cervical spine specimens by means of collisions. (Reproduced with permission of Kettler et al.)[28]

posture.[31,32] It has indeed been shown that degenerative alterations of the spine, for example, the ossification of the posterior longitudinal ligament (OPLL) and ossification of the flaval ligament (OFL), may induce the development of cervical myelopathy, possibly via pathological alterations of the strain patterns of the spinal cord associated with the ligament ossification.[33] The investigation of the strains in the spinal cord is indeed a subject of active research, both with imaging techniques such as contrast-enhanced radiography[34] and magnetic resonance imaging,[31] and from the biomechanical point of view.

In order to quantitatively investigate stresses and strains inside the spinal cord, the finite element method proved to be a very useful tool due to its ability in predicting the local values of such quantities, whereas the techniques allowing for such measurements *in vitro* do not currently exist. One example of such studies was published by Kim et al, who simulated the effect of OPLL and OFL on stresses in the spinal cord.[35] The authors predicted substantial increases in the cord stresses when the cross-sectional area of the spinal canal was reduced by 30 to 40% due to ligament ossification. Kato et al conducted a similar study in which spinal cord compression due to OPLL was simulated and also found a sharp increase in cord stresses between a degree of OPLL-induced compression of 20 and 40%.[36] The same research group investigated stresses in the spinal cord in cervical flexion myelopathy and found high stresses located in the gray matter, posterior funiculus, and in a region of the lateral funiculus under the simulation of 10° of flexion.[37] Another issue investigated with numerical simulations was the comparison of stresses in different spinal cord segments, which highlighted a substantial similarity in the stress distribution among the various levels, especially in the case of severe compression.[38]

Stresses in the spinal cord in traumatic injury scenarios have also been studied by means of finite element models, which allow access to results that cannot be measured

experimentally. Li et al built a finite element model of the cervical cord[39] and validated it by comparing the force-displacement response with *in vitro* data obtained in static tension and compression.[41,42] The model was then used to simulate a hyperextension injury scenario. The results of the simulations showed high localized stresses in the gray matter, and at the anterior and posterior horns (**Fig. 4.9**), which were consistent with previous observations on photomicrographs of the murine spinal cord under compression injury conditions.[42]

Another topic of investigation by means of numerical simulations was the age-related changes in the mechanical properties of the spinal cord.[43] By combining experimental measurements on bovine specimens and numerical simulations, the authors demonstrated that the biomechanical response of young and older spinal cords is evidently different; under the effect of the same compressive load, the older cords were subjected to higher internal stresses that may be associated with the development of CSM. In a subsequent paper, the same research group observed distinct mechanical properties between white and gray matter, resulting in different stresses that may also contribute to the development of tissue damage.[44]

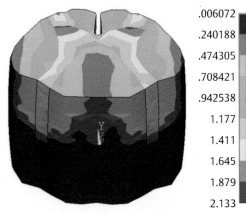

.006072
.240188
.474305
.708421
.942538
1.177
1.411
1.645
1.879
2.133

Fig. 4.9 Stresses (in Pa) in the cervical spinal cord under simulated compression, calculated with a finite element model. (Reproduced with permission of Li et al.)[42]

Conclusion

Although its clinical relevance is undoubted and many research questions remain unanswered, the biomechanics of the cervical spine has been relatively weakly investigated, significantly less than that of the lumbar spine. Especially, regarding the biomechanical effect of the degenerative changes, such as intervertebral disc degeneration, ossification of the ligaments, and facet arthrosis, the number of published studies remains markedly lower with respect to the abundance of extensive papers describing the degenerative disease in the lumbar spine. Nevertheless, several valuable papers are indeed available and have considerably advanced the knowledge about the biomechanics of the cervical spine and related disorders. Editors encourage authors to undertake projects in the field described in this chapter, in order to fill the remaining knowledge gaps, with the final aim of improving the clinical care of cervical disorders.

References

1. Knott PT, Mardjetko SM, Techy F. The use of the T1 sagittal angle in predicting overall sagittal balance of the spine. Spine J 2010; 10(11):994–998
2. Bogduk N, Mercer S. Biomechanics of the cervical spine. I: normal kinematics. Clin Biomech (Bristol, Avon) 2000;15(9):633–648
3. Wilke HJ, Wenger K, Claes L. Testing criteria for spinal implants: recommendations for the standardization of in vitro stability testing of spinal implants. Eur Spine J 1998; 7(2):148–154
4. Panjabi MM, Crisco JJ, Vasavada A, et al. Mechanical properties of the human cervical spine as shown by three-dimensional load-displacement curves. Spine 2001;26(24): 2692–2700
5. Ivancic P, Dvorak J, Goel VK, et al. Cervical spine kinematics and clinical instability. In: Benzel E, ed. The Cervical Spine. Wolters Kluwer - Lippincott Williams & Wilkins 2012; 53–72
6. Goel VK, Clark CR, McGowan D, Goyal S. An in-vitro study of the kinematics of the normal, injured and stabilized cervical spine. J Biomech 1984;17(5):363–376
7. Penning L. Normal movements of the cervical spine. AJR Am J Roentgenol 1978; 130(2):317–326
8. Kettler A, Marin F, Sattelmayer G, et al. Finite helical axes of motion are a useful tool to describe the three-dimensional in vitro kinematics of the intact, injured and stabilised spine. Eur Spine J 2004;13(6):553–559
9. Anderst WJ, Donaldson WF III, Lee JY, Kang JD. Three-dimensional intervertebral kinematics in the healthy young adult cervical spine during dynamic functional loading. J Biomech 2015;48(7):1286–1293
10. Macnab I. Cervical spondylosis. Clin Orthop Relat Res 1975; (109):69–77
11. Modic MT, Steinberg PM, Ross JS, Masaryk TJ, Carter JR. Degenerative disk disease: assessment of changes in vertebral body marrow with MR imaging. Radiology 1988; 166(1 Pt 1):193–199
12. Kettler A, Werner K, Wilke H-J. Morphological changes of cervical facet joints in elderly individuals. Eur Spine J 2007;16(7):987–992
13. Yang X, Karis DSA, Vleggeert-Lankamp CLA. Association between Modic changes, disc degeneration, and neck pain in the cervical spine: a systematic review of literature. Spine J 2019 (e-pub ahead of print). doi:10.1016/j. spinee.2019.11.002
14. Kettler A, Wilke H-J. Review of existing grading systems for cervical or lumbar disc and facet joint degeneration. Eur Spine J 2006;15(6):705–718
15. Kettler A, Rohlmann F, Neidlinger-Wilke C, et al. Validity and interobserver agreement of a new radiographic grading system for intervertebral disc degeneration: Part II. Cervical spine. Eur Spine J 2006;15(6): 732–741
16. Brooker AE, Barter RW. Cervical spondylosis. A clinical study with comparative radiology. Brain 1965;88(5):925–936
17. Friedenberg ZB, Miller WT. Degenerative disc disease of the cervical spine. J Bone Joint Surg Am 1963;45:1171–1178
18. Kellgren JH, Lawrence JS. Radiological assessment of osteo-arthrosis. Ann Rheum Dis 1957;16(4):494–502

19. Kumaresan S, Yoganandan N, Pintar FA, Maiman DJ, Goel VK. Contribution of disc degeneration to osteophyte formation in the cervical spine: a biomechanical investigation. J Orthop Res 2001;19(5):977–984

20. Hussain M, Natarajan RN, An HS, Andersson GBJ. Motion changes in adjacent segments due to moderate and severe degeneration in C5-C6 disc: a poroelastic C3-T1 finite element model study. Spine 2010;35(9):939–947

21. Hussain M, Natarajan RN, An HS, Andersson GBJ. Progressive disc degeneration at C5-C6 segment affects the mechanics between disc heights and posterior facets above and below the degenerated segment: A flexion-extension investigation using a poroelastic C3-T1 finite element model. Med Eng Phys 2012;34(5):552–558

22. Hussain M, Natarajan RN, Chaudhary G, An HS, Andersson GBJ. Posterior facet load changes in adjacent segments due to moderate and severe degeneration in C5-C6 disc: a poroelastic C3-T1 finite element model study. J Spinal Disord Tech 2012; 25(4):218–225

23. Hussain M, Natarajan RN, An HS, Andersson GBJ. Reduction in segmental flexibility because of disc degeneration is accompanied by higher changes in facet loads than changes in disc pressure: a poroelastic C5-C6 finite element investigation. Spine J 2010; 10(12):1069–1077

24. Hussain M, Natarajan RN, Chaudhary G, An HS, Andersson GBJ. Relative contributions of strain-dependent permeability and fixed charged density of proteoglycans in predicting cervical disc biomechanics: a poroelastic C5-C6 finite element model study. Med Eng Phys 2011;33(4):438–445

25. Cai X-Y, Sang D, Yuchi C-X, et al. Using finite element analysis to determine effects of the motion loading method on facet joint forces after cervical disc degeneration. Comput Biol Med 2020;116:103519

26. Simpson AK, Biswas D, Emerson JW, Lawrence BD, Grauer JN. Quantifying the effects of age, gender, degeneration, and adjacent level degeneration on cervical spine range of motion using multivariate analyses. Spine 2008;33(2):183–186

27. Richter M, Wilke HJ, Kluger P, Claes L, Puhl W. Load-displacement properties of the normal and injured lower cervical spine in vitro. Eur Spine J 2000;9(2):104–108

28. Kettler A, Schmitt H, Simon U, et al. A new acceleration apparatus for the study of whiplash with human cadaveric cervical spine specimens. J Biomech 2004; 37(10):1607–1613

29. Hartwig E, Kettler A, Schultheiss M, et al. In vitro low-speed side collisions cause injury to the lower cervical spine but do not damage alar ligaments. Eur Spine J 2004;13(7):590–597

30. Subramaniam V, Chamberlain RH, Theodore N, et al. Biomechanical effects of laminoplasty versus laminectomy: stenosis and stability. Spine 2009;34(16):E573–E578

31. Condon BR, Hadley DM. Quantification of cord deformation and dynamics during flexion and extension of the cervical spine using MR imaging. J Comput Assist Tomogr 1988;12(6):947–955

32. Breig A, el-Nadi AF. Biomechanics of the cervical spinal cord. Relief of contact pressure on and overstretching of the spinal cord. Acta Radiol Diagn (Stockh) 1966;4(6):602–624

33. Kotani Y, Takahata M, Abumi K, et al. Cervical myelopathy resulting from combined ossification of the ligamentum flavum and posterior longitudinal ligament: report of two cases and literature review. Spine J 2013;13(1):e1–e6

34. Dichiro G, Fisher RL. Contrast radiography of the spinal cord. Arch Neurol 1964;11: 125–143

35. Kim YH, Khuyagbaatar B, Kim K. Biomechanical effects of spinal cord compression due to ossification of posterior longitudinal ligament and ligamentum flavum: a finite element analysis. Med Eng Phys 2013;35(9):1266–1271

36. Kato Y, Kanchiku T, Imajo Y, et al. Biomechanical study of the effect of degree of static compression of the spinal cord in ossification of the posterior longi-tudinal ligament. J Neurosurg Spine 2010; 12(3):301–305

37. Kato Y, Kataoka H, Ichihara K, et al. Biomechanical study of cervical flexion myelopathy using a three-dimensional finite

element method. J Neurosurg Spine 2008; 8(5):436–441

38. Nishida N, Kanchiku T, Imajo Y, et al. Stress analysis of the cervical spinal cord: Impact of the morphology of spinal cord segments on stress. J Spinal Cord Med 2016;39(3):327–334

39. Li X-F, Dai L-Y. Three-dimensional finite element model of the cervical spinal cord: preliminary results of injury mechanism analysis. Spine 2009;34(11):1140–1147

40. Hung TK, Lin HS, Bunegin L, Albin MS. Mechanical and neurological response of cat spinal cord under static loading. Surg Neurol 1982;17(3):213–217

41. Maiman DJ, Coats J, Myklebust JB. Cord/spine motion in experimental spinal cord injury. J Spinal Disord 1989;2(1):14–19

42. Ma M, Basso DM, Walters P, Stokes BT, Jakeman LB. Behavioral and histological outcomes following graded spinal cord contusion injury in the C57Bl/6 mouse. Exp Neurol 2001;169(2):239–254

43. Okazaki T, Kanchiku T, Nishida N, et al. Age-related changes of the spinal cord: a biomechanical study. Exp Ther Med 2018; 15(3):2824–2829

44. Ichihara K, Taguchi T, Sakuramoto I, Kawano S, Kawai S. Mechanism of the spinal cord injury and the cervical spondylotic myelopathy: new approach based on the mechanical features of the spinal cord white and gray matter. J Neurosurg 2003; 99(3, Suppl):278–285

05 Clinical Tests and Differential Diagnosis of Cervical Spondylotic Myelopathy

Jesus Lafuente

Introduction

Cervical spondylotic myelopathy (CSM) is a disabling disease caused by a combination of mechanical compression and vascular compromise of the spinal cord. It is the most common cause of spinal dysfunction in older patients.[1] The onset is often insidious with long periods of episodic, stepwise progression and may present with different symptoms from one patient to another.[2] CSM is a clinical diagnosis that may involve broad-based gait disturbances first, associated with weakness of the legs, and then spasticity.[3] As spinal cord degeneration progresses, lower motor neuron findings in the upper extremities, such as loss of strength, atrophy, and difficulty in fine finger movements, may present.[3] Additional clinical findings may include: neck stiffness, shoulder pain, paresthesia in one or both arms or hands, radiculopathy, a positive Hoffman and/or Babinski sign, motor deficits, hyperreflexia, and bowel and bladder dysfunction.[3]

Physical examination findings are not always consistent with severity of disease in CSM; therefore, correlation to plain X-rays, MRI, and clinical symptoms is essential for a correct diagnosis. Anterior-posterior width reduction, cross-sectional evidence of cord compression, obliteration of the subarachnoid space, and signal intensity changes to the cord found on MR imaging are considered the most appropriate parameters for confirmation of a spinal cord compression myelopathy.[4] In some occasions when the diagnosis is still not clear, the use of other studies could help, such as diagnostic electrophysiology and cerebrospinal fluid (CSF) examination.

Clinical Tests

CSM is the most common cause of spinal cord dysfunction in the world. A meticulous physical examination of patients with cervical pathology can relatively make the distinction between radiculopathy or myelopathy easy. Routine physical examination of patients with cervical myelopathy should include special tests in addition to a thorough neurological examination. The relevant clinical examination tests are categorized in **Table 5.1**.

Table 5.1 Clinical examination tests used for cervical spondylotic myelopathy

Motor deficit	Sensory deficit	Upper motor neuron deficit	Provocative test	Gait and balance
Muscle weakness	Proprioception	Hoffman´s reflex	L´hermitte sign	Romberg test
Finger scape test	Vibratory test	Babinski reflex		Heel and toe walk
Grip and release	Pinprick	Sustained clonus		
		Inverted radial reflex		
		Scapulohumeral test		
		Hyperreflexia		

Muscle Weakness

The causes of lack of muscle strength are many; however, in CSM, the most common cause is due to a peripheral muscular fatigue, which represents the inability of a specific muscle to work, secondary to a loss or dysfunction on any of the motor neurological pathways. This can be caused by osteophytes or prolapsed discs that compress either the spinal cord directly or the spinal nerves. It is important to distinguish weakness from fatigue or asthenia, which are separate conditions with different etiologies that can coexist with, or be confused for, weakness.

Technique

The patient stays in a sitting position and the doctor tests the level of strength in all muscle groups, examining from upper to lower extremities and quantifying the severity of muscle weakness, according to the Medical Research Council (MRC) criteria[5]:

- **Grade 0**: No contraction or muscle movement.
- **Grade 1**: Trace of contraction but no movement at the joint.
- **Grade 2**: Movement at the joint with gravity eliminated.
- **Grade 3**: Movement against gravity but not against added resistance.
- **Grade 4**: Movement against external resistance with less strength than usual.
- **Grade 5**: Normal strength.

This grading is not only an excellent tool to determine muscle weakness but also a great tool to evaluate progression and recovery after treatment.

The Wartenberg´s Sign or Finger Scape Sign

It was first described by Robert Wartenberg in 1939. Wartenberg's sign refers to the slightly greater abduction of the fifth digit, due to paralysis of the abducting palmar interosseous muscle and unopposed action of the radial innervated extensor muscles (digiti minimi, digitorum communis).[6]

From the physiological standpoint, this sign is easily understandable. Adduction of the little finger is performed by the interosseous and abduction by the hypothenar muscles. Both groups of the muscles are innervated by the ulnar nerve. However, in abduction of the little finger, the extensor digiti minimi and the branch to the little finger of extensor digitorum communis also play a definite part; both are innervated by radial nerve. If the muscles innervated by the ulnar nerve are weak, those innervated by the intact radial nerve predominate in strength and abduct the little finger. Thus, it is understandable why this abduction of the little finger is best seen when extensor digitorum communis comes into action and extends the fingers and the hand. In cases with combined palsy of ulnar nerve and radial nerve, this sign would not be present.

The finger scape sign is not only seen in ulnar nerve palsies but also in patients with syringomyelia and is an important examination test in the myelopathic hand together with grip and release.

Technique

The patient is placed with the wrist in a neutral position, and forearm fully pronated and instructed to perform full extension of all the fingers. Once digits are extended, patient is asked to fully abduct all fingers and then adduct all fingers. A positive sign is indicated with the observation of abduction, along with the inability to adduct the 5th digit when extended (**Fig. 5.1**).

Grip and Release Test

Grip and release test is used to evaluate hand function in myelopathic patients. Grip and release tests are part of a group of quantitative clinical tests together with 10-step test and the 30 meters walking test.[7] They are all common, in that they can demonstrate an improvement numerically, comparing

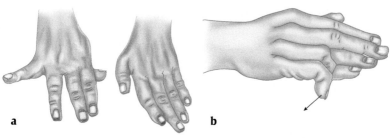

Fig. 5.1 Wartenberg scape test. 5th finger on abduction and flexion as the lesion does not allow the finger to adduct (radial nerve dominance).

a   b

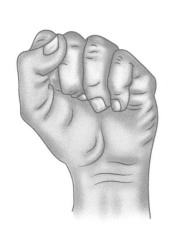

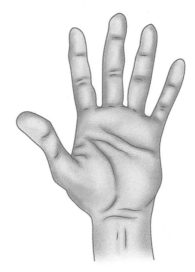

Fig. 5.2 Grip and release quantitative test. Opening and closing the hand. Normal value: > 20 in 10 seconds.

the performance before and after rehabilitation or surgery. This improvement normally coincides with better results in other clinical assessment subjective scales such as Japanese Orthopaedic Association (JOA), short form-36 (SF-36), neck disability index (NDI), and quality-adjusted life-years (QALY) and is reflection of a good management outcome.

It is believed that changes in grip aperture control are caused mainly by pyramidal tract damage in the spinal cord; however, recent studies confirm the importance of somatosensory inputs from the hand into grip aperture control.[8]

Technique

In this reflex, the patient is asked to form a fist and then extend the fingers, rapidly repeating the sequence. A normal response is more than 20 times in a 10-second period. Patients with cervical myelopathy (myelopathic hand) cannot achieve this goal (**Fig. 5.2**).

Proprioception

Proprioception, or kinesthesia, is the sense that lets us perceive the location, movement, and action of parts of the body. When we move, our brain senses the effort, force, and heaviness of our actions and positions and responds accordingly, for example, proprioception enables a person to close their eyes and touch their nose with their index finger. Proprioception includes a complex of sensations, including perception of joint position and movement, muscle force, and effort. In proprioception, the neuromuscular control is the efferent motor response to afferent (sensory) information, and it is a constant feedback loop that tells your brain what position you are in and what forces are acting upon your body at any given point in time.[9] Proprioception relies on the relationship between the body's central nervous system (CNS) and certain soft tissues, including muscles, tendons, and ligaments. Sensory receptors in the muscles are called muscle spindles, which are long proteins encapsulated in sheaths that lay parallel to muscle fibers. These muscle spindles are stretched on muscle extension and is the degree of this stretch effort that is delivered through the spinal nerves to the nervous system, which facilitates a signal sent to the muscle to contract or relax.

Proprioception sensory output ascends through the dorsal columns in the spinal cord. Normal proprioception lets you move freely without giving your movements a second thought. Abnormal proprioception causes symptoms that can interfere with even the simplest activities and even can cause you to fall in severe cases.[10] In upper extremity injuries like in CSM, you may have difficulty reaching properly, and you may have problems with fine motor tasks that require precision of movement (myelopathic hand). This is caused by a loss in proprioception.

Technique

The patient is positioned lying on the bed. He or she is asked to relax and close his or her eyes. The physician then moves the big toe up, down, or keeps it in neutral, asking the patient to recognize which is the position of the big toe (**Fig. 5.3**). Proprioception can also be done in the upper extremity, using the fingers phalanx and asking the patient to recognize what is the position of the finger or phalanx.

Vibratory Sensation

Assessment of vibration sense is the best clinical test of the dorsal column pathway. Vibration sense is tested with a tuning fork (normally 128 Hz) placed on predefined bony prominences (with the eyes closed), and the patient is asked to report when the vibration starts and stops. Sensory receptors (mostly Pacinian and Meissner corpuscles) convert the vibration into a neural signal. The temporal resolution of the neural information transfer (action potentials) should be at least equal to the frequency of the vibration. With age, the vibratory response might be lost in the ankle and both feet. Vibratory sensation is often diminished in peripheral neuropathy and myelopathy but spared in disease confined to the cerebral cortex, orientating the problem to a spinal one.

Technique

The patient is asked to lay on the couch. The examiner explains the procedure until the patient obtains a comprehensive understanding. He or she is then asked to close their eyes and after a gentle strike to the tuning fork, the examiner applies it on top of the big toe (**Fig. 5.4**), asking the patient if he or she feels the vibration and when does it stop. It is important to perform this procedure in both feet and arms to detect any discordance between both sides.

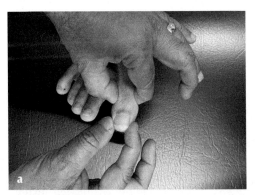
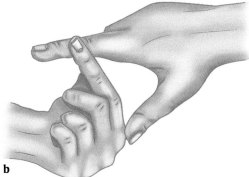

Fig. 5.3 Proprioception test in the phalanx of the big toe (**a**) and at the index finger (**b**).

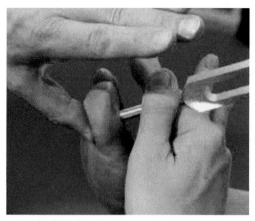

Fig. 5.4 Application of the tuning fork in the big toe in order to perform the vibration sense test.

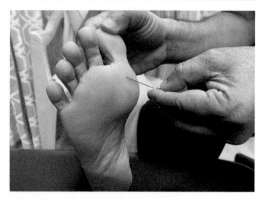

Fig. 5.5 Pinprick examination using a blunt needle or a pin, tapping in the skin and testing different areas of the body recognizing the dermatome involved.

Pinprick (PP) Test

The PP test is performed to test the numbness and pins and needles in a part of the body. The PP is a gross test that checks three variables: (1) the actual ability to feel a pinprick, (2) the ability to determine the difference between sharp and dull, and (3) the ability to locate the area where the pinprick has been tested on. Remember, pain and temperature sensory neurons entering the cord ascend ipsilaterally for two to three spinal segments in the dorsolateral tract of Lissauer before crossing just anterior to the central canal, in order to join the contralateral spinothalamic tract located in the lateral cord. Therefore, loss of pinprick or temperature sensation at a given level may indicate pathology two to three segments above the level detected on examination.

Technique

The patient is asked to lay on the couch. The examiner explains the procedure until the patient obtains a comprehensive understanding. Using a pin or a blunt needle and with the patient's eyes closed, the examiner begins targeting different areas in accordance with the relevant dermatome to be examined (**Fig. 5.5**). The pin should never penetrate the dermis, as it would render an invalid test. In examining the sensibility, the patient is not only asked if he or she can feel but also where he or she can feel it, as feeling the sensation is as relevant as localizing it.

Babinski Reflex

The Babinski reflex (plantar reflex) was described by the neurologist Joseph Babinski in 1899 and is considered normal for infants below the age of 2.[11,12] This reflex tests the integrity of the cortical spinal tract (CST). The CST or pyramidal tract (upper motor neuron) is a descending tract travelling from the eloquent motor area of the brain throughout the spinal cord until it synapses with the alfa motor neuron (lower motor neuron), facilitating a normal motor response.[4,11,12]

A normal Babinski results after stimulating the lateral side of the sole (S1 myotome) and obtaining a plantar flexor response from the toes. Stimulation at the sole (nociceptive fibers S1) travel in an ascending path through the sciatic nerve until the S1 region of the spine, where synapse with the anterior horn cells produce a descending response, which travels through sciatic and tibial nerve until S1 motor fibers and induce the toe plantar flexion.

An abnormal or positive Babinski occurs when stimulating the lateral plantar side of the sole, which leads to dorsiflexion (extension) of the big toe, and on occasions, fanning of the rest of the toes.[4] This is believed to be caused by overspreading of the S1 nociceptive response, reaching the L4 and L5 regions of the spine synapsing producing an overfiring of the anterior horn cells at that level, which descending cause and overwhelming extensor response through the peroneal nerve (extensor hallucis longus and extensor digitorum longus). An intact CST prevents this overspread.

A positive Babinski reflex is indicative of dysfunction of the CST, so not only does it reflect a problem in the cervical spinal cord but also all along the pyramidal tract from brain to lower thoracic spine.[4,11]

Technique

The patient has to be in supine position, relaxed with the legs resting on a couch. You need a pin or a blunt instrument, which has to be run up the lateral plantar side of the foot from the heel to the toes and across the metatarsal pads to the base of the big toe, watching for an extensor response (**Fig. 5.6**). Sharp instruments are not recommended.

There have been multiple variations to the Babinski sign, all eliciting same dorsiflexion response of the big toe. The most known include, Chaddock (stimulating under lateral malleolus), Gordon (squeezing calf), Oppenheim (applying pressure to the medial side of the tibia), and Throckmorton (hitting the metatarsophalangeal joint of the big toe).[12]

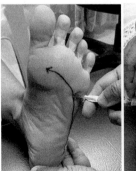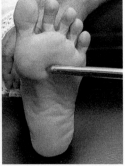

Fig. 5.6 Instructions in how to run the blunt instrument in the sole of the patient. Note the extensor response on the right.

Sustained Clonus

Clonus is a rhythmic, oscillating, repetitive stretch reflex; the cause of which is not totally known; however, it relates to lesions in upper motor neurons and therefore is generally accompanied by hyperreflexia. Like other signs of upper motor neuron syndrome clonus indicates some insult to the central rather than peripheral nervous system, so part of its utility as a clinical examination skill is in differentiating the two.[13]

The mechanism of this reflex is initiated by hyperexcitability produced in muscle stretch circuits when there is less tonic inhibition of motor neurons involved in the monosynaptic stretch reflex. This can occur when there is a lesion to descending motor nerves, predominantly the dorsal reticulospinal pathway, which can occur anywhere from the cortex to the spinal cord. The inhibitory dampening effect of these descending nerves on alpha and gamma motor neurons is removed, leading to a hyperexcitatory state in the muscle stretch reflex circuit.[13,14]

Technique

The patient is asked to relax with a passively flexed ankle to about 90 degrees and a passively flexed knee; this usually involves the examiner supporting the leg with the hand not performing clonus. Next, at the ankle, the examiner places their hand on the dorsum of the patient's forefoot and briskly dorsiflexes it, after which the former continues to maintain dorsiflexion pressure (**Fig. 5.7**). It is against this pressure that the clonus beats will be felt. Each beat will be felt as a plantar flexion followed by a relaxation. The initial beat is the longest, with decreasing duration of beats until the fourth beat, after which the beat frequency becomes equivalent from one to the next.[15] Count of three or over number of beats is considered pathological.

Hoffmann's Reflex

It was first described by the neurologist Johann Hoffmann.[16] This reflex is used to test

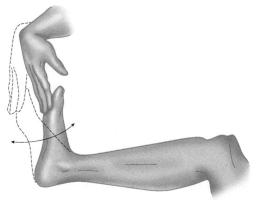

Fig. 5.7 Sustained clonus: In patients with cervical spondylotic myelopathy (CSM), after a brisk dorsiflexion on the foot, a sustained beat should be seen, confirming upper motorneurone damage.

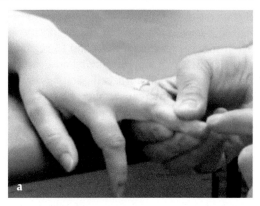

a

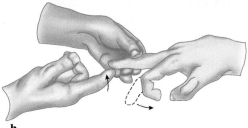

b

Fig. 5.8 On tapping the middle finger, the thumb and index fingers go on to flexion.

upper extremity reflexes and is considered a more reliable test when examining for suspected CSM compared to the Babinski reflex. Hoffmann's reflex has a different mechanism of reflex than Babinski, as it is a deep tendon reflex (spindle fiber) with a monosynaptic reflex pathway in Rexed lamina IX of the spinal cord, normally fully inhibited by descending input. Hoffman's reflex can be present on one side only, such as in Brown–Sequard syndrome in which only one-half of the spinal cord is affected.

Technique

The Hoffmann's reflex test itself involves loosely holding the middle finger and flicking the fingernail downward, allowing the middle finger to flick upward reflexively (**Fig. 5.8**). A positive response is seen when there is flexion and adduction of the thumb on the same hand, accompanied sometimes with flexion of the index or even all fingers.

Inverted Radial Reflex

The inverted supinator (brachioradialis) reflex is a sign that was introduced by Babinski in 1910.[11] The inverted radial reflex sign is commonly used in clinical practice to

assess cervical myelopathy. It is also indicative of a spinal cord lesion at C5 or C6, for example, due to trauma, syringomyelia, or disc prolapse and occurs because a lower motor neuron lesion of C5 is combined with an upper motor neuron lesion affecting reflexes below C5. There are two components of this abnormal reflex on tapping the lower end of the radius:

- Absent biceps and exaggerated triceps reflexes.
- A hyperactive response of the finger flexor muscles, causing finger flexion.

Technique

The supinator reflex is tested by striking the lower end of the radius (styloid process) just above the wrist with a tendon hammer (**Fig. 5.9**). This normally causes contraction of the brachioradialis and hence flexion of the elbow. If the only response is finger flexion, then this reflex is said to be inverted.[17]

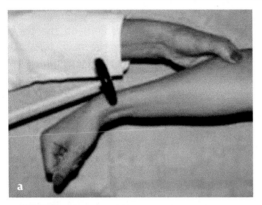

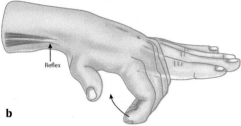

Fig. 5.9 Inverted brachial reflex. Tapping on the radius and unexpected finger flexion is obtained.

Scapulohumeral Reflex

The scapulohumeral reflex (SHR), which was first described by Shimizu in 1993, reflects damage in the upper cervical spine.[18] The reflex center of the SHR is clinically presumed to be located between the posterior arch of C1 and the caudal edge of the C3 body. A hyperactive SHR response was shown in 95% patients who exhibited neural compressive factors at the high cervical region.[18] Most of these cases had spastic symptoms and included several neurologic abnormalities (myelopathy, syrinx, EM). Hyperactive SHR provides useful information about dysfunctions of the upper motor neurons cranial to the C3 vertebral body level.

Technique

The SHR is elicited by tapping the tip of the spine of the scapula and acromion in a caudal direction. The SHR is classified as hyperactive only when an elevation of the scapula or an abduction of the humerus has been clearly defined after tapping at these points.

Hyperreflexia

Hyperreflexia is defined as overactive or overresponsive reflexes. Hyperactive deep tendon reflexes are a sign of upper motor neuron lesion and can be seen in normal but tense people. It can also be a consequence of loss of control ordinarily exerted by higher brain centers of lower neural pathways (disinhibition). Clonus is the higher representation of hyperreflexia. Diagnostic difficulty occurs when hyperreflexia and spasticity are the only findings. When hyperreflexia is found, it is wise to look for other features of upper motor neuron dysfunction such as positive Babinski sign and hypertonia, in order to determine a more clear diagnosis. Jaw clonus often indicates a lesion above the midpontine level.

Sensory nerve tracts eliciting the knee jerk reflex enter the spinal cord through L2, L3, and L4 spinal nerves. Synapse takes place between sensory and motor tracts in the spinal cord and immediately exits through the same spinal nerves. Hyperreflexia will occur when there is a lesion in the spinal cord which disrupts the inhibitory tract and originates in the brain and descends through the spinal cord, exiting via the spinal nerves of L2, L3, L4 to modulate the knee jerk reflex, or S1 to modulate the ankle jerk reflex.

The most common cause of hyperreflexia is spinal cord injury in which case the name changes onto autonomic hyperreflexia/dysreflexia. This condition results from chronic disruption of efferent impulses down the spinal cord, as seen in spinal trauma, neuromuscular diseases (amyotrophic lateral sclerosis [ALS]), or CSM. Autonomic hyperreflexia is uncommon if the level of the injury is below T5. Inciting stimuli such as bladder distention, bowel distention, or surgical stimulation can produce an exaggerated sympathetic response. This occurs because there is a loss of normal inhibitory impulses from areas above the level of the lesion.

Technique for Deep Tendon Reflexes

The patient has to be sitting with the legs hanging and completely relaxed. The physician uses a patellar hammer to gently strike the patellar ligament, eliciting the reflex (**Fig. 5.10**). Proper technique of reflexes examination and experience play a major role in eliciting and categorizing deep tendon reflexes. An overactive response should be considered hyperreflexia.

L'hermitte Sign

Lhermitte phenomenon was described in 1916 by the French neurologist Jean Lhermitte.[19] It is described as an uncomfortable sensation, resembling an electric shock, provoked by active or passive neck flexion or when the physician pounds on the cervical spine while it is flexed. This trigger gives Lhermitte's sign its alternative name of barber's chair syndrome, as this movement is similar to when you move your head forward to let the barber cut the back of your hair. This sensation runs throughout the spinal cord, radiating from arms to legs, and is a result of a dysfunction of the posterior columns at the cervical level. It usually lasts a few seconds but can be very intense.

Technique

Position the patient in a sitting or a standing position. Ask the patient to try and touch the chest with their chin (flexion) or gently apply some force, resting your hand on the back of the head and bending the neck forward (**Fig. 5.11**). The electric shock sensation will appear and the patient will regain his or her normal neck position (neutral).

Romberg Test

The Romberg test was first described in 1846 by the German neurologist Moritz H Romberg, which was originally described for the condition tabes dorsalis. The Romberg test is used for the clinical assessment of patients with imbalance or ataxia from sensory and motor disorders.[20]

Normal balance occurs when all acting forces (motor and sensory) are cancelled by each other, resulting in a stable balanced system. It is maintained through the sensory information from vestibular (VIII cranial nerve), somatosensory (dorsal columns of the spinal cord), and visual systems (II cranial nerve). A patient who has a problem with proprioception (somatosensory) can still maintain balance by compensating with vestibular function and vision. In the Romberg

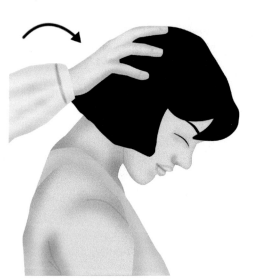

Fig. 5.11 L'hermitte sign. A positive result is obtained when flexing the neck and observing an "electric-like" sensation running down the back to arms and legs.

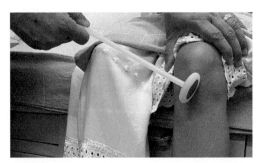

Fig. 5.10 Patellar reflex. With the leg resting, we tap the patellar ligament, obtaining a reflex.

test, the patient stands upright and is asked to close his eyes. A loss of balance is interpreted as a positive Romberg sign.[21]

Technique

The patient is kept in a standing position and legs are placed straight, with both feet touching each other and the head in a neutral position. A positive Romberg test results when the patient suddenly loses balance and has to be held to avoid a potential fall and/or injury when he or she is asked to close their eyes (**Fig. 5.12**).

Heel-to-Toe Walking

Heel-to-toe walking is another test to determine the integrity of the neurological pathways that control balance. The test result is considered positive when there is a demonstration of a loss of postural control.

Similar to Romberg's test, heel to toe positive test has been linked to all causes of proprioceptive deficits, including myelopathies of many causes, tabes dorsalis, and sensory neuropathies.

Technique

The patient is asked to walk in a straight line, touching the heel with the other's foot toes (**Fig. 5.13**). They are asked to do this for 8 to 10 steps, and contrary to Romberg's sign, the patient can keep their eyes open.

Nearly all of these tests are specific, versus sensitive, and are useful to rule in a suspected condition such as CSM. Furthermore, the tests, when used alone, may lead to a number of false negatives and, on rare occasions, false positives.

Differential Diagnosis

Only with a good history taking and physical examination can physicians derive appropriate differential diagnosis, which leads to proper imaging and other diagnostic tests that are cost-effective and minimally burdensome to patients. We can categorize the differential diagnosis broadly between compressive myelopathy, noncompressive myelopathy, and others (**Table 5.2**).

Compressive Myelopathies

Compression on to the spinal cord causes myelopathy. CSM with all its forms such as spondylosis, osteophyte formation, disc herniation, synovial cyst, ossification of posterior longitudinal ligament (OPLL), and subluxation, belong to this group of degenerative myelopathic diseases.

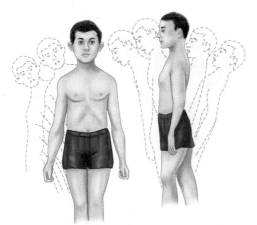

Fig. 5.12 Romberg test. On closing the eyes, the patient loses balance and has to widen the gait or advance a leg to avoid a fall.

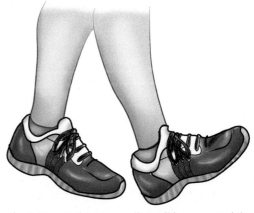

Fig. 5.13 Heel-to-toe walk. Walking on a straight line, heel to toe shows the status of the balance.

Table 5.2 Types of myelopathies

Compressive myelopathy	Noncompressive myelopathy	Others
Degenerative	Spinal cord infarct	AVM (vascular malformations)
Congenital malformation	Inflammatory/autoimmune	Dural fistula
Traumatic injury	MS	Retrovirus myelopathy (HIV)
Spinal tumors	Rheumatoid arthritis	Syringomyelia
Epidural hematoma	Acute infective myelitis	Subacute degeneration
Hematomyelia	Post-infection myelitis	(vitamin B deficiency)
Epidural abscess	Lupus/Sjögren	Tabes dorsalis
	Sarcoidosis	Familial spastic paraplegia
	Radiation myelopathy	Adrenomyeloneuropathy
	Discitis/osteomyelitis	
	ALS	
	Neuromyelitis optica	

Abbreviations: ALS, amyotrophic lateral sclerosis; AVM, arteriovenous malformations; HIV, human immunodeficiency virus; MS, multiple sclerosis.

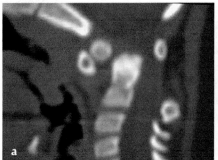 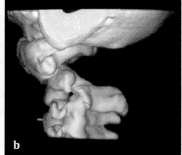 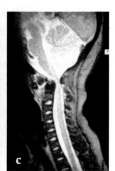

Fig. 5.14 Os odontoideum. (**a**): CT showing bony invasion of the cervical canal; (**b**): CT-3D spinal malalignment associated with os odontoideum; (**c**): MRI confirming severe compression to the spinal cord.

Spinal congenital malformations such as defects of the anterior or posterior arches of C1, occipital assimilation of the atlas, basilar invagination or impression, os odontoideum (**Fig. 5.14**), Klippel–Feil syndrome (**Fig. 5.15**), and cervical spine congenital stenosis can cause myelopathy by reducing the vertebral canal area and compressing the spinal cord. In congenital cervical stenosis, the average canal diameter, which produces the neurological symptoms, ranges from 7 to 9 mm[21]. In other congenital anomalies of the craniocervical junction such as Down´s syndrome, achondroplasia, and odontoid and atlas hypoplasia, the compression is caused by spinal malalignment associated with or without ligament laxity, which causes the area to be hypermobile, damaging the spinal cord on repetitive flexion and extension movements during normal living.[22] Chiari malformation, which is also a congenital disease, causes myelopathic symptoms on account of spinal cord compression caused by tonsillar descent, which occupies the vertebral canal, pressing the spinal cord posteriorly.

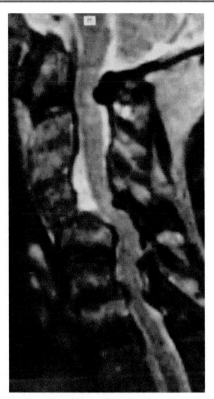

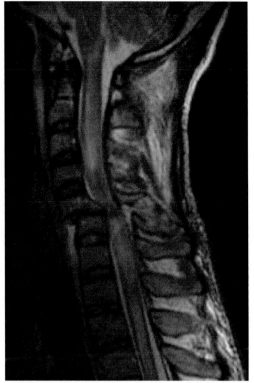

Fig. 5.15 MRI of a Klippel–Feil case. Spinal deformity; vertical translocation and staircase deformity, compressing the spinal cord on different levels.

Fig. 5.16 A 27-year-old man cervical MRI demonstrating an unstable fracture dislocation on C5/6 with severe cord compression and an incomplete tetraparesis.

Trauma to the cervical spine also causes myelopathy by compression of the bony fragments that had invaded the vertebral canal, compressing the spinal cord. Lesion to the spinal cord can be either a complete lesion (no function below the level of the injury) or an incomplete one (some useful motor function below the level of injury). In the event that no neurological deficit has occurred, classification of the cervical fracture is mandatory to determine its stability. On a stable fracture, a collar will suffice, while on an unstable fracture (**Fig. 5.16**), the management will include decompression, realignment, and stabilization.

A spinal tumor is an abnormal mass of tissue within or surrounding the spinal cord and/or spinal column. The tumors can be benign or malignant and can be classified according to their relation with the spine: extradural, intradural-extramedullary, and intradural intramedullary tumors.[23] They cause compression to the spinal cord by the presence of its mass, which competes with the spinal cord to space in the vertebral canal. The most common spinal tumors causing myelopathy are metastasis (lung, breast, and prostate), followed by meningiomas (**Fig. 5.17**) and schwannomas (intradural-extramedullary spinal tumors). Primary tumors of the bone and intramedullary tumors are infrequent.[24] On intramedullary tumors (**Fig. 5.18**), the presence of an intramedullary syrinx is common, which can extend to several levels, causing additional myelopathic symptoms and signs.

Cervical epidural hematoma (CEH) is a collection of blood between the dura mater and the bone, which can cause cord compression and myelopathy. CEH was first described by Jackson.[25] Hematomas can occur, following a cervical traumatic injury (venous), spontaneously in case of a clotting disorder (**Fig. 5.19**) or as a result of a postsurgical complication after a cervical laminectomy or an incomplete tumor removal.[26] Hematomyelia is the term used when the hemorrhage occurs inside the spinal cord. This hemorrhage is always

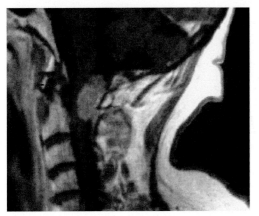

Fig. 5.17   MRI showing a meningioma at the C1–2 complex, compressing the spinal cord posteriorly.

due to a vascular anomaly or bleeding from a hemangioblastoma.

If the hematoma is confirmed by appropriate imaging and is causing a neurological deficit, the hematoma needs to be removed urgently; trying at the same time, to solve its cause.

Cervical epidural abscess (CEA) is a rare condition that leads to devastating neurological deficits and may be fatal. The classical triad of symptoms includes back pain, fever, and neurological deterioration. The infection often begins in the bone (osteomyelitis) and spreads inside the vertebral canal, causing myelopathy through two different mechanisms: direct compression on the spinal cord and due to a chemical reaction induced by pus and infectious pathogens (bacteria), which cause inflammation with local ischemia in the spinal cord, significantly worsening the symptomatology.[27,28] Abnormal blood inflammatory markers with fever and neurological deterioration would lead to a high suspicion of CEA. MRI with and without contrast and fat suppression is the imaging of choice with high sensitivity and specificity (**Fig. 5.20**).

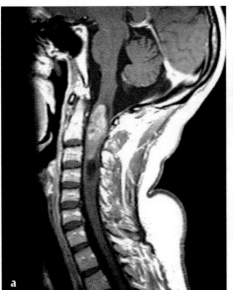
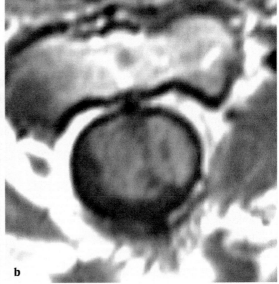

a   b

Fig. 5.18   MRI of an intramedullary tumor (ependymoma), causing severe cord compression and myelopathy.

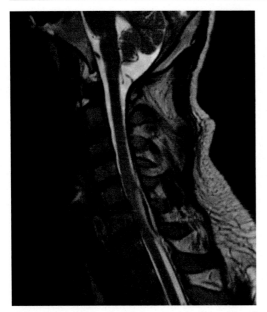

Fig. 5.19 MRI showing a spinal epidural hematoma (EDH) which is most common, as in this case, due to spontaneous venous bleeding, often in the setting of coagulopathy or over-anticoagulation.

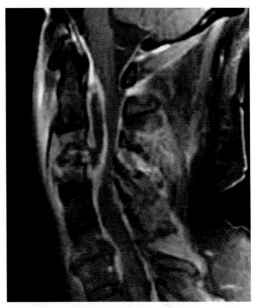

Fig. 5.20 MRI demonstrating anterior cervical epidural abscess following C3/4 discitis and osteomyelitis in C3 and C4, causing severe cord compression and tetraparesis.

Once the diagnosis is confirmed, urgent evacuation of the abscess is mandatory.

Noncompressive Myelopathies

Spinal cord dysfunction can result from noncompressive myelopathy that could be broadly grouped into inflammatory and non-inflammatory causes. The inflammatory group includes transverse myelitis, infections, and demyelinating and vasculitic diseases.[29] The noninflammatory groups comprise vascular, toxic and physical agents as well as degenerative, metabolic and inherited myelopathies.[30] Also, noncompressive myelopathies are clinically characterized by patterns of selective involvement of different anatomical structures of the spinal cord, and these patterns help the etiological diagnosis. Some of the classical syndromes with their most common causes are: Complete spinal cord syndrome (e.g., transverse myelitis), Brown–Sequard syndrome (e.g., multiple sclerosis), anterior spinal cord syndrome (e.g., anterior spinal artery infarct), posterolateral cord syndrome (e.g., vitamin B12 deficiency), central cord syndrome (e.g., neuromyelitis optica), and posterior syndrome (e.g., posterior spinal artery infarct and tractopathies or ALS).

Noncompressive myelopathy affects people across all age groups with a clear preponderance on patients in their middle age. Diagnosis of these conditions can be difficult, and it can be elusive in up to 1/3rd of the patients. Diagnostic tools to help to distinguish these syndromes include imaging (bone scan, MRI, fluorodeoxyglucose-positron emission tomography [FDG-PET]), CSF evaluation, blood cultures, and electromyography (EMG) studies.[31,32]

Transverse myelitis (TM) is an inflammation of the spinal cord, a major part of the CNS. The spinal cord carries nerve signals to and from the brain through nerves that extend from each side of the spinal cord and connect to nerves elsewhere in the body.

The term myelitis refers to inflammation of the spinal cord; transverse refers to the pattern of changes in sensation—there is often a band-like sensation across the trunk of the body, with sensory changes below.[29]

Causes of TM include infections, immune system disorders, and other disorders that may damage or destroy myelin, the fatty white insulating substance that covers nerve cell fibers. Inflammation within the spinal cord interrupts communications between nerve fibers in the spinal cord and the rest of the body, affecting sensation and nerve signaling below the injury. Symptoms include pain, sensory problems, weakness in the legs and possibly the arms, and bladder and bowel problems. The symptoms may develop suddenly (over a period of hours) or over days or weeks. Diagnosis of TM includes MRI (**Fig. 5.21**), blood tests looking for autoantibodies (antiaquaporin-4, antimyelin oligodendrocyte), and a host of antibodies associated with cancer (paraneoplastic antibodies), which may be found in people with TM and lumbar puncture, wherein CSF contains more protein than usual and an increased number of white blood cells among some people. A lumbar puncture also helps out to rule other infectious diseases.[32] Initial cases might render normal results through investigations; in such cases, repeating the MRI and CSF in 5 to 7 days is recommended. Treatment includes steroids, plasmapheresis, and immunoglobulins. Recovery can be long.

Spinal cord infarction usually results from ischemia and originates in an extravertebral artery. The first symptom of spinal cord infarction is usually sudden pain in the neck or the back, with tightness radiating circumferentially, followed within minutes by segmental bilateral flaccid weakness and sensory loss. Pain and temperature sensation are disproportionately impaired. Position and vibration sensation, conducted by the posterior columns, and often light touch are relatively spared.

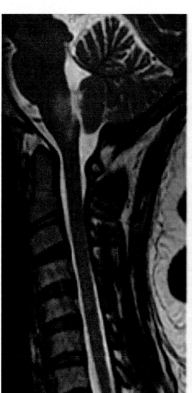 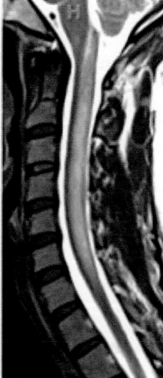

Fig. 5.21 MRI showing a case of transverse myelitis; please note the severe swelling of the spinal cord, affecting the entire cervical spine.

The main blood supply to the posterior third of the spinal cord is by two posterior spinal arteries; for the anterior 2/3 of the spinal cord, the anterior spinal artery is the only supply. The anterior spinal artery has only a few feeders from the cervical region and one large feeder in the lower thoracic region (artery of Adamkiewicz). All feeders originate from the aorta. Injury to an extravertebral feeder artery or the aorta (e.g., due to atherosclerosis, dissection, or clamping during surgery) causes infarction more commonly than intrinsic disorders of spinal arteries. Thrombosis is an uncommon cause, and polyarteritis nodosa is a rare cause.

Diagnosis of spinal cord infarction is conducted by good history taking and confirmed with an MRI (**Fig. 5.22**). If MRI is unavailable, CT myelography can be done.

The causes of Vitamin B12 and folate deficiency in author's patients were a combination of strict vegetarian diet, malnutrition, alcohol consumption, and phenytoin therapy. Vitamin B12 deficiency can also lead to symptoms similar to CSM, including sensory and motor deficiencies and gait ataxia. Deep tendon reflexes are usually absent or severely diminished, whereas pathological reflexes (Babinski sign) are present. Usually, these neurological findings are present with symptoms of dementia and/or other psychiatric symptoms. Patients with a history of pernicious anemia or gastrointestinal abnormalities who present with symptoms of gait ataxia and motor or sensory deficits should have a high index of suspicion for Vitamin B12 deficiency.[33] The patients afflicted with hepatic myelopathy had decompensated alcoholic liver disease with encephalopathy. The cause of spinal cord dysfunction could be multifactorial (toxic effect of adulterated alcohol, nutritional deficiency, nitrogenous breakdown products bypassing the liver through shunt, and venous hypertensive myelopathy).[34]

Spinal cord sarcoidosis usually affects the cervicodorsal cord. MRI of the spinal cord may be normal or show linear signal abnormality on T2-weighted imaging associated with patchy gadolinium enhancement, cord swelling with T2 hyperintensity without enhancement, subpial enhancement, or thickening with enhancement of the cauda equina. Isolated spinal cord sarcoidosis is extremely rare.[31] Serum angiotensin-converting enzyme (ACE) level is raised in only 50% of the patients. CSF ACE is less sensitive but relatively specific (94–95%) for CNS sarcoidosis.[35]

Multiple sclerosis (MS) is an autoimmune disease in which the body's immune system damages the myelin coating around the nerve fibers in the CNS and the nerve fibers themselves, interfering with the transmission

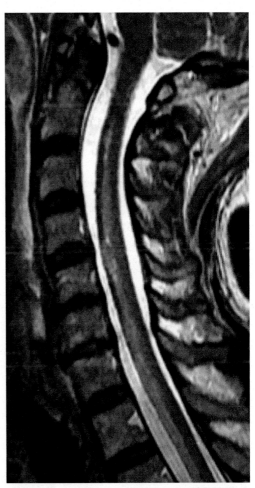

Fig. 5.22 Spinal cord infarction. Anterior spinal cord syndrome. Stroke on the anterior spinal artery territory causing flaccid tetraparesis.

of the nerve signals between the brain, spinal cord, and the rest of the body. MS is most commonly diagnosed in females aged between 20 to 40, but may occur at any age and among both genders, and contrary to ALS, often progresses slowly over many years (about 25 years). Patients with MS display relapsing symptoms involving the white matter tracts and, similarly to CSM, may present with L'hermitte phenomena, and motor, sensory, and bladder/bowel dysfunction.[33] Often, they show other symptoms that could help to distinguish CSM (visual defects, cognitive problems, epileptic fits).[33]

The diagnosis of MS usually involves a neurologist who will take the medical history, do blood tests, conduct tests to measure electrical activity in the brain and other areas, carry out an MRI (**Fig. 5.23**), and perform an analysis of CSF.

ALS, also known as motor neurone disease (MND) or Lou Gehrig's disease, is a neurodegenerative disease that causes death through gradual deterioration of neurons controlling voluntary muscles. Motor neurons are nerve cells that extend from the brain to the spinal cord and to muscles throughout the body. In ALS, both the upper motor neurons and the lower motor neurons degenerate or die and stop sending messages to the muscles. Unable to function, the muscles gradually weaken, start to twitch (fasciculations), and waste away (atrophy). Eventually, the brain loses its ability to initiate and control voluntary movements. Most people with ALS die from respiratory failure, usually within 3 to 5 years from when the symptoms first appear. However, about 10 percent of people with ALS survive for 10 or more years.

Electrophysiology tests are best to differentiate between ALS and CSM. Measuring motor-evoked potentials (MEP) from the trapezius muscle was found to be abnormal in all patients with ALS but normal in patients with CSM, whereas abnormal MEP's were found in all limbs in both CSM and ALS.[36] Furthermore, EMG resulted abnormal for both upper and lower limbs in patients with ALS-like symptoms, compared to abnormal EMG findings in only the upper limbs

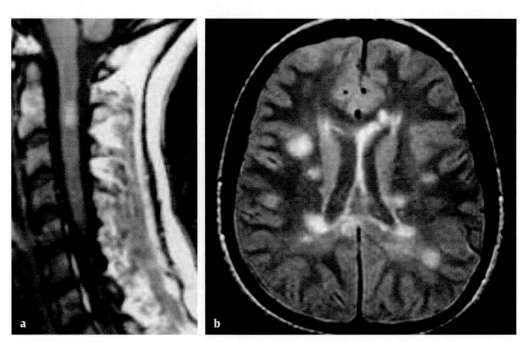

Fig. 5.23 Cervical and brain MRI showing some features of multiple sclerosis (MS). Typical MS plaque in the cervical spinal cord (**a**). Normally, it is accompanied with multiple plaques in the brain (**b**).

on the CSM group.[37] Another study recorded responses of masseter muscles to transcranial magnetic stimulation and found that the activation of corticobulbar descending fibers was absent or delayed in the majority of patients with ALS but normal in all patients with CSM, providing a means of distinguishing the two conditions.[38] CSF analysis can also help in the diagnosis of ALS.[32] The best biomarkers for distinguishing ALS from other neurodegenerative diseases and healthy subjects are erythropoietin (decreased),[39] hepatocyte growth factor (upregulated), monocytic chemotactic protein (increased),[40] neurofilament light and heavy subunits (upregulated), and cystatin C and transthyretin (reduced).[41]

Neuromyelitis optica (NMO) is an autoimmune, inflammatory, and demyelinating disorder of the CNS, with a predilection for the optic nerves and spinal cord often resulting in permanent blindness and/or paralysis and is characterized by the presence of serum aquaporin-4 immunoglobulin G antibodies (AQP4-IgG).[42] The pathological features of NMO include perivascular deposition of immunoglobulin and activated complement, loss of astrocytic AQP4, inflammatory infiltration with granulocyte and macrophage accumulation, and demyelination with axon loss. Immunosuppression and plasma exchange are the mainstays of therapy for NMO optic neuritis.

Syringomyelia refers to a disorder in which abnormal fluid-filled cavities or cysts form in the spinal cord.[43,44] This syrinx can get bigger and elongate over time, damaging the spinal cord and compressing and injuring the nerve fibers that carry information to the brain and from the brain to the rest of the body. The symptoms begin earlier than those of CSM, but, like CSM, its onset is insidious and progresses irregularly.[44] Symptoms include sensory loss, areflexic weakness and atrophy in the upper limb, leg spasticity, bladder and bowel dysfunction, and Horner syndrome.[44] The best diagnostic tool is an MRI (**Fig. 5.24**).

There are two major forms of syringomyelia:

Congenital syringomyelia (communicating syringomyelia): In most cases, syringomyelia is caused by a Chiari malformation, which may allow a syrinx to develop, mostly in the cervical region. Straining or coughing can force CSF into the ventricles, causing the person to develop headache or even lose consciousness (so-called cough syncope).

Acquired syringomyelia (noncommunicating syringomyelia): Causes of acquired syringomyelia include spinal cord injury, meningitis, arachnoiditis after intradural surgical operations, tethered cord syndrome, a spinal cord tumor, and bleeding into the cord (hemorrhage).

Vascular pathologies that have to be on the differential diagnosis of CSM include dural arteriovenous fistulas (DAVFs) and arterial venous malformations (AVMs).

Fistula means abnormal connection between two structures that are normally

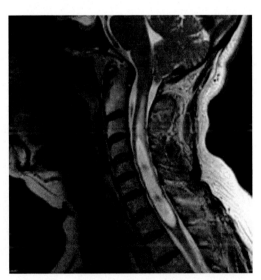

Fig. 5.24 MRI showing syringomyelia and Chiari malformation. Syrinx is a fluid-like cavity caused by the reopening of the congenital central canal, which is filled by cerebrospinal fluid (CSF) and expands the spinal cord, compressing the neuropathways and causing myelopathic symptoms.

not connected. An arteriovenous fistula is therefore an abnormal connection between an artery and a vein. When a fistula forms, blood from an artery under high pressure and flow goes directly into a vein, which is a low pressure and low flow structure. Even though the dural fistula is usually not directly on or within the spinal cord, it nevertheless causes dysfunction by interfering with normal spinal cord circulation, eventually producing severe and sometimes irreversible problems.[45] Spinal DAVFs are the spinal vascular malformations that are encountered most often, and they are usually encountered in the lower thoracic region. Cervical spine DAVFs are exceedingly rare and may be difficult to differentiate from radicular AVMs, epidural arteriovenous shunts, or perimedullary AVFs. Treatment includes embolization, surgical disconnection, or combined.[46,47]

Spinal AVMs **(Fig. 5.25)** are abnormal collections of blood vessels in the spinal canal that have a direct connection between the arterial system and the venous system without intervening capillaries.[48] Most of the AVMs will produce progressive neurological symptoms over months to years, especially back pain associated with progressive sensory loss and lower extremity weakness. They can be classified as: DAVF, the most common type; intradural AVMs, which are located between the spinal cord and the dura; and intramedullary AVMs, which are those located within the spinal cord. Diagnosis is made with MRI and spinal angiography, and treatment, as in DAVF, can be achieved through embolization, surgical excision, or a combination of both. Radiosurgery has also been used for some forms of AVM with promising results.

Conclusion

Physical examination findings are not always consistent with severity of disease in CSM, therefore, familiarizing with the clinical tests as an adjuvant to patient examination and correlating those findings with appropriate imaging are essential for arriving at the correct diagnosis. An MRI result is crucial in helping to distinguish between compressive and noncompressive myelopathic pathologies. In some cases where these imaging studies are still equivocal, use of other studies should be considered including electrodiagnostic studies as well as CSF examination.

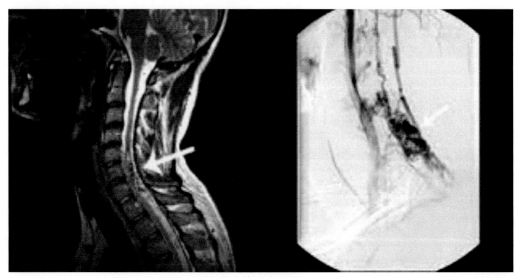

Fig. 5.25 Cervical AVM. Left: MRI demonstrating (arrow) a spinal arteriovenous malformation (AVM) with its classical "bag of worms" appearance. Right: Spinal angiography demonstrating the anatomical characteristics of the AVM.

Take-home Points

- Clinical tests are important tools to compliment a good anamnesis and neurological examination.
- The clinical tests mainly help to differentiate between CSM and radiculopathy.
- Clinical tests are cheap and easily done in the physician consulting rooms.
- MRI is an invaluable tool in the diagnosis of CSM together with plain X-rays (anteroposterior, lateral, and dynamic).
- Patients with bilateral sensory complaints in the hands should be presumed to have cervical cord pathology and should have cervical MR imaging, even if the EMG/NCS suggests bilateral carpal tunnel syndrome.
- Differential diagnosis in CSM can sometimes be extremely different, as many related pathologies can be present at the same time.
- ALS is distinct from CSM in the presence of cranial nerve involvement (CN XI) and the absence of pain or sensory changes.
- Electrodiagnostic studies demonstrate distinct characteristics in ALS and CSM.
- MS and NMO can be distinguished from CSM in the presence of visual symptomatology as well as the patient demographic is much younger.
- A good clinical examination together with a thoughtful investigation selection and good cooperation with our neurologist will help us to diagnose virtually all cases with myelopathy, providing patients with a professional and speedy solution to their problems.

References

1. Rovira M, Torrent O, Ruscalleda J. Some aspects of the spinal cord circulation in cervical myelopathy. Neuroradiology 1975; 9(4):209–214
2. Sadasivan KK, Reddy RP, Albright JA. The natural history of cervical spondylotic myelopathy. Yale J Biol Med 1993;66(3): 235–242
3. Harrop JS, Hanna A, Silva MT, Sharan A. Neurological manifestations of cervical spondylosis: an overview of signs, symptoms, and pathophysiology. Neurosurgery 2007; 60(1, Suppl 1):S14–S20
4. Cook C, Brown C, Isaacs R, Roman M, Davis S, Richardson W. Clustered clinical findings for diagnosis of cervical spine myelopathy. J Manual Manip Ther 2010;18(4):175–180
5. Ouellette H. Orthopedics Made Ridiculously Simple (Medmaster Ridiculously Simple). MedMaster Inc.; 2008
6. Wartenberg R. Studies of reflex. History, physiology, synthesis and nomenclature: study2. 1944
7. Singh A, Crockard HA. Quantitative assessment of cervical spondylotic myelopathy by a simple walking test. Lancet 1999; 354(9176):370–373
8. Omori M, Shibuya S, Nakajima T, et al. Hand dexterity impairment in patients with cervical myelopathy: a new quantitative assessment using a natural prehension movement. Behav Neurol 2018;2018:5138234
9. Han J, Waddington G, Adams R, Anson J, Liu Y. Assessing proprioception: A critical review of methods. J Sport Health Sci 2016;5(1): 80–90
10. Aman JE, Elangovan N, Yeh IL, Konczak J. The effectiveness of proprioceptive training for improving motor function: a systematic review. Front Hum Neurosci 2015;8:1075
11. Babinski J. Inversion du reflexe du radius. Bulletin et Memoires de la Societe de Medecine des Hopitaux de Paris,30,185–186. Archives of Neurology(Chic.) 1910;10:117–122
12. Ghosh D, Pradhan S. "Extensor toe sign" by various methods in spastic children with cerebral palsy. J Child Neurol 1998;13(5): 216–220

13. Young WF. Cervical spondylotic myelopathy: a common cause of spinal cord dysfunction in older persons. Am Fam Physician 2000; 62(5):1064–1070, 1073

14. Beres-Jones JA, Johnson TD, Harkema SJ. Clonus after human spinal cord injury cannot be attributed solely to recurrent muscle-tendon stretch. Exp Brain Res 2003; 149(2):222–236

15. Boyraz I, Uysal H, Koc B, Sarman H. Clonus: definition, mechanism, treatment. Med Glas (Zenica) 2015;12(1):19–26

16. Hoffmann P. Über eine Methode, den Erfolg einer Nervennaht zu beurteilen. Med Klin 1915b;11(13):359–360

17. Estanol BV, Marin OS. Mechanism of the inverted supinator reflex. A clinical and neurophysiological study. J Neurol Neurosurg Psychiatry 1976;39(9):905–908

18. Shimizu T, Shimada H, Shirakura K. Scapulohumeral reflex (Shimizu). Its clinical significance and testing maneuver. Spine 1993;18(15):2182–2190

19. Lhermitte JJ. Les formes douloureuses de la commotion de la moelle épinière. Rev Neurol (Paris) 1920;36:257–262

20. Findlay GFG, Balain B, Trivedi JM, Jaffray DC. Does walking change the Romberg sign? Eur Spine J 2009;18(10):1528–1531

21. Chau AM, Wong JH, Mobbs RJ. Cervical myelopathy associated with congenital C2/3 canal stenosis and deficiencies of the posterior arch of the atlas and laminae of the axis: case report and review of the literature. Spine 2009;34(24):E886–E891

22. Nishikawa K, Ludwig SC, Colón RJ, Fujimoto Y, Heller JG. Cervical myelopathy and congenital stenosis from hypoplasia of the atlas: report of three cases and literature review. Spine 2001;26(5):E80–E86

23. Nambiar M, Kavar B. Clinical presentation and outcome of patients with intradural spinal cord tumours. J Clin Neurosci 2012; 19(2):262–266

24. Kurzbuch AR, Rilliet B, Vargas MI, Boex C, Tessitore E. Coincidence of cervical spondylotic myelopathy and intramedullary ependymoma: a potential diagnostic pitfall. J Neurosurg Spine 2010;12(3):249–252

25. Jackson R. Case of spinal apoplexy. Lancet 1869;94:5–6

26. Phookan G, Lehman RA, Kuhlengel KR. Cervical spinal epidural haematoma: the double jeopardy. Ann Med 1996;28(5): 407–411

27. Khanna RK, Malik GM, Rock JP, Rosenblum ML. Spinal epidural abscess: evaluation of factors influencing outcome. Neurosurgery 1996;39(5):958–964

28. Curry WT Jr, Hoh BL, Amin-Hanjani S, Eskandar EN. Spinal epidural abscess: clinical presentation, management, and outcome. Surg Neurol 2005;63(4):364–371, discussion 371

29. Transverse Myelitis Consortium Working Group. Proposed diagnostic criteria and nosology of acute transverse myelitis. Neurology 2002;59(4):499–505

30. Kamble S, Sardana V, Maheshwari D, Bhushan B, Ojha P. Etiological Spectrum of Non-compressive Myelopathies in Tertiary Care Centre. J Assoc Physicians India 2019; 67(9):14–16

31. Sakushima K, Yabe I, Shiga T, et al. FDG-PET SUV can distinguish between spinal sarcoidosis and myelopathy with canal stenosis. J Neurol 2011;258(2):227–230

32. Thompson EJ, Thompson EJ. Proteins of the Cerebrospinal Fluid: Analysis and Interpretation in the Diagnosis and Treatment of Neurological Disease. Amsterdam: Elsevier Academic Press; 2005

33. Kim HJ, Tetreault LA, Massicotte EM, et al. Differential diagnosis for cervical spondylotic myelopathy: literature review. Spine 2013; 38(22, Suppl 1):S78–S88

34. Liao H, Yan Z, Peng W, Hong H. Hepatic myelopathy: case report and review of the literature. Liver Res Open J 2015;1:45–55

35. Khoury J, Wellik KE, Demaerschalk BM, Wingerchuk DM. Cerebrospinal fluid angiotensin-converting enzyme for diagnosis of central nervous system sarcoidosis. Neurologist 2009;15(2):108–111

36. Truffert A, Rösler KM, Magistris MR. Amyotrophic lateral sclerosis versus cervical spondylotic myelopathy: a study using transcranial magnetic stimulation with recordings from the trapezius and limb muscles. Clin Neurophysiol 2000;111(6): 1031–1038

37. Ishpekova B, Milanov I. Differential diagnosis of amyotrophic lateral sclerosis and similar syndromes. Electromyogr Clin Neurophysiol 2000;40(3):145–149

38. Trompetto C, Caponnetto C, Buccolieri A, Marchese R, Abbruzzese G. Responses of masseter muscles to transcranial magnetic stimulation in patients with amyotrophic lateral sclerosis. Electroencephalogr Clin Neurophysiol 1998;109(4):309–314

39. Brettschneider J, Widl K, Schattauer D, Ludolph AC, Tumani H. Cerebrospinal fluid erythropoietin (EPO) in amyotrophic lateral sclerosis. Neurosci Lett 2007;416(3):257–260

40. Wilms H, Sievers J, Dengler R, Bufler J, Deuschl G, Lucius R. Intrathecal synthesis of monocyte chemoattractant protein-1 (MCP-1) in amyotrophic lateral sclerosis: further evidence for microglial activation in neurodegeneration. J Neuroimmunol 2003; 144(1-2):139–142

41. Norgren N, Rosengren L, Stigbrand T. Elevated neurofilament levels in neurological diseases. Brain Res 2003;987(1):25–31

42. Levin MH, Bennett JL, Verkman AS. Optic neuritis in neuromyelitis optica. Prog Retin Eye Res 2013;36:159–171

43. Clark CR, Benzel EC, Currier BL, et al. The Cervical Spine. Philadelphia, PA: Lippincott Williams & Wilkins; 2005

44. Longo D, Fauci A, Kasper D, et al. Harrison's Principles of Internal Medicine. New York, NY: McGraw-Hill; 2011

45. Black P. Spinal vascular malformations: an historical perspective. Neurosurg Focus 2006;21(6):E11

46. Modi M, Bapuraj JR, Lal A, Prabhakar S, Khandelwal N. Vertebral arteriovenous fistula presenting as cervical myelopathy: a rapid recovery with balloon embolization. Cardiovasc Intervent Radiol 2010;33(6): 1253–1256

47. Takami T, Ohata K, Nishio A, et al. Microsurgical interruption of dural arteriovenous fistula at the foramen magnum. J Clin Neurosci 2005;12(5):580–583

48. Lad SP, Santarelli JG, Patil CG, Steinberg GK, Boakye M. National trends in spinal arteriovenous malformations. Neurosurg Focus 2009;26(1):1–5

06 Imaging Methods in Cervical Spondylotic Myelopathy

Mehmet Zileli, Onur Yaman, and Salman Sharif

Introduction

Cervical spondylosis is one of the most common spinal pathology in the elderly.[1] It usually occurs in the fifth decade of life and is often asymptomatic. It may progress to spinal cord compression and cervical spondylotic myelopathy (CSM).[2] CSM is caused by continuous cord compression and chronic spinal cord injury due to recurrent microtraumas.[3] Conventional imaging methods give only the anatomical findings. However, new advanced imaging techniques can detect the molecular changes and some pathologies at a reversible phase.[4]

Direct Radiograms

Canal Measurements

The first studies evaluating the canal diameter were based on direct radiographs.[5] They measured the size of the cervical spinal canal using a developmental segmental sagittal diameter (DSSD). This was done by measuring from the posterior surface of the vertebral body to the nearest point at the level of the pedicle in the spinolaminar line.[6] DSSD less than 10 mm was assessed with myelopathy.[7] However, differences in magnification and distance from the X-ray source to the film can confuse such measurements.[5] The ratio between canal diameter and vertebral body width was used to overcome this limitation (Torg–Pavlov ratio). If this rate is less than 0.8, it is considered as spinal canal stenosis.[5] However, this ratio has a low positive predictive value, due to positional false positives to the patient.[7] Direct radiographs were replaced by CT to evaluate the spinal canal.[8]

Functional Radiograms

Dynamic compression due to lower cervical instability (vertebral segments between C2–C7) is one of the most important pathogeneses of CSM.[9] Hayashi et al revealed that CSM is often caused by cervical instability.[10] Cervical disc degeneration leads to instability of adjacent discs.[11] A spontaneous fusion of some cervical segments may increase mobility at the adjacent segments. Cervical instability happens as a result of cervical spondylosis.[9]

Instability is measured by neutral and flexion-extension lateral radiograms. Translational instability is defined as more than 3.5-mm horizontal displacement of one vertebra in relation to an adjacent vertebra. Rotational instability is defined as more than 11° rotational difference from that of either adjacent vertebra (**Figs. 6.1 and 6.2**).

Instability further causes spinal cord damage by so-called dynamic compression.[12] In addition to segmental instability, longer duration of symptoms, lower preoperative Japanese Orthopaedic Association (JOA) score, and more preoperative physical signs were found to predict a poor surgical outcome.[12]

There is no consensus about the surgical intervention of the unstable segments. Some authors recommend surgical intervention for unstable segments if there is no increased signal intensity.[13] Some authors' suggestion is not to include the unstable level to the surgery. According to their suggestion, the cause of the symptoms is not related to unstable segment.[14] According to Zileli et al, instability of the cervical spine is predictive for outcomes. In patients with single segmental CSM with instability, longer duration of symptoms, lower preoperative JOA score, and

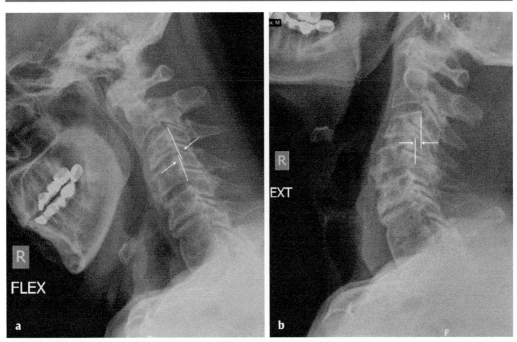

Fig. 6.1 **(a, b)** Translation instability: More than 3.5 mm displacement of one vertebra to the adjacent vertebrae.

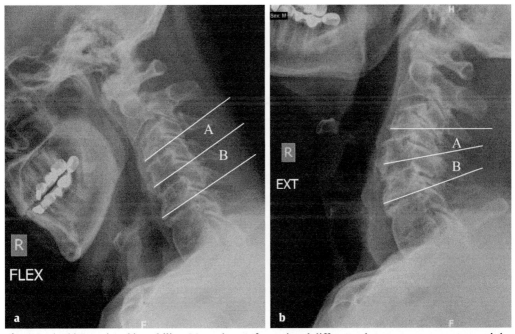

Fig. 6.2 **(a, b)** Rotational instability: More than 11° rotational difference between one segment and the adjacent segment (A-B > 11°).

more preoperative physical signs are highly predictive of a poor surgical outcome.[15]

Spinal Alignment and Balance

Importance of cervical sagittal balance has continued to evolve in the last years. The cervical spine has compensatory mechanisms to maintain the position of the head over the body and keep a horizontal gaze. Not only the shape of the cervical spine but the relationship between entire sagittal balance is also important. There is a paucity of information with regard to the cervical parameters, in order to determine good and pertinent clinical outcomes in patients.[15–17]

Cervical Sagittal Vertical Axis (SVA)

C2–7 SVA is the distance between two lines (midpoint of C2 vertebra drawn perpendicular to floor and posterior upper point of C7 drawn perpendicular to floor).[17]

C2–7 lordosis is the angle between the lower plate of C2 and the lower plate of C7.

C1 inclination is the angle between a line between the center of the C1 anterior and posterior arch and a horizontal reference line.

C2 slope is the angle between the C2 inferior endplate and a horizontal reference line.

C7 slope is the angle between a horizontal line and the superior endplate of C7 **(Fig. 6.3)**.[15,16]

The normal physiologic C2–C7 SVA has to be less than 4 cm. Measures of C2–C7 SVA greater than 4 cm have been correlated with worse outcomes following cervical spine surgery, as assessed by neck disability index (NDI).[18,19] Iyer et al mentioned that preoperative higher C2–C7 SVA values predict higher NDI values, while higher values of cervical lordosis and T1 slope correlated to lower NDI scores.[16,18,20] Another study showed that preoperative higher C2–7 SVA were associated with modified Japanese Orthopedic Association scores (mJOA).[17]

T1 slope correlates with sagittal alignment of the cervical spine. Larger T1 slopes provide

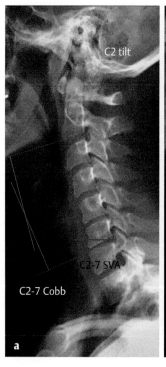
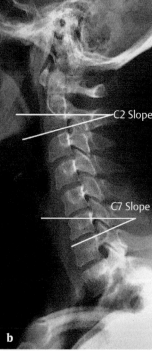

Fig. 6.3 (a, b) Measurements of cervical sagittal parameters: **C2–7 sagittal vertical axis (SVA)** is the distance between the midpoint of C2 vertebra drawn perpendicular to floor and superior posterior part of C7 (drawn with blue color on the left figure). **C2–7 Cobb angle** is the angle between the lower endplate of C2 and the lower endplate of C7 (on the left side with white color). **C2 tilt** is the angle between the posterior border of C2 vertebrae and the line perpendicular to floor (C2 tilt is the angle between two red lines on the left figure). **C2 slope** is the angle between the C2 inferior endplate and the horizontal reference line (C2 slope is the angle between two white lines shown on the right figure). **C7 slope** is the angle between a horizontal line and the superior endplate of C7 (C7 slope is the angle between two white lines shown on the right figure).

larger degrees of cervical lordosis, and thoracic inlet angle (TIA) provides a larger T1 slope.[21] So, we can say that there is a chain correlation with TIA and cervical lordosis. In a patient with positive global sagittal imbalance, the head tilts forward, and it increases T1 slope angle. Knott et al mentioned that T1 slope was correlated strongly with C2–7 SVA. They mentioned that patients with a high T1 slope (> 25°) who presented with pain all had at least 10 cm of sagittal imbalance (C2–C7 SVA), whereas those with a T1 slope of < 13° had a negative overall sagittal imbalance (C2 posterior to C7) of no clinical consequence.[20]

Kyphotic Cervical Spine

In elderly patients, SVA increases with time. Compensatory mechanism pelvic retroversion increases which, in turn, causes an upper thoracic kyphosis, and this cascade system increases the T1 slope.[20,22] In a kyphotic spine, increased cord tension and loss of spinal cord feeding cause myelopathy. Mohanty et al mentioned that preoperative sagittal malalignment is associated with abnormal spinal cord functional anatomy and also myelopathy.[23]

Structural compression, abnormal spinal alignment, and spinal cord excursion lead to dynamic compression and repetitive trauma.[24] According to Buell, patients with lordotic spine have more benefits following a surgical intervention.[22] Patients with kyphotic curvature have less clinical improvement after surgery.

The curvature of the cervical spine has been found to be one of the most important variables.[15] Cervical spine kyphosis predicts worse outcomes. Neurological improvement is significant in patients with normal cervical lordosis.[15]

Computed Tomography (CT)

CT axial sections are helpful to measure the bony canal diameters. CT is the most useful method for detecting ossification of the posterior longitudinal ligament (OPLL). Approximately 25% of patients with North American and Japanese cervical myelopathy have OPLL.[25] OPLL is divided into four types radiologically: (1) Continuous; a long lesion that extends to many levels, (2) Segmental; it is defined as multiple lesions, each containing a single level. (3) Mixed; it is a mixture of continuous and segmental type. (4) Limited; a solitary lesion covering one level.[26]

All dimensions of cervical canal stenosis can be fully demonstrated on CT.[27] In axial CT sections, the mushroom or crest-shaped OPLL, with a sharp radiolucent line between the posterior vertebral body and the ossifying ligament, is also characteristic.[28] In axial CT section, it provides evaluation of the type and degree of central canal stenosis; > 60% stenosis, ≤ 6 mm area for cord and ossification pattern in the lateral plane are associated with the risk of developing myelopathy.[29] In reconstructed 2D and 3D CT scan, myelo-CT scan provides great advantage in showing spinal cord compression caused by ventral OPLL. Dynamic studies more often show kyphosis or dorsal compression, due to yellow ligament hypertrophy, facet arthropathy, or laminar roof ossification.[29]

Magnetic Resonance Imaging (MRI)

The benefit of MRI is its ability to measure soft-tissue components that contribute to canal stenosis. AP diameter, transverse area (TA), and compression ratio (CR) are the preferred measurements for evaluating spondylotic cord compression.[30–32] CSM is mainly caused by narrowing of the spinal canal. This condition is caused by intervertebral disc hernia, osteophyte, and OPLL. However, only the presence of cord compression on MRI is insufficient for the diagnosis of CSM, as it can be demonstrated in about 5% of asymptomatic patients.[33,34] The specificity of cord compression revealed in MRI is limited for the diagnosis of CSM.

Since the degree of segmental pathological changes and cord compression are present in a spectrum, the need to assess the severity of these processes has resulted in the development of classification systems. Kang et al classified cervical stenosis including signal intensity changes in T2WI.[35]

Kang classification

Grade 0: absence of spinal canal stenosis.

Grade 1: subarachnoid space obliteration exceeding 50%.

Grade 2: presence of spinal cord deformity.

Grade 3: presence of spinal cord signal intensity (SI) change.

In their study, Kang et al have revealed that there is a positive correlation with the degree of stenosis, neurological impairment, and percent of patients undergoing surgery.[35]

Spinal Canal Measurements on MRI

AP diameter: The distance between posterior edge of the vertebral body and the spinolaminar line is defined as AP diameter. However, there is no significant association between the AP diameter and prognosis.[36,37]

CR: The ratio of the AP diameter to the transverse diameter of the spinal cord in axial sections is defined as CR.[37] Bednarik et al found a negative prognostic association with CR which is less than 0.436.[30] They also mentioned that there is a limitation in the cases that have peripheral cord compression. There is no high-quality study linking CR to postoperative outcomes.[38]

Cross-sectional area (CSA): The CSA of the spinal cord on axial images is one of the prognostic factors. Fukushima has found that patients with CSA less than 45 mm² have poorer functional results. Patients with higher CSA have better neurological outcomes.[37,39,40]

Maximum spinal canal compromise (MSCC): The ratio of the AP diameter of the spinal canal to the average of the AP diameter of the normal areas above and below of the spinal canal is defined as MSCC.[32] Nouri et al have found that patients with MSCC have

poorer clinical outcomes, especially at the 6 months follow-up.[32]

CR, MSCC, and CSA are important parameters that change postoperative surgical outcome, so every parameter has to be considered before the surgery.

SI Changes on MRI: T2 and/or T1-weighted signal changes on MRI are attributed to myelomalacia, edema, gliosis, and ischemic white matter changes.[31,41,42] Edema, inflammation, gliosis, and myelomalacia may cause hyperintensity on T2-weighted, while cyclic necrosis and syrinx may decrease the signals on T1-weighted MRI.[41] According to spinal cord compression there are changes on T1- and T2-weighted signals. Patients may be significantly symptomatic with only mild cervical stenosis without hyperintensity in T2WI, while others may have severe stenosis with myelomalacia and minimal symptoms.[43] Some classification systems have been described about spinal cord signal changes, but this topic is still controversial.[42,44–46]

Okada et al mentioned that there is no relationship with the SI and clinical symptoms.[46–48] On the contrary, there is a strong correlation between the intensity on T2WI and surgical outcomes, and that hypointensity in T1WI is not a predictor for surgical outcome. Hypointensity in T1-weighted imaging and hyperintensity in T2-weighted imaging worsen the surgical outcomes.[46] Many studies admit that patients with strong hyperintensity changes in T2WI have poorer results.[36,48–51] Only increase of intensity in T2WI is not a predictor of surgical outcome.[52]

The most widely used grading system for high SI changes in T2-weighted images has been proposed by You et al **(Fig. 6.4)**[53]:

- **Type 1:** A fuzzy margin of intramedullary T2 hyperintensity may reflect acute and currently active injury to the spinal cord, which is related to cord edema or inflammation.
- **Type 2:** This is similar in concept to the previously reported snake-eye

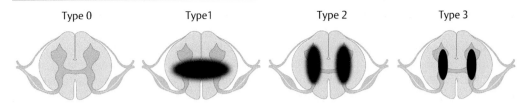

Fig. 6.4 Types of MRI cord signal intensity (SI) according to You et al.[53] Type 0, normal signal intensity of spinal cord without any intramedullary T2 hyperintensity; type 1, diffuse pattern of intramedullary T2 hyperintensity occupying more than two-thirds of axial dimension of spinal cord with an obscure and faint border; and types 2 and 3, focal patterns of intramedullary T2 hyperintensity occupying less than two-thirds of axial dimension of spinal cord.

appearance, and it is not associated with a poor prognosis.

- **Type 3:** A discrete margin of intramedullary T2 hyperintensity may reflect a chronic and poor prognosis that is related to gliosis or cystic cavitation.

T2 hyperintensity presents in approximately one-third of the patients with CSM.[54] Long tract signs and pathologic reflexes are also correlated with SI changes.[36,46]

Many studies have investigated the relationship of SI changes and outcomes of CSM, and most of them have reported a worse relation with the degree of SI.[7,30,31] Zileli et al mentioned that high SI on T2-weighted MR images is a negative predictor for prognosis.[34]

The outcomes are worse in presence of hypointensity on T1-weighted imaging (T1WI).[7,46] Persistence of T2 hyperintensity after decompressive surgery may also show a worse outcome.[34,55] However, some researchers have reported that in mild CSM, presence of hyperintensity on T2 can subside over time with conservative treatment.[50] In general, T2 hyperintensity is not specific and may be reversible, but T1 hypointensity is irreversible. T1 hypointensity is a sign of significant tissue loss or cord atrophy. In case there is a weak signal hyperintensity on T2 without clear border, it would reflect reversible changes due to edema, demyelination, and ischemia. If there is strong signal hyperintensity with sharp, clear border on T2, it is largely irreversible, reflecting potential cavitation, neural tissue loss, myelomalacia, necrosis, and gray matter changes.[32]

In general, we can predict worse outcomes if there are one of the following conditions: (a) sharp bordered T2-weighted SI changes, (b) long, multiple level T2-weighted SI changes, (c) persisting T2-weighted SI changes after surgery.

According to Zileli et al, among the many variables assessed using MRI, CR, MSCC, and TA are most importantly correlated with functional outcomes following surgery in patients with CSM. Each parameter has its own strengths and limitations and thus a combined assessment of MR parameters has a greater predictive yield.[34]

Advanced MRI Techniques

MRI plays an essential role in the management of patients with CSM. Improvements in MR technology like diffusion tensor imaging (DTI), MR spectroscopy (MRS), and functional MRI can give more details about spinal cord structure.[56–58]

Dynamic MRI

All the radiological imaging methods involve morphological changes, rather than giving functional information.[59,60] Both the mechanical pressure and vascular lesion increase during flexion and extension as a result of hypermotility. The spinal cord stretches during flexion. In addition, the anterior compression of the osteophyte is marked, and the anterior feeding of the cord is reduced.[4] During the extension, however, the canal narrows, the cord shortens and thickens, and the compression of the posterior ligament becomes marked, while the compression increases with the retrolisthesis of the hypermobile segment, and a pincer effect is seen.[60,61] It is possible to measure the canal diameter, which changes depending on the ligaments and discs, as well as the sagittal bony diameter of the canal, and the diameter of the spinal cord can be measured using dynamic MRI, in contrast to the ordinary X-rays obtained during flexion and extension.[4] It is possible to image the compression of the cord, as it changes with movement to measure the transverse cord area, which is the most important indicator of the prognosis in spinal pathologies, and to image the effect of movement on the unstable segment with dynamic axial images **(Fig. 6.5)**.[60]

Diffusion Tensor Imaging (DTI)
Water molecules diffuse along the spinal cord tracts. Displacement of the water molecules cause a signal change during diffusion MR imaging. Because of the direction-dependent diffusion of water molecules, according to neutral structures, it causes anisotropy.[62] Affection of the diffusion of water molecules help us in detecting spinal cord pathologies. DTI was used for neurological diseases, spinal cord injury, and spinal cord tumors.[63] DTI is more specific and more sensitive than

conventional MR. DTI gives better information on demyelination and axonal damage in the spinal cord.[64]

Both animal and human-being studies showed that degenerative compressive myelopathy also demonstrated significant changes in fractional anisotropy (FA) and apparent diffusion coefficient (ADC) values of the affected stenotic segment.[65] Acute compression of spinal cord tissue may result in a focal decrease in ADC as well as a focal increase in FA. Chronic compression increases ADC and decreases FA. Bhosole et al established that there is a significant decrease in FA and increase in ADC values at the stenotic level of the cervical spine and had improvement after decompressive surgery.[65] Also, FA was correlated strongly with mJOA. Guan et al mentioned that FA at level of maximal compression (LMC) is a useful tool to identify the severity of myelopathy.[43,66] Another study showed that if preoperative FA was high in the compression region, these patients experienced better functional recovery.[64] FA may play a particular role as a biomarker in predicting postoperative outcome.[43]

MR Spectroscopy (MRS)
MRS can provide metabolic information about the spinal cord.[58] It can give important clues about early stages of cell failure.

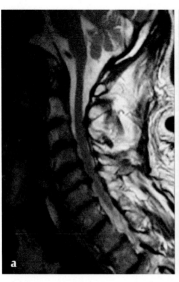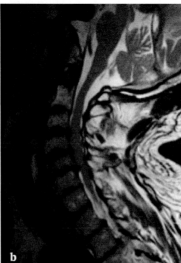

Fig. 6.5 The spinal cord stretches during flexion (**a**). In addition, the anterior compression of the osteophytes become marked. During extension (**b**), however, the canal narrows, the cord shortens and thickens, and the compression of the posterior ligament becomes marked.

MRS is sometimes called "virtual biopsy."[7] Biochemical markers such as N-acetyl aspartate (NAA), lactate, choline (Cho), glutamine-glutamate complex (Glx), and creatinine (Cr) can be used to assay. These small molecules give different resonance signals.[57,67,68] Related to ischemia, lactate plays a key role in spinal cord injury. Some studies have indicated that NAA is only found in axons and neurons and is considered an indicator of axonal integrity.[56] Holly et al mentioned that the NAA/Cr ratio was significantly lower in CSM due to increased neuronal and axonal injury.[69] They also found increased lactate signals.[69]

Myo-inositol (Myo-I) is an early marker for spinal cord inflammation and increases before neurological symptoms. In the late period, choline/creatinine (Cho/Cr) ratio increases with spinal cord changes along with clinical symptoms. Salamon et al showed increased Myo-I levels in cervical stenosis patients.[2] They also mentioned that high choline/creatinine (Cho/CR) is strongly correlated with JOA scores and surgical outcomes.[2]

Take-home Points

- Magnetic resonance imaging is the gold standard for diagnosis of cervical spondylotic myelopathy.

- Computerized tomography is necessary for OPLL diagnosis.

- Kang classification of cervical stenosis, including signal intensity changes in T2WI, is useful for grading the stenosis.

- Cervical sagittal parameters, especially C2–7 sagittal vertical axis (SVA) and C2–7 Cobb angle must be measured in cervical spondylotic myelopathy.

References

1. Zhang JT, Meng FT, Wang S, Wang LF, Shen Y. Predictors of surgical outcome in cervical spondylotic myelopathy: focusing on the quantitative signal intensity. Eur Spine J 2015;24(12):2941–2945

2. Salamon N, Ellingson BM, Nagarajan R, Gebara N, Thomas A, Holly LT. Proton magnetic resonance spectroscopy of human cervical spondylosis at 3T. Spinal Cord 2013;51(7):558–563

3. Shamji MF, Ames CP, Smith JS, Rhee JM, Chapman JR, Fehlings MG. Myelopathy and spinal deformity: relevance of spinal alignment in planning surgical intervention for degenerative cervical myelopathy. Spine 2013; 38(22, Suppl 1):S147–S148

4. Yu L, Zhang Z, Ding Q, Li Y, Liu Y, Yin G. Relationship between signal changes on T2-weighted magnetic resonance images and cervical dynamics in cervical spondylotic myelopathy. J Spinal Disord Tech 2015;28(6):E365–E367

5. Pavlov H, Torg JS, Robie B, Jahre C. Cervical spinal stenosis: determination with vertebral body ratio method. Radiology 1987; 164(3):771–775

6. Edwards WC, LaRocca H. The developmental segmental sagittal diameter of the cervical spinal canal in patients with cervical spondylosis. Spine 1983;8(1):20–27

7. Arvin B, Kalsi-Ryan S, Karpova A, et al. Postoperative magnetic resonance imaging can predict neurological recovery after surgery for cervical spondylotic myelopathy: a prospective study with blinded assessments. Neurosurgery 2011;69(2):362–368

8. Sureka B, Mittal A, Mittal MK, Agarwal K, Sinha M, Thukral BB. Morphometric analysis of cervical spinal canal diameter, transverse foramen, and pedicle width using computed tomography in Indian population. Neurol India 2018;66(2):454–458

9. Eck JC, Humphreys SC, Lim TH, et al. Biomechanical study on the effect of cervical spine fusion on adjacent-level intradiscal pressure and segmental motion. Spine 2002;27(22):2431–2434

10. Hayashi H, Okada K, Hamada M, Tada K, Ueno R. Etiologic factors of myelopathy. A radiographic evaluation of the aging changes in the cervical spine. Clin Orthop Relat Res 1987; (214):200–209

11. Wang B, Liu H, Wang H, Zhou D. Segmental instability in cervical spondylotic myelopathy with severe disc degeneration. Spine 2006;31(12):1327–1331

12. Lu K, Gao X, Tong T, Miao D, Ding W, Shen Y. Clinical predictors of surgical outcomes

and imaging features in single segmental cervical spondylotic myelopathy with lower cervical instability. Med Sci Monit 2017; 23:3697–3705

13. Katsuura A, Hukuda S, Saruhashi Y, Mori K. Kyphotic malalignment after anterior cervical fusion is one of the factors promoting the degenerative process in adjacent intervertebral levels. Eur Spine J 2001; 10(4):320–324

14. Kawakami M, Tamaki T, Ando M, Yamada H, Matsumoto T, Yoshida M. Preoperative instability does not influence the clinical outcome in patients with cervical spondylotic myelopathy treated with expansive laminoplasty. J Spinal Disord Tech 2002; 15(4):277–283

15. Zileli M, Maheshwari S, Kale SS, Garg K, Menon SK, Parthiban J. Outcome Measures and Variables Affecting Prognosis of Cervical Spondylotic Myelopathy: WFNS Spine Committee Recommendations. Neurospine 2019;16(3):435–447

16. Ling FP, Chevillotte T, Leglise A, Thompson W, Bouthors C, Le Huec JC. Which parameters are relevant in sagittal balance analysis of the cervical spine? A literature review. Eur Spine J 2018; 27(Suppl 1):8–15

17. Smith JS, Lafage V, Ryan DJ, et al. Association of myelopathy scores with cervical sagittal balance and normalized spinal cord volume: analysis of 56 preoperative cases from the AOSpine North America Myelopathy study. Spine 2013; 38(22, Suppl 1):S161–S170

18. Iyer S, Nemani VM, Nguyen J, et al. Impact of cervical sagittal alignment parameters on neck disability. Spine 2016;41(5):371–377

19. Ames CP, Blondel B, Scheer JK, et al. Cervical radiographical alignment: comprehensive assessment techniques and potential importance in cervical myelopathy. Spine 2013; 38(22, Suppl 1):S149–S160

20. Tang R, Ye IB, Cheung ZB, Kim JS, Cho SK. Age-related changes in cervical sagittal alignment: a radiographic analysis. Spine 2019;44(19):E1144–E1150

21. Lee SH, Son ES, Seo EM, Suk KS, Kim KT. Factors determining cervical spine sagittal balance in asymptomatic adults: correlation with spinopelvic balance and thoracic inlet alignment. Spine J 2015;15(4):705–712

22. Buell TJ, Buchholz AL, Quinn JC, Shaffrey CI, Smith JS. Importance of sagittal alignment of the cervical spine in the management of degenerative cervical myelopathy. Neurosurg Clin N Am 2018;29(1):69–82

23. Mohanty C, Massicotte EM, Fehlings MG, Shamji MF. Association of preoperative cervical spine alignment with spinal cord magnetic resonance imaging hyperintensity and myelopathy severity: analysis of a series of 124 cases. Spine 2015;40(1):11–16

24. Shamji MF, Mohanty C, Massicotte EM, Fehlings MG. The association of cervical spine alignment with neurologic recovery in a prospective cohort of patients with surgical myelopathy: analysis of a series of 124 cases. World Neurosurg 2016;86:112–119

25. Takatsu T, Ishida Y, Suzuki K, Inoue H. Radiological study of cervical ossification of the posterior longitudinal ligament. J Spinal Disord 1999;12(3):271–273

26. Tetreault L, Nakashima H, Kato S, et al. A systematic review of classification systems for cervical ossification of the posterior longitudinal ligament. Global Spine J 2019; 9(1):85–103

27. Saetia K, Cho D, Lee S, Kim DH, Kim SD. Ossification of the posterior longitudinal ligament: a review. Neurosurg Focus 2011; 30(3):E1

28. Soo MY, Rajaratnam S. Symptomatic ossification of the posterior longitudinal ligament of the cervical spine: pictorial essay. Australas Radiol 2000;44(1):14–18

29. Matsunaga S, Nakamura K, Seichi A, et al. Radiographic predictors for the development of myelopathy in patients with ossification of the posterior longitudinal ligament: a multicenter cohort study. Spine 2008;33(24):2648–2650

30. Bednarik J, Kadanka Z, Dusek L, et al. Presymptomatic spondylotic cervical myelopathy: an updated predictive model. Eur Spine J 2008;17(3):421–431

31. Nouri A, Tetreault L, Zamorano JJ, et al. Role of magnetic resonance imaging in predicting surgical outcome in patients with cervical spondylotic myelopathy. Spine 2015;40(3):171–178

32. Nouri A, Martin AR, Mikulis D, Fehlings MG. Magnetic resonance imaging assessment of degenerative cervical myelopathy: a review of structural changes and measurement techniques. Neurosurg Focus 2016;40(6):E5

33. Kato F, Yukawa Y, Suda K, Yamagata M, Ueta T. Normal morphology, age-related changes and abnormal findings of the cervical spine. Part II: Magnetic resonance imaging of over 1,200 asymptomatic subjects. Eur Spine J 2012;21(8):1499–1507

34. Zileli M, Borkar SA, Sinha S, et al. Cervical Spondylotic Myelopathy: Natural Course and the Value of Diagnostic Techniques -WFNS Spine Committee Recommendations. Neurospine 2019;16(3):386–402

35. Kang Y, Lee JW, Koh YH, et al. New MRI grading system for the cervical canal stenosis. AJR Am J Roentgenol 2011;197(1): W134-40

36. Karpova A, Arun R, Kalsi-Ryan S, Massicotte EM, Kopjar B, Fehlings MG. Do quantitative magnetic resonance imaging parameters correlate with the clinical presentation and functional outcomes after surgery in cervical spondylotic myelopathy? A prospective multicenter study. Spine 2014; 39(18):1488–1497

37. Kovalova I, Kerkovsky M, Kadanka Z, et al. Prevalence and imaging characteristics of nonmyelopathic and myelopathic spondylotic cervical cord compression. Spine 2016; 41(24):1908–1916

38. Karpova A, Arun R, Cadotte DW, et al. Assessment of spinal cord compression by magnetic resonance imaging–can it predict surgical outcomes in degenerative compressive myelopathy? A systematic review. Spine 2013;38(16):1409–1421

39. Fukushima T, Ikata T, Taoka Y, Takata S. Magnetic resonance imaging study on spinal cord plasticity in patients with cervical compression myelopathy. Spine 1991; 16(10, Suppl):S534–S538

40. Waly FJ, Abduljabbar FH, Fortin M, Nooh A, Weber M. Preoperative computed tomography myelography parameters as predictors of outcome in patients with degenerative cervical myelopathy: results of a systematic review. Global Spine J 2017; 7(6):521–528

41. Wada E, Yonenobu K, Suzuki S, Kanazawa A, Ochi T. Can intramedullary signal change on magnetic resonance imaging predict surgical outcome in cervical spondylotic myelopathy? Spine 1999;24(5):455–461, discussion 462

42. Yukawa Y, Kato F, Yoshihara H, Yanase M, Ito K. MR T2 image classification in cervical compression myelopathy: predictor of surgical outcomes. Spine 2007;32(15): 1675–1678, discussion 1679

43. Rindler RS, Chokshi FH, Malcolm JG, et al. Spinal diffusion tensor imaging in evaluation of preoperative and postoperative severity of cervical spondylotic myelopathy: systematic review of literature. World Neurosurg 2017;99:150–158

44. Chen CJ, Lyu RK, Lee ST, Wong YC, Wang LJ. Intramedullary high signal intensity on T2-weighted MR images in cervical spondylotic myelopathy: prediction of prognosis with type of intensity. Radiology 2001;221(3):789–794

45. Flanagan EP, Krecke KN, Marsh RW, Giannini C, Keegan BM, Weinshenker BG. Specific pattern of gadolinium enhancement in spondylotic myelopathy. Ann Neurol 2014; 76(1):54–65

46. Nouri A, Tetreault L, Dalzell K, Zamorano JJ, Fehlings MG. The relationship between preoperative clinical presentation and quantitative magnetic resonance imaging features in patients with degenerative cervical myelopathy. Neurosurgery 2017; 80(1):121–128

47. Okada Y, Ikata T, Yamada H, Sakamoto R, Katoh S. Magnetic resonance imaging study on the results of surgery for cervical compression myelopathy. Spine 1993;18(14):2024–2029

48. Vedantam A, Rajshekhar V. Does the type of T2-weighted hyperintensity influence surgical outcome in patients with cervical spondylotic myelopathy? A review. Eur Spine J 2013;22(1):96–106

49. Vedantam A, Jonathan A, Rajshekhar V. Association of magnetic resonance imaging signal changes and outcome prediction after surgery for cervical spondylotic myelopathy. J Neurosurg Spine 2011;15(6):660–666

50. Oshima Y, Seichi A, Takeshita K, et al. Natural course and prognostic factors in patients with mild cervical spondylotic myelopathy with increased signal intensity on T2-weighted magnetic resonance imaging. Spine 2012;37(22):1909–1913

51. Uchida K, Nakajima H, Takeura N, et al. Prognostic value of changes in spinal cord signal intensity on magnetic resonance

imaging in patients with cervical compressive myelopathy. Spine J 2014;14(8):1601–1610

52. Tetreault LA, Dettori JR, Wilson JR, et al. Systematic review of magnetic resonance imaging characteristics that affect treatment decision making and predict clinical outcome in patients with cervical spondylotic myelopathy. Spine 2013; 38(22, Suppl 1): |S89–S110

53. You JY, Lee JW, Lee E, Lee GY, Yeom JS, Kang HS. MR classification system based on axial images for cervical compressive myelopathy. Radiology 2015;276(2):553–561

54. Harrop JS, Naroji S, Maltenfort M, et al. Cervical myelopathy: a clinical and radiographic evaluation and correlation to cervical spondylotic myelopathy. Spine 2010;35(6):620–624

55. Mastronardi L, Elsawaf A, Roperto R, et al. Prognostic relevance of the postoperative evolution of intramedullary spinal cord changes in signal intensity on magnetic resonance imaging after anterior decompression for cervical spondylotic myelopathy. J Neurosurg Spine 2007;7(6):615–622

56. Martin AR, Aleksanderek I, Cohen-Adad J, et al. Translating state-of-the-art spinal cord MRI techniques to clinical use: A systematic review of clinical studies utilizing DTI, MT, MWF, MRS, and fMRI. Neuroimage Clin 2015;10:192–238

57. Ellingson BM, Salamon N, Hardy AJ, Holly LT. Prediction of neurological impairment in cervical spondylotic myelopathy using a combination of diffusion mri and proton mr spectroscopy. PLoS One 2015;10(10): e0139451

58. Ellingson BM, Salamon N, Holly LT. Advances in MR imaging for cervical spondylotic myelopathy. Eur Spine J 2015;24(Suppl 2): 197–208

59. Kim CH, Chung CK, Kim KJ, et al. Cervical extension magnetic resonance imaging in evaluating cervical spondylotic myelopathy. Acta Neurochir (Wien) 2014;156(2):259–266

60. Dalbayrak S, Yaman O, Firidin MN, Yilmaz T, Yilmaz M. The contribution of cervical dynamic magnetic resonance imaging to the surgical treatment of cervical spondylotic myelopathy. Turk Neurosurg 2015;25(1): 36–42

61. Joaquim AF, Baum G, Tan LA, et al. Dynamic cord compression causing cervical myelopathy. Neurospine 2019 (e-pub ahead of print). doi:10.14245/ns.1938202.101

62. Nakamura M, Fujiyoshi K, Tsuji O, et al. Clinical significance of diffusion tensor tractography as a predictor of functional recovery after laminoplasty in patients with cervical compressive myelopathy. J Neurosurg Spine 2012;17(2):147–152

63. Avadhani A, Rajasekaran S, Shetty AP. Comparison of prognostic value of different MRI classifications of signal intensity change in cervical spondylotic myelopathy. Spine J 2010;10(6):475–485

64. Jones JG, Cen SY, Lebel RM, Hsieh PC, Law M. Diffusion tensor imaging correlates with the clinical assessment of disease severity in cervical spondylotic myelopathy and predicts outcome following surgery. AJNR Am J Neuroradiol 2013;34(2):471–478

65. Bhosale S, Ingale P, Srivastava S, Marathe N, Bhide P. Diffusion tensor imaging as an additional postoperative prognostic predictor factor in cervical myelopathy patients: An observational study. J Craniovertebr Junction Spine 2019;10(1):10–13

66. Nilsson M, Lätt J, Ståhlberg F, van Westen D, Hagslätt H. The importance of axonal undulation in diffusion MR measurements: a Monte Carlo simulation study. NMR Biomed 2012;25(5):795–805

67. Wyss PO, Hock A, Kollias S. The application of human spinal cord magnetic resonance spectroscopy to clinical studies: a review. Semin Ultrasound CT MR 2017;38(2):153–162

68. Zhang C, Das SK, Yang DJ, Yang HF. Application of magnetic resonance imaging in cervical spondylotic myelopathy. World J Radiol 2014;6(10):826–832

69. Holly LT, Freitas B, McArthur DL, Salamon N. Proton magnetic resonance spectroscopy to evaluate spinal cord axonal injury in cervical spondylotic myelopathy. J Neurosurg Spine 2009;10(3):194–200

Electrophysiological Techniques for Cervical Spondylotic Myelopathy

Krešimir Rotim and Marina Zmajević Schönwald

Introduction

Cervical spondylotic myelopathy (CSM) includes a series of symptoms caused by repeated compression of the cervical spinal cord. CSM prognosis is connected to the patient's age, duration of symptoms, and severity of the myelopathy.[1] Neurophysiological techniques can be used to evaluate cervical spinal cord and radicular (peripheral nerve) functions in CSM.[2] These techniques can be modified and used in intraoperative monitoring of CSM surgeries.

Background

Neurophysiological diagnostic in CSM has three main tasks: The first task is to confirm the diagnosis. Neurophysiological methods that are commonly applied for that purpose are as follows: somatosensory evoked potentials (SSEPs), transcranial magnetic stimulation (TMS), motor evoked potentials (MEPs), electromyography (EMG), and nerve conduction studies (NCS). Information obtained through these methods aids in discerning concrete, temporal steps for surgical intervention. The second task is to use neurophysiological methods as a tool for intraoperative monitoring in order to reduce possible postoperative neurological deficits in CSM surgeries that carry a higher risk for spinal cord and peripheral (radicular) neural injury. Spinal cord is anatomically small but functionally condensed. Hence, multimodal neurophysiological methods are combined and sometimes used simultaneously during the intraoperative monitoring of spinal cord functions. Most commonly we use SSEPs, transcranial electrical stimulation (TES), MEPs, electrical direct nerve (radicular) stimulation MEPs, and intraoperative EMG. The third task of the neurophysiological diagnostic involves evaluating the patient postoperatively.

Preoperative and Postoperative Diagnostics and Intraoperative Neurophysiological Monitoring

Preoperative and Postoperative Diagnostics

Severity and duration of CSM symptoms are the primary variables for predicting the outcome of the disease.[1] Neurophysiological methods are used to clarify differential diagnosis, especially if there is suspicion of possible motor neuron system disease (MND), that is, amyotrophic lateral sclerosis (ALS). The primary aim of postoperative diagnostics is to lead the patient's individual rehabilitation process in the right direction.

Somatosensory Evoked Potentials (SSEPs)

SSEP uses peripheral electrical stimulation to excite large myelinated sensory fibers of somatosensory pathways. Elicited evoked potentials are recorded along the afferent sensory pathways on their way to the primary sensory cortex. Upper limb SSEPs enable recording of N9 potentials at Erb point (EP), N11, P/N13 potentials generated in the cervical spinal cord, P14 in the medial lemniscus and the lower pons, and N20 (N25) cortical response potentials in the parietal lobe. Decreased N9 is an additional finding in some CSM patients, since a dorsal ganglion dysfunction can be noted. The absence of N11 potential is a frequent finding in CSM caused by the dysfunctions of gray matter in dorsal horns and cervical root entry.[3,4] According to previous research, the activity of the dorsal column nuclei (nucleus cuneatus) generates P/N13 potentials, and dysfunction of spinal cord in CSM is often marked by absence or significant wave deformation of spinal N13 potential findings, which are functionally and anatomically more close to cervical gray matter.[5,6,7-11] The prolongation of the EP-P/N13 interpeak latency has been found in 70% to 100% of patients with CSM.[12,13] SSEPs showed abnormal N13 recording in 95% CSM patients after radial nerve stimulation, in 90% after median, and in 54% after ulnar stimulation.[14] Frequently decreased N13 correlates with MRI confirmed spinal cervical damage at C5 level.[15] Decreased amplitude of N13 potential more often presents in CSM patients with spinal cord compression at multiple levels than in patients with a single level compression (C4–C5 or C5–C6).[16] Potential P14, generated as a scalp positive activity in the medial lemniscus and lower pons, is usually normal in CSM.[17-19] Median nerve SSEP recordings, using noncephalic references, better distinguishes N13 from P14 response. The interpeak latency is supposed to be the transit time for the ascending volley up to the level of the lower brainstem.[15-20] Some authors confirm that the tibial SSEP was better in detecting CSM, with the confirmation of the same abnormal findings in 75% of patients.[21-23] However, in lower limbs, SSEP sensory potentials must pass longer distances to the structures in the cervical spinal cord (N30 response) and cortex (P37, P40 response). This causes a temporal dispersion of action potential discharge and diminishes the potential amplitude. In CSM patients, N30 cervical potential is frequently absent.

However, the absence of N30 is also recorded in older healthy adults. A more reliable recording for the diagnosis of CSM is that of the N22 potential (generated in dorsal roots, dorsal root entry zone, and by postsynaptic activity in the lumbar cord enlargement), the P37 cortical potential, and the measurement of N22–P37 interpeak latency prolongation.[24] Many authors who use cephalic reference montages can confirm dorsal column dysfunction using lower limb SSEP in 43 to 100% of patients. By using upper limb SSEP, the dysfunction was found in 57 to 74% of patients after n. ulnaris stimulation, and 24 to 59% after median nerve stimulation.[22,23,25,26] However, in some cases the SSEP appeared to be too sensitive, so when there were cases of normal MRI findings, SSEP recordings were found to be abnormal.[27] In severe CSM cases, the analysis of the whole N9–N20 interval can predict the postoperative functional outcome.[28,29] However, in patient follow-ups after the spinal cord operative decompression SSEP sometimes produces false-positive results, that is, it is possible to have a successful operation and patient recovery with persisting SSEP abnormalities in postoperative recordings.[30]

Transcranial Magnetic Stimulation Motor Evoked Potentials

TMS is used as a noninvasive motor cortex stimulation. Recordings of TMS-MEP can be used for the evaluation of the corticospinal tract in cervical spine segments.[31,32] The measurement of central motor conduction time (CMCT) is an accepted way of evaluating the grade of dysfunction of the central motor pathways in cervical myelopathy.[33-35] Prolonged CMCT recordings in different muscles better locate compressions in the cervical spinal segments. In compression at C3/C4 CMCT prolongation is recorded in biceps brachii muscles. At the cervical level rostral to C6–C7, CMCT was prolonged in abductor hallucis muscle, and caudal segments of cervical compression were recorded as an abductor digiti minimi CMCT prolongation.[36] Therefore, authors recommend inclusion of abductor hallucis CMCT in the screening for and confirmation of CSM.[37] TMS MEP and CMCT measurement is useful in predicting the CSM postoperative outcome.[34,38,39] In follow-ups after CSM surgeries, the recorded improvement in CMCT recordings was noticed.[34,40] TMS MEPs can also be very useful in preoperative differential diagnostics with regard to distinguishing CSM from early stages of amyotrophic lateral sclerosis (ALS). Bilateral TMS-MEPs recorded from the trapezius muscle can be used to exclude patients in early stages of ALS.[41]

Electromyography and Nerve Conduction Study

EMG evaluates peripheral motor nerve pathologies and can help in differentiating diagnosis of CSM from radiculopathies, compressive neural (bilateral carpal tunnel) syndromes, or MND (ALS) at early stages. EMG is used in cases when combined radiculopathy and myelopathy are recorded in older CSM patients.[42] In addition to SSEP pathological recordings, 41% of CSM patients have also abnormal EMG, confirming radicular lesions.[43] Based on that knowledge, Liu et al evaluated preoperative EMG and MRI diagnostic with a postoperative outcome in 94 patients with CSM. The best prognosis was recorded for patients who had negative mild symptoms and pathological findings in EMG, with absence of increased signal intensity on T2-weighed MRI. The most challenging postoperative recovery was found in patients with positive pathological findings in both diagnostic methods.[44] When defining possible radicular/segmental disorders using EMG, one should keep in mind that the majority of the muscles do not only accept innervation from a single radix/segment. F wave variables are more precise compared to MRI findings in the same patients and showed 100% similarity and 55% sensitivity in detecting cervical radiculopathy at precise segments.[45] EMG combined with NCS can better define peripheral nerve from radicular lesion and also estimate motor neuron damage degree as in patients with CSM and bilateral carpal tunnel syndrome at the same time.[46] Statistically

significant appearance of CSM, together with carpal tunnel syndrome was confirmed, without explanation for the unified genesis and clear connection between both disorders.[47] Although not practiced routinely, method of cutaneous silent period (CSP) recording after noxious stimuli has 95% sensitivity in detecting spinal cord compression and is therefore recommended as an additional tool in confirming suspected CSM.[48] CSP was sensitive in CSM detection as much as TMS MEPs.[49] A relatively new method of contact heat-evoked potentials (CHEPs) was also used to confirm spinal cord compression in CSM with 95% sensitivity to discover at-level impairments in CSM patients. Clinical worsening of the CSM status correlates to the impairment of CHEPs.[50] EMG analysis using surface electrodes during patient's walk and gait can also be useful in the evaluation of CSM and development in rehabilitation, because it gives more information about the specific muscle paresis in the gait impairment.[51]

The Value of Neurophysiological Diagnostics in Comparison to Neuroimaging Findings

Analysis of neuroimaging variables is essential in the evaluation of CSM patients and their prognosis.[1] The aim of preoperative neurophysiological diagnostic is not to compete with neuroimaging in CSM, but to add functional information about the severity of cervical cord compression and/or possible radicular conflict. MRI is frequently used as the standard reference while studying the effectiveness of neurophysiology methods as in Lo et al prospective TMS MEP study. The results showed a strong correlation between TMS MEP variables and MRI findings, with 98% sensitivity and 98% specificity in confirming the severity of spinal cord compression.[52] In the other 2-year follow-up study, TMS MEP and MRI values were compared in 16 CSM patients. The group with normal CMCT but with significant stenosis on MRI was treated conservatively without any clinical deterioration during those 2 years. This suggests that TMS MEP can be an important additional tool, that can help in deciding whether to choose an operative approach in treatment or not.[53] In later research, the same author performed 414 consecutive TMS MEP evaluations in CSM patients, comparing them with MRI-measured sagittal and parasagittal diameters of the spinal canal and cord T2 hyperintensities. In patient group with CMCT pathology detected in the arms, all patients had T2 hyperintensities, compared to none in patient groups with abnormal CMCT legs measurement. The authors suggest that the close correlation between MRI and TMS MEP findings can be detected when direct mechanical spinal cord compression and therefore segmental demyelination of central motor pathways occur.[54] Other authors used SSEP as neurophysiological method of choice in comparison to MR neuroimaging. Liu et al analyzed quantitative MRI and pathological SSEP in CSM patients. Myelin water fraction (MWF) reduction in MRI linearly correlates with SSEP pathology. Microstructural changes in white matter result in spinal cord functional deterioration, which is measured as impaired SSEPs and evidence of demyelination.[55] The studies use diffusion tensor imaging (DTI) to evaluate the microstructural damage of the somatosensory tract, and SSEP for functional evaluation at the same time. The results showed that pathological changes in DTI could have greater sensitivity outlining the focal or extensive lesions in CSM patients, which cause the abnormal SSEP in the first place.[56] Transcranial magnetic (TCM) MEP and SSEP are still often used in cervical cord compression graduation.[57]

Differential Diagnosis and/or Comorbidities with ALS

CSM and early stages of ALS can sometimes give a similar clinical picture. Needle EMG recording that will confirm lower motoneuron involvement in initial ALS diagnosis is sometimes not immediately positive; however, needle EMG recording for ALS prevails.[58,59] CSM is present as a complication in 50% of ALS patients. Some authors use apparent diffusion coefficients (ADCs) of intracranial corticospinal tracts to distinguish

between ALS and CSM patient deficit.[60] When using triple stimulation technique, the upper motoneuron degeneration was confirmed in 1 of every 2,25 patients.[61] EMG recorded from sternocleidomastoid and tongue muscles and dermatomal somatosensory evoked potential (DSSEP) can be used for distinguishing ALS from CSM patients.[62] Single-fiber electromyography can be performed in patients with early stage ALS and/or CSM.[63] TMS MEPs using trapezius muscle recording can also be utilized in differential diagnosis.[41] In SSEP, CSM has prolonged EP-P/N13 interpeak interval, which is usually normal in ALS.[12,13] However, abnormalities of central conduction time of SSEP could be recorded in ALS. In case of an abnormal central conduction SSEP recording in CSM, an alternative diagnosis should be considered.[64,65]

In the preoperative approach to the CSM patient, neurological examination is carefully focused on detecting motor and/or sensory disabilities. **Table 7.1** shows key characteristics of the above-discussed preoperative neurophysiological diagnostic techniques used for functional evaluation of CSM patients. Those techniques are specified, focused, and tailored individually for each patient, according to the previously obtained neurological examination result. Each of the techniques (see first column of **Table 7.1**) is connected with a different functional anatomical area (second column of **Table 7.1**) and serves for selective, focused additional diagnostic information (see third column of **Table 7.1**). Therefore, it is very difficult to emphasize which of them should prevail or be favored as more specific or sensitive. The established patient clinical pathology should lead in choosing the appropriate neurophysiological method.

Intraoperative Neurophysiological Monitoring

While intraoperative neurophysiological monitoring (IONM) is well-established in spinal tumor surgeries, the question remains whether it is justifiable for CSM surgeries.

Table 7.1 Neurophysiological methods commonly used by neurologist and neurophysiologist for cervical spondylotic myelopathy (CSM) diagnostic. Neurophysiological techniques (first column): somatosensory evoked potential (SSEP), transcranial magnetic (TCM) motor evoked potential (MEP), and electromyography (EMG) combined with nerve conduction studies (NCS) (F wave inclusive) distinguished according to functional areas (second column) and usefulness in CSM diagnostics (third column).

Neurophysiological method	Anatomical areas of functional evaluation:	Useful for:
SSEP	Complete somatosensory tract from peripheral nerve to primary sensory cortex for CSM analysis usually focused on dorsal column of the spinal cord: (upper extremity nerves SSEP on cuneate fasciculus, lower extremity nerves SSEP on gracile fasciculus)	1) Functional graduation of cervical spinal cord stenosis severity, focused on dorsal columns pathology 2) Confirmation of additional demyelination process located in cervical cord 3) Differential diagnosis of demyelination diseases (multiple sclerosis)
TMS MEP	Complete corticospinal tract from primary motor cortex to muscle fibers response for CSM analysis, usually focused on spinal cord: lateral corticospinal tract (posterior part of funiculus lateralis) and anterior corticospinal tract (spinal cord's anterior, ventral parts)	1) Functional graduation of spinal cord stenosis severity, focused on alfa motoneuron damage in lateral, and anterior (ventromedial) parts of spinal cord 2) Differential diagnostic in detecting ALS at early disease stages.
EMG combined with NCS F wave	2nd motor neuron	1) Additional diagnostic and/or verification of proximal or distal 2nd motoneuron damage: cervical radiculopathies, brachial plexopathies, mononeuropathies (most frequently compressive peripheral nerves syndromes), polyneuropathies 2) Differential diagnostic in detecting motoneuron damage connected with MND, especially ALS at early disease stages

Abbreviations: ALS, amyotrophic lateral sclerosis; CSM, cervical spondylotic myelopathy; EMG, electromyography; MND, motor neuron disease; NCS, nerve conduction studies; SSEP, somatosensory evoked potentials; TMS MEP, transcranial magnetic stimulation motor evoked potentials.

There is a lack of scientifically proven evidence of IONM benefits. Highly graduated evidence-based medicine (EBM) trials are difficult to achieve in this particular branch of neurophysiology.[66-68] EBM criteria demands controlled, prospective clinical trials, which are designed with a large number of participants, and control groups, that is, equal number of patients in similar conditions who are receiving identical surgical treatment and who are either monitored or not monitored. There lies also an ethical dilemma. A treatment should be proposed despite the reasonable risk of iatrogenic intraoperative deficit that could be avoided by IONM. Hence, the question lies in whether it is ethically justifiable to have patients of similar conditions (preoperatively) be assigned to a "control group" without the chance to benefit from intraoperative monitoring? So far, no such trial has been performed.

However, there are clinical studies, case reports, and scientific reviews that highly support IONM during CSM surgeries. It is important to distinguish the neural functional areas that can be monitored only by rightly chosen, certain IONM techniques, so the misunderstandings about the effectiveness and usefulness of IONM, in general, can be avoided.

During CSM surgeries, multimodal IONM techniques are strongly recommended. Intraoperative SSEP, TES MEPs, and free-running EMG together with electrically triggered EMG are combined and performed.

Intraoperative Somatosensory Evoked Potentials

SSEP was the first evoked response registration technique used in IONM during scoliosis surgeries.[69] Later on, SSEP became popular and accepted in spinal surgeries as the standard monitoring method for corrective spinal deformity surgery and posterior approach surgery, for example, scoliosis surgery.[70] To keep simplicity and speed in monitoring, intraoperative SSEP has its characteristics kept in record. After peripheral stimulation,

cortical response is the main variable that has to be monitored to record the somatosensory impulse values at the end of the somatosensory pathway. Therefore, in the intraoperative SSEP monitoring, cortical corkscrew electrodes are situated in the projection of primary sensory cortex. **Fig. 7.1** shows the placement scheme of transcranial electrodes on the scalp during IONM.[71,72]

The disadvantage of SSEP as a method is its delay in providing information, due to the time required to average the recorded results. If not averaged, the recorded SSEP amplitudes will be very low.[72] To have the clearest recording while running SSEP, the noise from the operating room should be reduced as much as possible. SSEP recordings could also be disturbed by the body temperature, partial pressure of alveolar carbon dioxide, anesthetic drugs, and blood pressure.[73] In their intraoperative SSEP evaluation, May et al concluded that the method does not lack

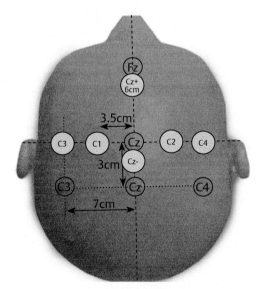

Fig. 7.1 Position of basic transcranial electrodes used during intraoperative monitoring according to the 10/20 EEG system. In the rows from anterior to posterior, the electrodes are marked for: (**a**) TES: Cz + 6cm, Cz-, C1, C2, C3, C4, (**b**) SSEP projections: Cz ' for the legs, C3' for the right hand, C4 ' for the left hand, and Fz as the midfrontal reference.

the sensitivity (99%); however, it is not specific enough (27%).[74] Because of the ascendent pathways that are stimulated distally in the neural peripheral system, the monitoring approach through SSEP can give the information not only about spinal cord function but also of peripheral stimulated nerves and/or roots. This could be very valuable regarding the positioning of patients before cervical surgery.[74] During surgery in cervical CSM operations, SSEP nerve stimulation monitoring from all limbs is required. Median SSEP has high sensitivity to acute insults that can appear during the cervical spinal surgeries.[75] **Fig. 7.2** presents bilateral median SSEP intraoperative monitoring during cervical disk decompressive operation on C5/C6 and C6/C7 levels. Cortical N20 (P25) waves are shown recorded on C4'-Fz (Fpz) and C3'-Fz (Fpz) channels. Baseline values are marked in red. There is a 50% amplitude drop and prolonged latency of N20 cortical response recorded on C3'-Fz channel. A warning was issued, and surgical measures applied. After 10 minutes, N20 amplitude recovers to baseline values

but latency remains prolonged. The patient woke up with slight paresis of the right arm, which recovered during a 1-week period.

Ulnar nerve stimulation is still recommended by some authors because of a higher possibility for ulnar nerve to be injured during patient positioning.[76] While tibial SSEP is a very sensitive tool for CSM preoperative graduation, the same placed recording in IONM is degraded because of additional noise of the operating room and/or anesthesia.[77]

In CSM surgery, there is higher risk of additional spinal cord compression and/or radicular nerve damage during the patient's (prone or supine) positioning. With SSEP recordings during the patient's positioning, these postoperative deficits can be avoided.[74,78–80] Reversible, position-related peripheral arm nerve injuries (brachial plexus injuries inclusive) can be also detected through SSEP waveform changes.[81–83] In their retrospective IONM study, Schwartz et al analyzed 3806 patients who underwent anterior cervical spine surgery. Intraoperative warning due to the impending injury secondary

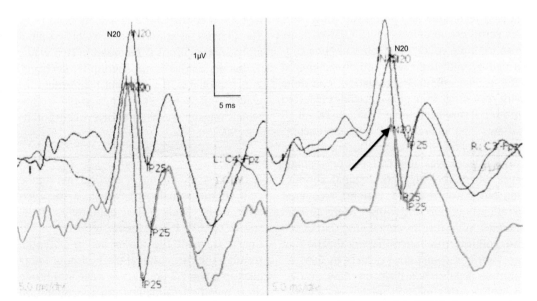

Fig. 7.2 Recording of bilateral median somatosensory evoked potential (SSEP) intraoperative monitoring during cervical disk decompressive operation on C5/C6 and C6/C7 levels. Cortical responses are recorded on C4'-Fz (Fpz) and C3'-Fz (Fpz) channels. Baseline values are marked in red. Average (800) values in green and single pass recording in black. There is 50% amplitude drop and prolonged latency of N20 cortical response recorded on C3'-Fz channel (shown with the *black arrow*).

to positioning was issued in 69 patients. Progression of spinal cord injury due to neck extension was detected in 19% of cases, while brachial plexus injury in 65% of cases. Ulnar nerve injury caused by tightly fixated arms was observed in 16% of cases. Because of this, ulnar SSEP stimulation montage was recommended. Multimodal IONM (SSEP and MEP) should be performed at the time of patient positioning.[76] MEP recording is difficult to obtain at first, due to the myorelaxants given during the intubation, and SSEP is not sufficient to give complete information about spinal cord functioning.[84–86] After some authors reported unchanged intraoperative SSEP in patients with postoperative anterior spinal artery syndrome[69,87] using only SSEP during IONM of the spinal cord operations is considered highly inappropriate.[88] In order to improve SSEP usefulness, there are techniques which were developed in spinal cord operations for estimation of the location of the dorsal fissure. Then, a particular form of somatosensory mapping of the dorsal columns was used.[89] Tani et al reported usefulness of the spinal cord evoked potentials (SCEPs) technique in finding the most serious compressive defects in 16 CSM patients with multiple spinal cord compressions confirmed by MRI. The evaluation of spinal cord after caudal epidural stimulation was done with recordings in needle electrodes inserted into serial cervical intervertebral disks. All 16 patients had operation of anterior decompression followed by fusion. During that, the surgical team was able to focus on a single level where the suggestive spinal conduction block was revealed. Patients recovered excellently within 6 months.[90] More authors shared similar results, concluding that SCEPs can confirm the functional localization of most serious spinal cord defects in CSM on multiple levels.[35,91,92] It is on new studies to evaluate this method further on a larger patient sample.

Intraoperative Motor Evoked Potentials

Spine surgeries can be demanding due to the very small anatomical area of the corticospinal tract which should be functionally preserved. Therefore, in spinal operations with high risk of postoperative motor deficit using MEP as the IONM method is inevitable.[88,93–95] Thus, various techniques of MEP have evolved, differing in place of stimulation and site,[96–101] and confirmed TES MEP as very useful[102–105] and most sensitive, even in comparison with SSEP and SCEPs.[94] Merton and Morton conducted the first TES after placing electrodes on the cranium skin in the projection of the primary motor cortex (according to the 10/20 EEG system). The TES electrodes function as bipolar (in pairs) and generate MEP in the white matter of the brain. The intensity of TES stimulation determines the depth from the surface of the cortex at which motor fibers will be aroused.[106] Later high frequency (250 Hz) short train stimuli (STS) technique was able to induce MEP in anesthetized patient.[107] The location of TES electrodes is pointed out in **Fig. 7.1**. The pair of stimulation electrodes where stimulation results in minimal twitching and cramping of the trunk, neck, and shoulder muscles should be chosen. Lower extremity montage Cz/Cz + 6 cm or C1–C2 is usually used.[102–110] The activity of stimulated fast corticospinal alpha motoneurons is recorded in two ways: 1. by an epidural (or subdural) electrode, which produces D wave and I (interneuron) waves, and 2. by needle muscle electrodes, which register muscle motor evoked potential (MMEP).

D-Wave

It is direct excitation of cortical pyramidal cells in the spinal cord, which is recorded with an electrode placed epidurally on the spinal cord.[111] It represents total orthodromic passage of the motor action potential through the corticospinal tract without lateralization. **Fig. 7.3** presents D wave amplitude drop recorded caudally from the operation field (caudal D wave) in higher thoracic segments.[108,112] While recorded proximal from neuromuscular junction, D wave is resistant to neuromuscular blockage, and independent of inhalation anesthetics.[109,113]

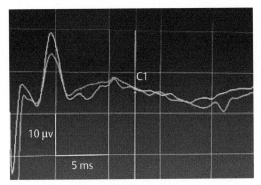

Fig. 7.3 D wave amplitude drop recording from the epidural electrode located caudally from the operated field.

During the orthodromic propagation, D wave's amplitude gradually drops and becomes low in the caudal part of the thoracic spine (below the Th10–Th11 level). The normal variation of the D wave amplitude with regard to the segmental level of the electrode placing is 10%.[114] However, during IONM, the D wave amplitude decrease for 20% from the baseline value is considered as the first warning of possible corticospinal tract injury.[110] During unilateral hemispheric TES, the decrease in D wave amplitude by more than 30% is connected with severe contralateral motor deficit.[115] During bilateral hemispheric TES, the D wave amplitude drop of 50% is a warning of a permanent motor deficit. Complete disappearance of D wave, dependable of spinal recording site, results in postoperative quadriplegia or paraplegia.[116,117] Therefore, the transcutaneous epidural electrode insertion technique during anterior cervical spinal surgery was introduced.[118] However, this technique of epidural electrode insertion increases risks of iatrogenic injuries. Therefore, D wave monitoring is not routinely applied during CSM surgeries.[119] Still, in complicated cases with adopted and unusual operative approach and spine exposure, D wave recording MEP technique is always recommended.

Muscle Motor Evoked Potentials Registration
MMEP is muscular response registered by two monopolar needle electrodes placed in the effective muscle. This type of registration involves IONM of central and peripheral motoneurons.[120–122] Due to the proximity and vulnerability of the pyramidal path within the spinal cord, during manipulation (traction, use of ultrasound aspiration apparatus, use of bipolar electrode), MMEP may be completely dropped. If MMEP registration is lost (uni or bilaterally) with unaltered (or not significantly altered) D wave registration (same amplitude or amplitude drop between 30–50%), the patient is likely to have only transient motor weakness, which will recede over several hours to several weeks.[94,123] The worst possible combination is if the MMEP is lost bilaterally and at the same time the D wave amplitude was decreased (50% less than its initial value) or not registered at all. This is always a sign of a permanent motor deficit.[124–126] If not D wave is used in spinal cord surgery with MMEP, permanent damage to the pyramidal tract cannot be identified with certainty. Scientific and professional opinions are divided on whether MEP as IONM technique should be used in CSM operations. The recommendation of the majority of authors is to use TES MEP in spinal surgeries' IONM including CSM surgery.[127–130] Others believe that spinal decompression surgery in cervical segments does not need IONM.[131] Clark et al conducted a large retrospective study comparing MEP monitoring in patients with degenerative[102] and nondegeneative[42] causes of CSM. MEP predicted and prevented permanent postoperative damage and was more sensitive in degenerative CSM cases surgeries.[131] Kim et al searched for the benefits of MEP monitoring in 200 patients during anterior cervical discectomy and fusion (ACDF) and found it useful in detection of possible segmental and long tract injury.[132]

In following 160 cases of cervical laminoplasty, the TES MEP was found very good in predicting acute postoperative segmental upper extremity palsy—a common complication of C5 nerve root. However, the delayed palsy (onset 2 days after the operation) was not detectible.[133] **Fig. 7.4a** shows significant

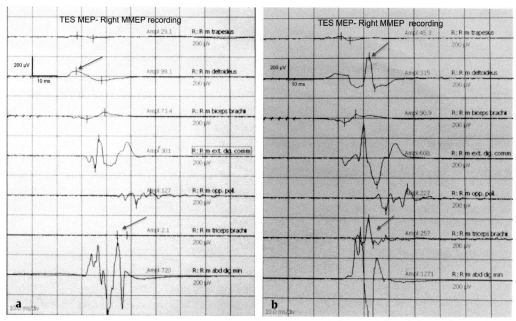

Fig. 7.4 Intraoperative transcranial electrical stimulation (TES) muscle motor evoked potential (MMEP) recording during the cervical operation (posterior approach): **(a)** significant MMEP amplitude decrease recorded in channels for right deltoid and right triceps brachii muscles **(b)** MMEP amplitude increase after corrective measures application.

decrease of the MMEP amplitude for right deltoideus muscle and right triceps brachii muscle together with general decrease of MMEP amplitudes for right arm muscles during the cervical operation (posterior approach). The warning was issued, and surgical measures applied. MMEPs reappeared later as seen in **Fig. 7.4b** and patient awoke without postoperative deficit.

Combining of SSEP and MEP in IONM
Searching for the ultimate modality that will monitor all functionally different spinal pathways or planning IONM on the wrong functional anatomy premises leads to the patient postoperative deficit with normal values of wrongly chosen IONM technique. The examples for that are described as cases of "false negative SSEPs" during anterior cervical decompression (ACD). The authors monitored SSEP solely, which gave them selective information about the dorsal columns' functioning. Unfortunately, they reported patients postoperative motor deficit, emphasizing that

"SSEP recording was normal." MEP corticospinal tract monitoring functionally connected with anterior spinal parts and spinal artery irrigation was not performed in those patients.[85,134] However, sometimes SSEP can be "indirectly sensible" in ACD and deteriorate just in time to prevent postoperative motor deficit. In both reported cases, the SSEP alteration started even before the beginning of the operation and was caused by hyperextension of the neck.[85] Further retrospective review of IONM was done on 119 patients during instrumented anterior cervical fusion during CSM surgery. MEP and SSEP were evaluated, focused on warnings that caused the surgical intervention. The authors concluded that there is usefulness of the MEP and SSEP, which is connected to the control of head positioning and spinal cord blood perfusion monitoring. The review confirms that cervical spinal surgery with surgery for CSM included demands of multimodal IONM, with at least MEP and SSEP modalities. The authors also supported adding the free-running EMG technique to multimodal IONM in order to have more information about possible radicular iatrogenic injuries.[135]

Intraoperative Free Running EMG and Triggered EMG

Intraoperative technique for recording spontaneous EMG activity—free-running EMG began in the 1980s, with continuous registration of spontaneous EMG activity in facial muscles during operations with a high risk of postoperative facial nerve lesions.[136,137] The method is transferable to all other muscle groups, and it is recommended to be used together with MEP in all cases where corticospinal tract could be intraoperatively compromised and where the speed of alert is important.[138,139] Both SSEP and MEP are intermittent monitoring methods, and frequency of their activation as well as the focus on each of them is determined according to the decision of the neurophysiologist who is accompanying the surgery. In contrast, free-running EMG is a continuous, real-time recording method. This is why many researchers are beginning to use it as the first detection of possible disorders, especially at the radicular level. The aim is to gain better control in monitoring of possible iatrogenic radicular lesions due to the muscle location and analysis of spontaneous discharges. Activity outbreaks that should be distinguished during initial spontaneous EMG recording and considered during monitoring are motor unit and endplate potential outbreaks, fibrillation

potentials, complex repetitive, myotone, myochemical outbreaks, etc. The location of surgery and the risk of possible postoperative deficits also determine the muscles in which intraoperative spontaneous EMG activity is registered. In spinal operations, muscles are then monitored for compromised myotomes.[140] For cervical spine operations, Balzer et al recommend bilateral free-running EMG recording in several muscle groups as follows: deltoid (C5), biceps (C5–C6), extensor carpi radialis (C6), triceps brachii and flexor carpi radialis (C7) and abductor pollicis brevis (C8–Th1).[141] **Fig. 7.5** presents free EMG recording of neurotonic discharges in left deltoid muscle during cervical decompressive surgery at C4/C5. The reason was mechanical manipulation of left C5 nerve root.

In cervical spinal surgery done for segmental decompression, there is a higher incidence (up to 30%) of iatrogenic C5 nerve root palsy regardless of surgical approach (anterior, posterior). A large study on 508 patients who have had anterior cervical fusion with single-level or multilevel corpectomies, Khan et al confirmed that most frequent postoperative deficit was radicular C5 weakness recorded at deltoid muscle.[142] Therefore, many authors suggest involvement of free EMG monitoring to detect possible irritation or lesion of radix C5 at the start of being damaged.[143,144] On 200 patients who underwent cervical laminectomy, Fan et al studied deltoid and biceps brachii muscle responses trough MMEPs and free-running EMG. They reported sudden appearance of free-running EMG pattern characterized as asynchronous neurotonic discharge and connected it with changes in MMEPs recording. Patients in question had postoperative transient C5 palsy.[145] Jimenez et al analyzed 161 patients and compared two groups, with and without free-running EMG monitoring. No postoperative C5 palsy was found in patients who had a still EMG recording during the operation. In four patients who had postoperative C5 palsy, the surgeon was always warned and took appropriate actions, so only one ended with a radicular C5 motor deficit.[146] The consensus

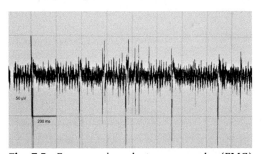

Fig. 7.5 Free-running electromyography (EMG) recording of neurotonic discharges in left deltoid muscle during cervical decompressive surgery at C4/C5, while left C5 nerve root was mechanically manipulated.

group for spinal surgeries of Sutter and colleagues agreed that IONM should be applied in extensive anterior and/or posterior decompression procedures and that free-running and triggered EMG should be included in multimodal monitoring.[147] However free-running EMG without proper interpretation could be too sensitive and a burden for the surgeon and his team. Spontaneous activity could be caused also with minimal surgical manipulation, which will not cause any postoperative damage. Therefore, it is very convenient to combine it and use it as a comparison to MMEP recordings. **Fig. 7.6** presents recordings from the free EMG channels and MEP channels during the C5/C6 cervical discectomy. On the left side is free-running EMG with noticeable spikes and bursts of B-train spontaneous activity[148] recorded in left biceps brachii muscle and left extensor carpi radialis muscle. Those activities were connected with slight mechanical root manipulation and

evaluated as unharmful while MEPs remained unchanged. The patient awoke without any neurological deficit.

In stabilization and fusion of cervical spinal segments to detect the malposition of the pedicle screw, indirect nerve root (spinal cord) stimulation methods are used. If the muscular response registered as a triggered EMG is obtained after very low electrical stimulation in the stabilization screw hole, then the conductivity is too high, and the screw is incorrectly positioned. The warning of lowest stimulation limit varies according to the author and is 6 mA to 10 mA.[149] Djurasovic et al used triggered EMG on 147 screws and established stimulation thresholds of 10 to 15 mA and higher for rightly placed ones.[150] Using free-running EMG and triggered EMG for pedicle screw placement monitoring are recommended in the position statement of American Society of Neurophysiological Monitoring.[151]

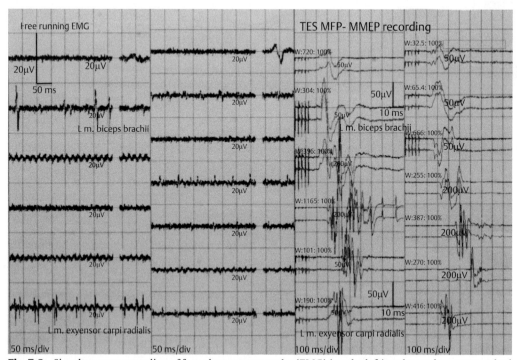

Fig. 7.6 Simultaneous recording of free electromyography (EMG) (on the left) and muscle motor evoked potential (MMEP) (on the right) recording during the C5–6 cervical discectomy. There is a recording of slight spontaneous activity in left biceps brachii and left extensor carpi radialis during the minimal mechanical C6 nerve root manipulation. MMEP recording remains unchanged.

Anesthesia during Intraoperative Neurophysiological Monitoring

Difficulties in interpreting intraoperative evoked potentials are often associated with general anesthesia and neuromuscular blockage. Halogen anesthetics act as neuronal depressants, eliciting MMEPs and SSEP response.[152–156] Therefore, the best solution compatible with IONM is total intravenous anesthesia (TIVA), with target-controlled infusion (TCI) of propofol and opiates.[157,158] The combination of propofol and remifentanil is often successfully used. Anesthesia can gradually affect the amplitude of MMEP, depending on the dose of anesthetic and the duration of surgery.[159] This effect was called "anesthetic fade" effect. Therefore, referral value of compound muscle action potential (CMAP) can be recorded in facial muscles after TES stimulation of corticobulbar motor evoked potentials (CoMEPs).[160] Application of neuromuscular relaxants during the patient intubation causes diminishing of MMEPs due to the blockage of neuromuscular synapses. Therefore, neuromuscular relaxants should be used only once, at the beginning of surgery, and avoided later during the surgery.[161] Its effect can be controlled by the "train of four stimulus technique." Other disorders may interfere with TES and aggravate MMEP registration such as head skin edema, and systemic hypotension and hypothermia or peripheral ischemic compression of the arm or leg at the site where MMEP is registered.[121]

IONM techniques in spinal surgery are advancing rapidly. **Table 7.2** shows key characteristics of mostly used IONM modalities that can be applied during CSM operations.

Additional Corrective Measures—TIP

Spinal surgery especially when spinal cord is involved is very difficult to perform without IONM, because traction, manipulation, overheating with a bipolar/monopolar electrode, or the use of CUSA can cause a permanent neural lesion. Sensitivity to possible ischemia and/or permanent damage of neural tissue is individual for each patient. In the case of a neurophysiological intraoperative warning,

additional corrective measures to alleviate possible postoperative iatrogenic injury will be implemented. Corrective measures are remembered by "time, irrigation, pressure/papaverine" (TIP).

Time: Surgical interventions can be carried out quickly, or at a slower pace, by using "stop and go strategies," where the neurosurgeon stops work in case of a motor response failure or a significant D-wave amplitude decrease. If the surgery is rushed after warning, a reversible injury is likely to become irreversible.[95]

Irrigation: The next emergency measure after warning of the possibility of damage to the corticospinal tract is irrigating the operative field with warm saline. In traumatic ischemic spinal cord injury, damage to the cell membrane further leads to penetration of K ions into extracellular spaces and impairs axonal repolarization, therefore nerve fiber conduction is limited.[162] Irrigation with saline should also flush out extracellular K and accelerate recovery of spinal conduction pathways. The role of mild hyperthermia, which should have a beneficial effect on neural tissue and improve conduction, remains open if there is irrigation with warm fluid, but this theory has not yet been fully explored.

Pressure: A third factor in the correction of possible injury is a slight increase in systemic blood pressure to achieve better medullovascular perfusion. Local neurovascular vasodilators such as papaverine or nimodipine could be applied locally in the operative field, especially when it comes to suspected insufficiencies in smaller blood vessels irrigation.

Conclusion

CSM as a clinical entity has witnessed a rising incidence among middle aged, randomly selected, population. There is a need to define variables that are affecting the prognosis in most cases of this slowly progressive disease. The main neurophysiological diagnostic methods that should be used for that are SSEP, TMS MEP, and EMG with NCS.

Table 7.2 Characteristics of some methods used for IONM during CSM surgery

Neurophysiological method (stimulation/recording)	Advantages	Disadvantages	Anesthesia
SSEP Stimulation: peripheral sensory nerve Recording: transcutaneous projections on somatosensory pathway	Intraoperative monitoring of: 1. dorsal columns 2. possible neck hyperextension 3. Very sensitive to neural tissue hypoxia	1. Requires averaging[a] 2. Sensitive to systemic blood pressure alterations and temperature 3. Requires uncompromised peripheral nerves as stimulation site	TIVA
TES MEP Stimulation: TES Recording: MMEP (muscle recording)	Intraoperative detection of motor deficit: 1. Cortex and spinal cord with lateralization 2. On radicular level, detects insufficiency in irrigation of anterior spinal artery.	1. Movement of the operation field during the TES MEP stimulation [b] 2. Diminishing of MMEP recording during spinal cord traction that can be interpreted as possible postoperative deficit (false positive results)	1. TIVA 2. Muscle relaxants allowed only during intubation period 3. "Anesthetic fade effect" in longer operations
D wave Stimulation: low-intensity TES Recording: D wave (spinal, epidural, rostral and caudal from op field)	1. Monitoring of bilateral corticospinal tracts 2. Recording without false positive results 3. Low-intensity TES stimulation without operation field movement	1. Inability to differentiate the lateralization in motor deficit 2. Difficulties in placing the D wave subdural electrode in CSM operations	TIVA and halogenous anesthetics
Direct Electrical Spinal Cord Stimulation: direct low intensity Recording: 1. spinal sub/epidural 2. muscle recording	Direct mapping of motor function in spinal cord segment that is at risk during the operation	1. Modest prolongation of operation duration. 2. Operation team should be educated to perform direct stimulation motor tract correctly	1. TIVA 2. For muscle recording muscle relaxants are allowed only during intubation period

(*Continued*)

Table 7.2 (*Continued*) Characteristics of some methods used for IONM during CSM surgery

Neurophysiological method (stimulation/recording)	Advantages	Disadvantages	Anesthesia
Direct electrical nerve root/ plexus/ peripheral nerve stimulation Stimulation: direct low intensity current electrical nerve root/ plexus/peripheral nerve stimulation applied on its most proximal parts in op field Recording: triggered EMG (muscle recording)	Motor nerve root identification/ exact definition of myotomes/precise evaluation in case of root overlapping	1. Modest prolongation of operation duration. 2. Operation team should be educated to perform direct stimulation motor tract correctly	1. TIVA 2. For muscle recording relaxants are allowed only during intubation period
Indirect spinal cord nerve root/ stimulation Stimulation: pedicle screw probe applied in pedicle screw hole Recording: muscle	Pedicle screw correct placement control	Prolongation of operation duration.	TIVA Muscle relaxants allowed only during intubation period
Free-running EMG Recording: muscle recording	Warning in real time of possible radicular iatrogenic injuries (most common C5 level)	The artefacts during recording should be not wrongly interpreted (false positive warnings possible)	1. TIVA 2. Muscle relaxants allowed during intubation period

Abbreviations: CSM, cervical spondylotic myelopathy; EMG, electromyography; IONM, intraoperative neurophysiological monitoring; SSEP, somatosensory evoked potentials; TIVA, total intravenous anaesthesia; TMS MEP, transcranial magnetic stimulation motor evoked potentials.
[a] It is also possible to follow each propagation of single SSEP stimuli without averaging.
[b] Could be diminished by adjusted TES electrode scalp placing and coordination of stimulation timing with the work of surgical team.

To evaluate potential deficit in spinal cord dorsal columns CSM, upper and lower limbs' SSEP should be used. For possible corticospinal tract dysfunction within the spinal cord, TMS MEP should be performed. If there is cervical radicular nerve comorbidity combined with CSM, EMG diagnostic will be included. EMG will find and graduate severity of compressive radiculopathy attached to CSM. The most dysfunctional segments of spinal cord can be indirectly revealed that way. IONM is efficient in prevention of serious neurological deficit in spine surgery, and therefore should be performed in complicated CSM surgeries (multiple levels surgery, greater degree of spinal cord compression).

Multimodal neurophysiological monitoring should be the only way to monitor CSM operations. Combined in one monitoring SSEP, TES MEP, free-running EMG and triggered EMG should be used to detect cervical spine and/or peripheral nerve injury. Special focus should be on SSEP and free-running EMG during the head and neck positioning in surgery for CSM. Later on, C5 and C6 spinal segments should be monitored. Triggered EMG should be used for the control of correct pedicle screw placement during the cervical spine stabilization surgeries. IONM should be individually tailored according to the preoperative patient examination and diagnostics. A neurophysiologist should be keeping the record of monitored cases for further evaluations and possible new directions in patient's surgical treatment.

Take-home Points

- The main neurophysiological diagnostic methods for evaluating CSM are as follows: upper and lower limbs' SSEPs, TMS MEPs, and EMG with NCS.

- Intraoperative neurophysiological monitoring should be performed in complicated surgeries for CSM to monitor the spinal cord and/or peripheral nerve injuries.

- Multimodal neurophysiological monitoring is the only proper way to monitor CSM surgeries: intraoperative SSEP, TES MEP, and free-running EMG and triggered EMG should be used mutually.

- For prevention of postoperative deficit connected to motoneuron lesion, TES MEP should be applied, and MMEP should be recorded.

- SSEP and free-running EMG techniques should be monitored during head and neck positioning in CSM surgeries.

References

1. Zileli M, Maheshwari S, Kale SS, Garg K, Menon SK, Parthiban J. Outcome measures and variables affecting prognosis of cervical spondylotic myelopathy: WFNS spine committee recommendations. Neurospine 2019;16(3):435–447

2. Zileli M, Borkar SA, Sinha S, et al. Cervical spondylotic myelopathy: natural course and the value of diagnostic techniques – WFNS spine committee recommendations. Neurospine 2019;16(3):386–402

3. Daube JR. Somatosensory evoked potentials. In: Daube JR, ed. Clinical Neurophysiology. 2nd ed. New York: Oxford University Press; 2002:194–195

4. Jones SJ. Investigation of brachial plexus traction lesions by peripheral and spinal somatosensory evoked potentials. J Neurol Neurosurg Psychiatry 1979;42(2):107–116

5. Restuccia D, Di Lazzaro V, Lo Monaco M, Evoli A, Valeriani M, Tonali P. Somatosensory evoked potentials in the diagnosis of cervical spondylotic myelopathy. Electromyogr Clin Neurophysiol 1992;32(7-8):389–395

6. Chiappa KH, Hill R. Short latency somatosensory evoked potentials: interpretation. In: Chiappa KH, ed. Evoked Potentials in Clinical Medicine. 3rd ed. Philadelphia: Lippincott-Raven; 1997:341–352

7. Emerson RG, Pedley TA. Effect of cervical spinal cord lesions on early components of the median nerve somatosensory evoked potential. Neurology 1986;36(1):20–26

8. Urasaki E, Wada S, Kadoya C, Matsuzaki H, Yokota A, Matsuoka S. Absence of spinal N13-P13 and normal scalp far-field P14 in a patient with syringomyelia. Electroencephalogr Clin Neurophysiol 1988;71(5):400–404

9. Restuccia D, Mauguière F. The contribution of median nerve SEPs in the functional assessment of the cervical spinal cord in syringomyelia. A study of 24 patients. Brain 1991;114(Pt 1B):361–379

10. Mauguière F, Restuccia D. Inadequacy of the forehead reference montage for detecting abnormalities of the spinal N13 SEP in cervical cord lesions. Electroencephalogr Clin Neurophysiol 1991;79(6):448–456

11. Ibáñez V, Fischer G, Mauguière F. Dorsal horn and dorsal column dysfunction in intramedullary cervical cord tumours. A somatosensory evoked potential study. Brain 1992;115(Pt 4):1209–1234

12. Oh SJ, Sunwoo IN, Kim HS, Faught E. Cervical and cortical somatosensory evoked

potentials differentiate cervical spondylotic myelopathy from amyotrophic lateral sclerosis. Neurology 1985;35:147–148

13. Bosch EP, Yamada T, Kimura J. Somatosensory evoked potentials in motor neuron disease. Muscle Nerve 1985;8(7):556–562

14. Restuccia D, Di Lazzaro V, Valeriani M, Tonali P, Mauguière F. Segmental dysfunction of the cervical cord revealed by abnormalities of the spinal N13 potential in cervical spondylotic myelopathy. Neurology 1992; 42(5):1054–1063

15. Restuccia D, Valeriani M, Di Lazzaro V, Tonali P, Mauguière F. Somatosensory evoked potentials after multisegmental upper limb stimulation in diagnosis of cervical spondylotic myelopathy. J Neurol Neurosurg Psychiatry 1994;57(3):301–308

16. Kaneko K, Kawai S, Taguchi T, Fuchigami Y, Ito T, Morita H. Correlation between spinal cord compression and abnormal patterns of median nerve somatosensory evoked potentials in compressive cervical myelopathy: comparison of surface and epidurally recorded responses. J Neurol Sci 1998;158(2):193–202

17. Morioka T, Shima F, Kato M, Fukui M. Direct recording of somatosensory evoked potentials in the vicinity of the dorsal column nuclei in man: their generator mechanisms and contribution to the scalp far-field potentials. Electroencephalogr Clin Neurophysiol 1991;80(3):215–220

18. Mavroudakis N, Brunko E, Delberghe X, Zegers de Beyl D. Dissociation of P13-P14 far-field potentials: clinical and MRI correlation. Electroencephalogr Clin Neurophysiol 1993;88(3):240–242

19. Restuccia D. Anatomic origin of P13 and P14 scalp far-field potentials. J Clin Neurophysiol 2000;17(3):246–257

20. Mehalic TF, Pezzuti RT, Applebaum BI. Magnetic resonance imaging and cervical spondylotic myelopathy. Neurosurgery 1990;26(2):217–226, discussion 226–227

21. Yiannikas C, Shahani BT, Young RR. Short-latency somatosensory-evoked potentials from radial, median, ulnar, and peroneal nerve stimulation in the assessment of cervical spondylosis. Comparison with conventional electromyography. Arch Neurol 1986;43(12):1264–1271

22. Veilleux M, Daube JR. The value of ulnar somatosensory evoked potentials (SEPs) in cervical myelopathy. Electroencephalogr Clin Neurophysiol 1987;68(6):415–423

23. Yu YL, Jones SJ. Somatosensory evoked potentials in cervical spondylosis. Correlation of median, ulnar and posterior tibial nerve responses with clinical and radiological findings. Brain 1985;108(Pt 2):273–300

24. Chiappa KH. Short latency somatosensory evoked potentials: methodology. In: Chiappa KH, ed. Evoked Potentials in Clinical Medicine. 3rd ed. Philadelphia: Lippincott-Raven; 1997:283–339

25. El Negamy E, Sedgwick EM. Delayed cervical somatosensory potentials in cervical spondylosis. J Neurol Neurosurg Psychiatry 1979;42(3):238–241

26. Ganes T. Somatosensory conduction times and peripheral, cervical and cortical evoked potentials in patients with cervical spondylosis. J Neurol Neurosurg Psychiatry 1980;43(8):683–689

27. Berthier E, Turjman F, Mauguière F. Diagnostic utility of somatosensory evoked potentials (SEPs) in presurgical assessment of cervical spondylotic myelopathy. Neurophysiol Clin 1996;26(5):300–310

28. Lyu RK, Tang LM, Chen CJ, Chen CM, Chang HS, Wu YR. The use of evoked potentials for clinical correlation and surgical outcome in cervical spondylotic myelopathy with intramedullary high signal intensity on MRI. J Neurol Neurosurg Psychiatry 2004;75(2):256–261

29. Ma Y, Hu Y, Valentin N, Geocadin RG, Thakor NV, Jia X. Time jitter of somatosensory evoked potentials in recovery from hypoxic-ischemic brain injury. J Neurosci Methods 2011;201(2):355–360

30. de Noordhout AM, Myressiotis S, Delvaux V, Born JD, Delwaide PJ. Motor and somatosensory evoked potentials in cervical spondylotic myelopathy. Electroencephalogr Clin Neurophysiol 1998;108(1):24–31

31. Barker AT, Jalinous R, Freeston IL. Non-invasive magnetic stimulation of human motor cortex. Lancet 1985;1(8437):1106–1107

32. Tavy DL, Wagner GL, Keunen RW, Wattendorff AR, Hekster RE, Franssen H. Transcranial magnetic stimulation in patients with cervical spondylotic myelopathy: clinical

and radiological correlations. Muscle Nerve 1994;17(2):235–241

33. Takahashi J, Hirabayashi H, Hashidate H, et al. Assessment of cervical myelopathy using transcranial magnetic stimulation and prediction of prognosis after laminoplasty. Spine 2008;33(1):E15–E20

34. De Mattei M, Paschero B, Sciarretta A, Davini O, Cocito D. Usefulness of motor evoked potentials in compressive myelopathy. Electromyogr Clin Neurophysiol 1993;33(4): 205–216

35. Fujimoto K, Kanchiku T, Imajo Y, et al. Use of central motor conduction time and spinal cord evoked potentials in the electrophysiological assessment of compressive cervical myelopathy. Spine 2017; 42(12):895–902

36. Ofuji A, Kaneko K, Taguchi T, Fuchigami Y, Morita H, Kawai S. New method to measure central motor conduction time using transcranial magnetic stimulation and T-response. J Neurol Sci 1998;160(1):26–32

37. Funaba M, Kanchiku T, Imajo Y, et al. Transcranial magnetic stimulation in the diagnosis of cervical compressive myelopathy: comparison with spinal cord evoked potentials. Spine 2015;40(3):E161–E167

38. Chang CW, Lin SM. Measurement of motor conduction in the thoracolumbar cord. A possible predictor of surgical outcome in cervical spondylotic myelopathy. Spine 1996;21(4):485–491

39. Capone F, Tamburelli FC, Pilato F, et al. The role of motor-evoked potentials in the management of cervical spondylotic myelopathy. Spine J 2013;13(9):1077–1079

40. Jaskolski DJ, Laing RJ, Jarratt JA, Jukubowski J. Pre- and postoperative motor conduction times, measured using magnetic stimulation, in patients with cervical spondylosis. Br J Neurosurg 1990;4(3):187–192

41. Truffert A, Rösler KM, Magistris MR. Amyotrophic lateral sclerosis versus cervical spondylotic myelopathy: a study using transcranial magnetic stimulation with recordings from the trapezius and limb muscles. Clin Neurophysiol 2000; 111(6):1031–1038

42. Epstein NE, Epstein JA. Individual and coexistent lumbar and cervical canal stenosis. Spine: State of the art Reviews 1987;1:401–402

43. Yiannikas C. Cervical radiculopathies In: Chiappa KH, ed. Evoked Potentials in Clinical Medicine. New York: Raven Press; 1997:441–449

44. Liu FJ, Sun YP, Shen Y, Ding WY, Wang LF. Prognostic value of magnetic resonance imaging combined with electromyography in the surgical management of cervical spondylotic myelopathy. Exp Ther Med 2013;5(4):1214–1218

45. Lo YL. How has electrophysiology changed the management of cervical spondylotic myelopathy? Eur J Neurol 2008;15(8): 781–786

46. Epstein NE, Epstein JA, Carras R. Coexisting cervical spondylotic myelopathy and bilateral carpal tunnel syndromes. J Spinal Disord 1989;2(1):36–42

47. Bednarik J, Kadanka Z, Vohánka S. Median nerve mononeuropathy in spondylotic cervical myelopathy: double crush syndrome? J Neurol 1999;246(7):544–551

48. Lo YL, Tan YE, Dan YF, et al. Cutaneous silent periods in the evaluation of cord compression in cervical spondylosis. J Neurol 2007;254(1):14–19

49. Stetkarova I, Kofler M. Cutaneous silent periods in the assessment of mild cervical spondylotic myelopathy. Spine 2009;34(1): 34–42

50. Jutzeler CR, Ulrich A, Huber B, Rosner J, Kramer JLK, Curt A. Improved diagnosis of cervical spondylotic myelopathy with contact heat evoked potentials. J Neurotrauma 2017;34(12):2045–2053

51. Malone A, Meldrum D, Gleeson J, Bolger C. Electromyographic characteristics of gait impairment in cervical spondylotic myelopathy. Eur Spine J 2013;22(11):2538–2544

52. Lo YL, Chan LL, Lim W, et al. Transcranial magnetic stimulation screening for cord compression in cervical spondylosis. J Neurol Sci 2006;244(1-2):17–21

53. Defteros SN, Kechagias E, Ioakeimidou C, Georgonikou D. Transcranial magnetic stimulation but not MRI predicts long-term clinical status in cervical spondylosis: a case series. Spinal Cord 2015;53(Suppl 1):S16–S18

54. Defteros SN. Abnormal central motor conduction at the upper but not lower limbs correlates with severe cervical spondylosis: discussion of an unexpected observation. Spinal Cord Ser Cases 2017;3:17009

55. Liu H, MacMillian EL, Jutzeler CR, et al. Assessing structure and function of myelin in cervical spondylotic myelopathy: Evidence of demyelination. Neurology 2017;89(6): 602–610

56. Wen CY, Cui JL, Mak KC, Luk KD, Hu Y. Diffusion tensor imaging of somatosensory tract in cervical spondylotic myelopathy and its link with electrophysiological evaluation. Spine J 2014;14(8):1493–1500

57. Nardone R, Höller Y, Brigo F, et al. The contribution of neurophysiology in the diagnosis and management of cervical spondylotic myelopathy: a review. Spinal Cord 2016;54(10):756–766

58. Inghilleri M, Iacovelli E. Clinical neurophysiology in ALS. Arch Ital Biol 2011; 149(1):57–63

59. Eisen A, McComas AJ. Motor neuron disorders. In: Brown WF, Bolton CF, eds. Clinical Electromyography. 2nd ed. Boston: Butterworths Heineman; 1987:427–440

60. Koike Y, Kanazawa M, Terajima K, et al. Apparent diffusion coefficients distinguish amyotrophic lateral sclerosis from cervical spondylotic myelopathy. Clin Neurol Neurosurg 2015;132:33–36

61. Furtula J, Johnsen B, Frandsen J, et al. Upper motor neuron involvement in amyotrophic lateral sclerosis evaluated by triple stimulation technique and diffusion tensor MRI. J Neurol 2013;260(6):1535–1544

62. Kang DX, Fan DS. The electrophysiological study of differential diagnosis between amyotrophic lateral sclerosis and cervical spondylotic myelopathy. Electromyogr Clin Neurophysiol 1995;35(4):231–238

63. Liu M, Cui L, Guan Y, Li B, Du H. Single-fiber electromyography in amyotrophic lateral sclerosis and cervical spondylosis. Muscle Nerve 2013;48(1):137–139

64. Cascino GD, Ring SR, King PJ, Brown RH, Chiappa KH. Evoked potentials in motor system diseases. Neurology 1988;38(2):231–238

65. Radtke RA, Erwin A, Erwin CW. Abnormal sensory evoked potentials in amyotrophic lateral sclerosis. Neurology 1986;36(6): 796–801

66. Hadley MN, Shank CD, Rozzelle CJ, Walters BC. Guidelines for the use of electrophysiological monitoring for surgery of the human spinal column and spinal cord. Neurosurgery 2017;81(5):713–732

67. Sala F, Skinner SA, Arle JE, et al. Letter: guidelines for the use of electrophysiological monitoring for surgery of the human spinal column and spinal cord. Neurosurgery 2018;83(2):E82–E84

68. Nasi D, Ghadirpour R, Servadei F. Letter: guidelines for the use of electrophysiological monitoring for surgery of the human spinal column and spinal cord. Neurosurgery 2019;84(2):E127–E128

69. Nash CL Jr, Lorig RA, Schatzinger LA, Brown RH. Spinal cord monitoring during operative treatment of the spine. Clin Orthop Relat Res 1977;126(126):100–105

70. Nuwer MR, Dawson EG, Carlson LG, Kanim LE, Sherman JE. Somatosensory evoked potential spinal cord monitoring reduces neurologic deficits after scoliosis surgery: results of a large multicenter survey. Electroencephalogr Clin Neurophysiol 1995;96(1):6–11

71. Moller AR. Monitoring of Somatosensory evoked potentials-SSEP in monitoring of spinal cord. In: Moller AR, ed. Intraoperative Neurophysiological Monitoring. 2nd ed. Totowa New Jersey: Humana Press; 2006: 125–144

72. Simon Mirela V. Neurophysiologic tests in the operating room. In: Deletis V, Shils JL, eds. Intraoperative Neurophysiology: A Comprehensive Guide to Monitoring and Mapping. New York: Demos Medical Publishing; 2010:1–44

73. Cui H, Luk KDK, Hu Y. Effects of physiological parameters on intraoperative somatosensory-evoked potential monitoring: results of a multifactor analysis. Med Sci Monit 2009;15(5):CR226–CR230

74. May DM, Jones SJ, Crockard HA. Somatosensory evoked potential monitoring in cervical surgery: identification of pre- and intraoperative risk factors associated with neurological deterioration. J Neurosurg 1996;85(4):566–573

75. Baumann SB, Welch WC, Bloom MJ. Intraoperative SSEP detection of ulnar nerve compression or ischemia in an obese patient: a unique complication associated with a specialized spinal retraction system. Arch Phys Med Rehabil 2000;81(1):130–132

76. Schwartz DM, Sestokas AK, Hilibrand AS, et al. Neurophysiological identification of position-induced neurologic injury during

anterior cervical spine surgery. J Clin Monit Comput 2006;20(6):437–444

77. Epstein NE, Danto J, Nardi D. Evaluation of intraoperative somatosensory-evoked potential monitoring during 100 cervical operations. Spine 1993;18(6):737–747

78. Kamel I, Barnette R. Positioning patients for spine surgery: avoiding uncommon position-related complications. World J Orthop 2014;5(4):425–443

79. Than KD, Mummaneni PV, Smith ZA, et al. Brachial plexopathy after cervical spine surgery. Global Spine J 2017; 7(1, Suppl) 17S–20S

80. Ofiram E, Lonstein JE, Skinner S, Perra JH. "The disappearing evoked potentials": a special problem of positioning patients with skeletal dysplasia: case report. Spine 2006;31(14):E464–E470

81. Kamel IR, Drum ET, Koch SA, et al. The use of somatosensory evoked potentials to determine the relationship between patient positioning and impending upper extremity nerve injury during spine surgery: a retrospective analysis. Anesth Analg 2006; 102(5):1538–1542

82. Uribe JS, Kolla J, Omar H, et al. Brachial plexus injury following spinal surgery. J Neurosurg Spine 2010;13(4):552–558

83. Jones SC, Fernau R, Woeltjen BL. Use of somatosensory evoked potentials to detect peripheral ischemia and potential injury resulting from positioning of the surgical patient: case reports and discussion. Spine J 2004;4(3):360–362

84. Minahan RE, Sepkuty JP, Lesser RP, Sponseller PD, Kostuik JP. Anterior spinal cord injury with preserved neurogenic 'motor' evoked potentials. Clin Neurophysiol 2001;112(8):1442–1450

85. Jones SJ, Buonamassa S, Crockard HA. Two cases of quadriparesis following anterior cervical discectomy, with normal perioperative somatosensory evoked potentials. J Neurol Neurosurg Psychiatry 2003;74(2):273–276

86. Pelosi L, Jardine A, Webb JK. Neurological complications of anterior spinal surgery for kyphosis with normal somatosensory evoked potentials (SEPs). J Neurol Neurosurg Psychiatry 1999;66(5):662–664

87. Zornow MH, Grafe MR, Tybor C, Swenson MR. Preservation of evoked potentials in a case of anterior spinal artery syndrome. Electroencephalogr Clin Neurophysiol 1990; 77(2):137–139

88. Deletis V, Sala F. Intraoperative neurophysiological monitoring of the spinal cord during spinal cord and spine surgery: a review focus on the corticospinal tracts. Clin Neurophysiol 2008;119(2):248–264

89. Kržan MJ. Intraoperative neurophysiological mapping of the spinal cords dorsal columns. In: Deletis V, Shils JL, eds. Neurophysiology in Neurosurgery. Amsterdam: Academic press; 2002:153-164

90. Tani T, Ushida T, Yamamoto H. Surgical treatment guided by spinal cord evoked potentials for tetraparesis due to cervical spondylosis. Paraplegia 1995;33(6):354–358

91. Tadokoro N, Tani T, Kida K, et al. Localization of the primary sites of involvement in the spinal sensory and motor pathways for multilevel MRI abnormalities in degenerative cervical myelopathy. Spinal Cord 2018; 56(2):117–125

92. Azuma Y, Kato Y, Taguchi T. Etiology of cervical myelopathy induced by ossification of the posterior longitudinal ligament: determining the responsible level of OPLL myelopathy by correlating static compression and dynamic factors. J Spinal Disord Tech 2010;23(3):166–169

93. Kothbauer K. Motor evoked potential monitoring for intramedullary spinal cord tumor surgery. In: Deletis V, Shils J, ed. Neurophysiology in Neurosurgery: A Modern Intraoperative Approach. Amsterdam: Academic Press; 2002:73–89

94. Sala F, Palandri G, Basso E, et al. Motor evoked potential monitoring improves outcome after surgery for intramedullary spinal cord tumors: a historical control study. Neurosurgery 2006;58(6):1129–1143, discussion 1129–1143

95. Sala F, Lanteri P, Bricolo A. Motor evoked potential monitoring for spinal cord and brain stem surgery. Adv Tech Stand Neurosurg 2004;29:133–169

96. Tamaki T, Takano H, Nakagawa T. Evoked spinal cord potentials elicited by spinal cord stimulation and its use in spinal cord monitoring. In: Cracco RQ, Bodis-Wollner I, eds. Evoked Potentials. New York: Alan Liss; 1986:428–33

97. Tamaki T, Takano H, Takakuwa K. Spinal cord monitoring: basic principles and experimental aspects. Cent Nerv Syst Trauma 1985;2(2):137–149

98. Owen JH, Bridwell KH, Grubb R, et al. The clinical application of neurogenic motor evoked potentials to monitor spinal cord function during surgery. Spine 1991; 16(8, Suppl)S385–S390

99. Toleikis JR, Skelly JP, Carlvin AO, Burkus JK. Spinally elicited peripheral nerve responses are sensory rather than motor. Clin Neurophysiol 2000;111(4):736–742

100. North RB, Drenger B, Beattie C, et al. Monitoring of spinal cord stimulation evoked potentials during thoracoabdominal aneurysm surgery. Neurosurgery 1991;28(2):325–330

101. Humphrey DR. Re-analysis of the antidromic cortical response. I. Potentials evoked by stimulation of the isolated pyramidal tract. Electroencephalogr Clin Neurophysiol 1968;24(2):116–129

102. Langeloo DD, Journée HL, de Kleuver M, Grotenhuis JA. Criteria for transcranial electrical motor evoked potential monitoring during spinal deformity surgery A review and discussion of the literature. Neurophysiol Clin 2007;37(6):431–439

103. Bartley K, Woodforth IJ, Stephen JP, Burke D. Corticospinal volleys and compound muscle action potentials produced by repetitive transcranial stimulation during spinal surgery. Clin Neurophysiol 2002; 113(1):78–90

104. Langeloo DD, Lelivelt A, Louis Journée H, Slappendel R, de Kleuver M. Transcranial electrical motor-evoked potential monitoring during surgery for spinal deformity: a study of 145 patients. Spine 2003;28(10): 1043–1050

105. Lang EW, Chesnut RM, Beutler AS, Kennelly NA, Renaudin JW. The utility of motor-evoked potential monitoring during intramedullary surgery. Anesth Analg 1996; 83(6):1337–1341

106. Merton PA, Morton HB. Stimulation of the cerebral cortex in the intact human subject. Nature 1980;285(5762):227

107. Taniguchi M, Cedzich C, Schramm J. Modification of cortical stimulation for motor evoked potentials under general anesthesia: technical description. Neurosurgery 1993;32(2):219–226

108. Szelényi A, Kothbauer KF, Deletis V. Transcranial electric stimulation for intraoperative motor evoked potential monitoring: Stimulation parameters and electrode montages. Clin Neurophysiol 2007;118(7):1586–1595

109. Deletis V. Intraoperative neurophysiology and methodologies used to monitor the functional integrity of the motor system. In: Deletis V, Shils J, eds. Neurophysiology in Neurosurgery: A Modern Intraoperative Approach. Amsterdam: Academic Press; 2002:25–51

110. Burke D, Hicks RG. Surgical monitoring of motor pathways. J Clin Neurophysiol 1998; 15(3):194–205

111. Patton HD, Amassian VE. Single and multiple-unit analysis of cortical stage of pyramidal tract activation. J Neurophysiol 1954;17(4):345–363

112. Deletis V. Intraoperative neurophysiology of the corticospinal tract of the spinal cord. Suppl Clin Neurophysiol 2006;59: 107–112

113. Scheufler KM, Reinacher PC, Blumrich W, Zentner J, Priebe HJ. The modifying effects of stimulation pattern and propofol plasma concentration on motor-evoked potentials. Anesth Analg 2005;100(2):440–447

114. Burke D, Hicks R, Stephen J, Woodforth I, Crawford M. Trial-to-trial variability of corticospinal volleys in human subjects. Electroencephalogr Clin Neurophysiol 1995; 97(5):231–237

115. Yamamoto T, Katayama Y, Nagaoka T, Kobayashi K, Fukaya C. Intraoperative monitoring of the corticospinal motor evoked potential (D-wave): clinical index for postoperative motor function and functional recovery. Neurol Med Chir (Tokyo) 2004;44(4):170–180, discussion 181–182

116. Morota N, Deletis V, Constantini S, Kofler M, Cohen H, Epstein FJ. The role of motor evoked potentials during surgery for intramedullary spinal cord tumors. Neurosurgery 1997; 41(6):1327–1336

117. Kitagawa H, Itoh T, Takano H, et al. Motor evoked potential monitoring during upper cervical spine surgery. Spine 1989;14(10): 1078–1083

118. Gokaslan ZL, Samudrala S, Deletis V, Wildrick DM, Cooper PR. Intraoperative monitoring of spinal cord function using motor evoked potentials via transcutaneous epidural electrode during anterior cervical spinal surgery. J Spinal Disord 1997;10(4): 299–303

119. Yamada T, Tucker M, Husain AM. Spinal cord surgery. In: Husain AM, ed. A Practical Approach to Neurophysiologic Intra-operative Monitoring. 2nd ed. New York: Demos Medical Publishing; 2015:106–26

120. MacDonald DB, Janusz M. An approach to intraoperative neurophysiologic monitoring of thoracoabdominal aneurysm surgery. J Clin Neurophysiol 2002;19(1):43–54

121. Macdonald DB, Al Zayed Z, Al Saddigi A. Four-limb muscle motor evoked potential and optimized somatosensory evoked potential monitoring with decussation assessment: results in 206 thoracolumbar spine surgeries. Eur Spine J 2007;16(Suppl 2):S171–S187

122. Calancie B, Molano MR. Alarm criteria for motor-evoked potentials: what's wrong with the "presence-or-absence" approach? Spine 2008;33(4):406–414

123. Kothbauer KF, Deletis V, Epstein FJ. Motor-evoked potential monitoring for intra-medullary spinal cord tumor surgery: correlation of clinical and neurophysi-ological data in a series of 100 consecutive procedures. Neurosurg Focus 1998;4(5):e1

124. Deletis V, Isgum V, Amassian VE. Neurophysiological mechanisms under-lying motor evoked potentials in anesthet-ized humans. Part 1. Recovery time of corticospinal tract direct waves elicited by pairs of transcranial electrical stimuli. Clin Neurophysiol 2001;112(3):438–444

125. Deletis V, Rodi Z, Amassian VE. Neurophysiological mechanisms underlying motor evoked potentials in anesthetized humans. Part 2. Relationship between epi-durally and muscle recorded MEPs in man. Clin Neurophysiol 2001;112(3):445–452

126. Novak K, de Camargo AB, Neuwirth M, Kothbauer K, Amassian VE, Deletis V. The refractory period of fast conducting corticospinal tract axons in man and its implications for intraoperative monitor-ing of motor evoked potentials. Clin Neurophysiol 2004;115(8):1931–1941

127. Nuwer MR, Emerson RG, Galloway G, et al; American Association of Neuromuscular and Electrodiagnostic Medicine. Evidence-based guideline update: intraoperative spinal monitoring with somatosensory and transcranial electrical motor evoked potentials. J Clin Neurophysiol 2012;29(1): 101–108

128. Fehlings MG, Brodke DS, Norvell DC, Dettori JR. The evidence for intraoperative neurophysiological monitoring in spine surgery: does it make a difference? Spine 2010; 35(9, Suppl)S37–S46

129. Stecker MM. A review of intraoperative monitoring for spinal surgery. Surg Neurol Int 2012;3(Suppl 3):S174–S187

130. Gavaret M, Jouve JL, Péréon Y, et al; French Society of Spine Surgery SFCR. Intraoperative neurophysiologic monitoring in spine surgery. Developments and state of the art in France in 2011. Orthop Traumatol Surg Res 2013; 99(6, Suppl):S319–S327

131. Traynelis VC, Abode-Iyamah KO, Leick KM, Bender SM, Greenlee JD. Cervical decom-pression and reconstruction without intra-operative neurophysiological monitoring. J Neurosurg Spine 2012;16(2):107–113

132. Kim DG, Jo SR, Park YS, et al. Multi-channel motor evoked potential monitoring during anterior cervical discectomy and fusion. Clin Neurophysiol Pract 2017;2:48–53

133. Fujiwara Y, Manabe H, Izumi B, Tanaka H, Kawai K, Tanaka N. The efficacy of intra-operative neurophysiological monitoring using transcranial electrically stimulated muscle-evoked potentials (TcE-MsEPs) for predicting postoperative segmental upper extremity motor paresis after cervical laminoplasty. Clin Spine Surg 2016;29(4): E188–E195

134. Taunt CJ Jr, Sidhu KS, Andrew SA. Somatosensory evoked potential monitor-ing during anterior cervical discectomy and fusion. Spine 2005;30(17):1970–1972

135. Bose B, Sestokas AK, Schwartz DM. Neurophysiological monitoring of spinal cord function during instrumented anterior cervical fusion. Spine J 2004;4(2):202–207

136. Prass RL, Kinney SE, Hardy RW Jr, Hahn JF, Lüders H. Acoustic (loudspeaker) facial EMG monitoring: II. Use of evoked EMG activity during acoustic neuroma resection.

Otolaryngol Head Neck Surg 1987;97(6): 541–551

137. Prass RL, Lüders H. Acoustic (loudspeaker) facial electromyographic monitoring: Part 1. Evoked electromyographic activity during acoustic neuroma resection. Neurosurgery 1986;19(3):392–400

138. Takeda M, Yamaguchi S, Mitsuhara T, Abiko M, Kurisu K. Intraoperative neurophysiologic monitoring for degenerative cervical myelopathy. Neurosurg Clin N Am 2018;29(1):159–167

139. Kelleher MO, Tan G, Sarjeant R, Fehlings MG. Predictive value of intraoperative neurophysiological monitoring during cervical spine surgery: a prospective analysis of 1055 consecutive patients. J Neurosurg Spine 2008;8(3):215–221

140. Fotakopoulos G, Alexiou GA, Pachatouridis D, et al. The value of transcranial motor-evoked potentials and free-running electromyography in surgery for cervical disc herniation. J Clin Neurosci 2013;20(2): 263–266

141. Balzer JR, Crammond D, Habeych M, Sclabassi R. Intraoperative EMG during spinal pedicle screw instrumentation. In: Nuwer MR, ed. Intraoperative Monitoring of Neural Function Handbook of Clinical Neurophysiology. Amsterdam: Elsevier; 2008:407

142. Khan MH, Smith PN, Balzer JR, et al. Intraoperative somatosensory evoked potential monitoring during cervical spine corpectomy surgery: experience with 508 cases. Spine 2006;31(4):E105–E113

143. Sakaura H, Hosono N, Mukai Y, Ishii T, Yoshikawa H. C5 palsy after decompression surgery for cervical myelopathy: review of the literature. Spine 2003;28(21): 2447–2451

144. Epstein N. Anterior approaches to cervical spondylosis and ossification of the posterior longitudinal ligament: review of operative technique and assessment of 65 multilevel circumferential procedures. Surg Neurol 2001;55(6):313–324

145. Fan D, Schwartz DM, Vaccaro AR, Hilibrand AS, Albert TJ. Intraoperative neurophysiologic detection of iatrogenic C5 nerve root injury during laminectomy for cervical compression myelopathy. Spine 2002;27(22):2499–2502

146. Jimenez JC, Sani S, Braverman B, Deutsch H, Ratliff JK. Palsies of the fifth cervical nerve root after cervical decompression: prevention using continuous intraoperative electromyography monitoring. J Neurosurg Spine 2005;3(2):92–97

147. Sutter M, Deletis V, Dvorak J, et al. Current opinions and recommendations on multimodal intraoperative monitoring during spine surgeries. Eur Spine J 2007;16(Suppl 2):S232–S237

148. Sala F. Take the A train. Clin Neurophysiol 2015;126(9):1647–1649

149. Isley MR, Pearlman RC, Bridwell KH, Gelb DE. Recent advances in intraoperative neuromonitoring of spinal cord function: Pedicle screw stimulation techniques. Am J Electroneurodiagn Technol 1997;37: 93–126

150. Djurasovic M, Dimar JR II, Glassman SD, Edmonds HL, Carreon LY. A prospective analysis of intraoperative electromyographic monitoring of posterior cervical screw fixation. J Spinal Disord Tech 2005;18(6): 515–518

151. Leppanen RE. Intraoperative monitoring of segmental spinal nerve root function with free-run and electrically-triggered electromyography and spinal cord function with reflexes and F-responses. A position statement by the American Society of Neurophysiological Monitoring. J Clin Monit Comput 2005;19(6):437–461

152. Kalkman CJ, Drummond JC, Ribberink AA. Low concentrations of isoflurane abolish motor evoked responses to transcranial electrical stimulation during nitrous oxide/opioid anesthesia in humans. Anesth Analg 1991;73(4):410–415

153. Haghighi SS, Madsen R, Green KD, Oro JJ, Kracke GR. Suppression of motor evoked potentials by inhalation anesthetics. J Neurosurg Anesthesiol 1990;2(2):73–78

154. Zentner J, Albrecht T, Heuser D. Influence of halothane, enflurane, and isoflurane on motor evoked potentials. Neurosurgery 1992;31(2):298–305

155. Zhou HH, Zhu C. Comparison of isoflurane effects on motor evoked potential and F wave. Anesthesiology 2000;93(1):32–38

156. Rehberg B, Grünewald M, Baars J, Fuegener K, Urban BW, Kox WJ. Monitoring of immobility to noxious stimulation during

sevoflurane anesthesia using the spinal H-reflex. Anesthesiology 2004;100(1): 44–50

157. Sloan TB, Heyer EJ. Anesthesia for intraoperative neurophysiologic monitoring of the spinal cord. J Clin Neurophysiol 2002; 19(5):430–443

158. Schmidt J, Hering W, Albrecht S. [Total intravenous anesthesia with propofol and remifentanil. Results of a multicenter study of 6,161 patients]. Anaesthesist 2005; 54(1):17–28

159. Lyon R, Feiner J, Lieberman JA. Progressive suppression of motor evoked potentials during general anesthesia: the phenomenon of "anesthetic fade". J Neurosurg Anesthesiol 2005;17(1):13–19

160. Tanaka S, Kobayashi I, Sagiuchi T, et al. Compensation of intraoperative transcranial motor-evoked potential monitoring by compound muscle action potential after peripheral nerve stimulation. J Clin Neurophysiol 2005;22(4):271–274

161. Fujiki M, Furukawa Y, Kamida T, et al. Intraoperative corticomuscular motor evoked potentials for evaluation of motor function: a comparison with corticospinal D and I waves. J Neurosurg 2006;104(1): 85–92

162. Chesler M, Young W, Hassan AZ, Sakatani K, Moriya T. Elevation and clearance of extracellular K+ following graded contusion of the rat spinal cord. Exp Neurol 1994; 125(1):93–98

08 Conservative Nonoperative Treatment or Follow-up for Mild Cervical Spondylotic Myelopathy

Nobuyuki Shimokawa and Toshihiro Takami

Introduction

Cervical degenerative conditions, such as cervical spondylosis, disc herniation, and ossification of the posterior longitudinal ligament (OPLL), are common causes of neurological disorders. They usually progress slowly with age, might worsen acutely after minor falls or trauma, and are recognized typically as cervical spondylotic myelopathy (CSM). The clinical condition of CSM can be classified into three grades and two subgrades based on the modified Japanese Orthopedic Association scale (mJOA): mild (grade 1) myelopathy is defined as a mJOA score of 15 to 17, moderate myelopathy (grade 2) as a score of 12 to 14, and severe (grade 3) as a mJOA score of 0 to 11, with each grade subdivided into the subgrades of (i) myelopathy signs but no symptoms, and (ii) no symptoms but with significant stenosis (premyelopathic condition).[1–5] Regarding surgical intervention for CSM, while there is a global consensus on the treatment strategy for moderate-to-severe CSM, the choice between surgical intervention or conservative nonoperative treatment for modest or mild CSM, or even for the premyelopathic condition, is not well established.[3–11] Treatment options for modest or mild CSM vary, based on available resources and local practices. The Spine Committee of the World Federation of Neurosurgical Societies (WFNS) organized a consensus meeting on the management of CSM in Nagpur, India, in September 2018, to develop recommendations for global applicability.[11,12] At that consensus meeting, each speaker was tasked with suggesting questions related to the topic, found answers

to those questions, and finally made recommendation statements for the management of CSM. At the end of each talk, the statements were voted on by committee members using the Delphi method, and approved statements were declared as recommendations of the WFNS Spine Committee. This chapter provides a comprehensive review about conservative nonoperative therapy and follow-up for mild CSM, based on previously published systemic reviews, clinical studies, and WFNS Spine Committee recommendations.[9–12]

Imaging to Assess Spinal Cord Condition in CSM

Value of Prognostic Imaging

Although it is not always easy to accurately assess the spinal cord condition in CSM, careful imaging-based diagnosis would enable estimation of prognostic factors. Shimomura et al retrospectively evaluated seventy patients with mild CSM.[13] The follow-up rate was 80%. Possible prognostic factors that might exacerbate clinical symptoms of CSM, such as age, gender, follow-up period, developmental or dynamic factors on plain lateral radiograph, high-signal intensity area on T2-weighted sagittal MR images, and the extent of maximum cord compression, that is, partial or circumferential spinal cord compression on axial MR images, were examined. Univariate and multivariate logistic regression analyses were conducted to examine significant prognostic factors. They found that 19.6% of patients deteriorated after conservative nonoperative treatment. Conversely, 80% of patients were stable during a 3-year follow-up. They concluded that the only factor that was significantly associated with exacerbation of clinical symptoms of CSM was evidence of circumferential spinal cord compression on axial MR images. Evaluation showed that 30.3% of CSM patients with circumferential spinal cord compression on axial MR images deteriorated after nonoperative treatment. Sumi et al examined the functional prognosis of patients with mild CSM.[14] They classified those patients into two study groups, based on the findings of MR images: ovoid deformity and angular-edge deformity of the spinal cord shape on T1-weighted axial MR images. They suggested that the overall tolerance rate for patients with mild CSM was 70%, but that angular-edge deformity on T1-weighted axial MR images was the image findings with poor prognosis (tolerance rate 58%). They proposed that surgical treatment for mild CSM should be considered when patients with mild CSM demonstrate an angular-edge deformity on MR images. The presence of increased signal intensity on T2-weighted MR images is considered to reflect various intramedullary lesions. It has been reported that increased signal intensity on T2-weighted MR images might reflect irreversible changes of the spinal cord and, thus, might indicate a poor prognosis for CSM.[15-18] Matsumoto et al retrospectively examined whether increased signal intensity on T2-weighted MR images can be the image findings to predict the outcome of patients with CSM.[19] Fifty-two patients with mild CSM receiving nonoperative conservative treatment were examined. Satisfactory outcomes were confirmed in 78% of patients without increased signal intensity, in 70% of those with multisegmental increased signal intensity, and in 63% of those with focal increased signal intensity. They suggested that increased signal intensity on T2-weighted MR images may not necessarily be the imaging findings to predict the outcome of CSM with nonoperative treatment. Salem et al examined 93 patients with CSM who were operated on by either the anterior or posterior

approach, and found that signal changes on T1-weighted MR images predicted worse outcomes after surgery.[20] Another study showed that increased signal intensity on T2-weighted MR images alone cannot be considered as a predictor of worse outcome.[21] Strong and sharp signal changes with a clear border on T2-weighted MR images, low-signal intensity on T1-weighted MR images, or both can be considered as negative predictors of surgical outcome. These signal changes on MR images might reflect more severe histological changes and worse outcomes after surgery.[9] Oshima et al reported a retrospective comparative study to investigate the natural course in 45 patients with mild CSM.[22] Twenty patients (60%) demonstrated the stable course during a mean follow-up period of 78 months. They suggested that a large range of motion, segmental kyphosis, and instability at the narrowest part of the spinal canal may be the adverse prognostic factors. Kong et al evaluated a total of 90 patients with mild CSM.[23] All their patients initially received conservative nonoperative treatment and were followed-up periodically. Seventy-eight of the 90 patients were available for data analysis, among whom only 21 patients (26.9%) deteriorated and underwent surgery, while the remaining 57 patients (73.1%) were treated conservatively throughout. They suggested that segmental instability and cervical spinal stenosis were factors correlating with a poor prognosis. Matsunaga et al reported 323 OPLL patients with significant cervical stenosis, but with no symptoms.[24] They found that during an average follow-up period of 17.6 years, only 17% developed myelopathy. So far, only two studies have examined the rate of progression to myelopathy in patients with significant canal stenosis having no symptoms.[3,24]

Considering the results of many of these papers, approximately 20% of patients with mild CSM who received initial conservative treatment might need surgical treatment during follow-up. The following factors are possible predictors of deterioration during nonoperative management: circumferential compression in axial MRI, angular-edged deformity, high-signal intensity on T2-weighted MRI/low-signal intensity on T1-weighted MRI of the spinal cord, hypermobility/instability of the spinal segment, kyphosis, and presence of OPLL and cervical stenosis. For these reasons, careful analysis of imaging characteristics, as well as consideration of individual patient factors, is important in determining treatment strategies for mild CSM.

Innovative Technology to Assess CSM

Diffusion tensor imaging (DTI) is an MRI-based technology that is recently being increasingly used.[25-29] It can provide not only fiber tracking images, but also quantitative imaging parameters such as apparent diffusion coefficient (ADC), mean diffusivity (MD), and fractional anisotropy (FA). These imaging parameters may be applied for quantitative evaluation of the spinal cord condition and be more sensitive for the recognition of early-stage CSM. Uda et al analyzed the DT parameters of MD and FA in patients with CSM using a 3.0T MR system.[29] They demonstrated that most cases of CSM demonstrated an increase in MD or decrease in FA. Although both an MD increase and FA decrease had diagnostic validity for myelopathy, receiver operating characteristic (ROC) analysis demonstrated a higher sensitivity and specificity for prediction by an MD increase than an FA decrease. They concluded that CSM can be predicted with high accuracy with DT parameters. Gaun et al conducted a meta-analysis to explore the potential role of DT imaging as a diagnostic biomarker for CSM.[30] They cited a total of 14 studies involving 479 CSM patients and 278 controls. FA was significantly reduced and ADC was significantly increased at the level of greatest compression in CSM patients compared to controls. They proposed the possible use of DTI parameters in differentiating CSM patients from healthy subjects. Banaszek et al reviewed the current role of DTI in the diagnosis and management of CSM.[31] They suggested that DTI might detect the condition of the spinal cord in the course of CSM earlier than any other method and might also be useful in predicting surgical outcomes in CSM patients. Zheng et al examined DTI parameters using a 3.0T MR system in 61 patients with CSM who required surgical decompression.[32] They divided patients into four groups, based on a JOA recovery rate after surgery. They suggested that DTI parameters were closely related to the severity of CSM and were useful for surgeons to predict surgical outcomes in patients with CSM. These recent studies clearly suggested that DTI parameters might quantitatively reflect the pathology of spinal cord condition and can be used for evaluation of the functional status of the spinal cord in patients with CSM. However, the clinical use of DTI is still limited because of anatomical disadvantages, such as the relatively small size of the spinal cord. Further technical innovation is truly desired to accurately assess the spinal cord condition in CSM.

Surgical Indications for Mild CSM

Neo et al suggested that decompression surgery might be indicated for carefully selected patients with only slight myelopathy, because the surgery can relieve their symptoms and persistent anxiety.[33] Stoffman et al examined a total of 89 patients with CSM and suggested that higher depression scores were associated with worse myelopathy than the arm, sphincter, or sensory symptoms.[34] They concluded that walking disability might exacerbate the mental anxiety in patients with CSM. AOSpine North America prospective multicenter study recently indicated that the surgery of CSM not only arrested the clinical symptoms, but also improved functional status, and finally the quality of life (QOL) of patients regardless of the severity of myelopathy.[35] AOSpine International and North America multicenter study demonstrated that patients with depression or bipolar disorder have fewer functional and QOL improvements after surgery compared to patients without psychiatric comorbidities.[36] Additionally, Badhiwala et al conducted an international prospective multicenter study to explore the efficacy and safety of surgical decompression in 193 patients with mild CSM.[37] They concluded that mild CSM is associated with significant impairment of QOL, and that surgery results in significant gains in terms of functional status, level of disability, and QOL.

■ Illustrative Case 1

A 37-year-old man presented with mild neck stiffness. He had a transient episode of acute scapular pain caused by cervical radiculopathy. Neurological evaluation demonstrated that his functional condition estimated using the JOA score was 16. MRI demonstrated the disc herniation at C5/6 with moderate compression of the spinal cord (**Fig. 8.1a**). The patient demonstrated a significantly anxious mood and decreased functional ability. He underwent anterior cervical discectomy and fusion (ACDF). His postoperative course was satisfactory. He is now without significant symptoms or limitations even 15 years after surgery (**Figs. 8.1b-d**).

Adjacent disc degeneration has been observed during postoperative follow-up, but it is still tolerable.

■ Illustrative Case 2

A 52-year-old man presented with bilateral clumsy hands. Neurological evaluation demonstrated that his functional condition estimated using the JOA score was 15. MRI demonstrated spinal cord compression at the level of C4/5/6/7 caused by cervical OPLL (**Figs. 8.2a, 8.3a**). The patient demonstrated a significantly anxious mood and decreased functional ability. He underwent posterior decompression and fusion. His postoperative course was uneventful for 17 years. His JOA score long after surgery was still 15 (**Fig. 8.3b-d**). Serial long-term follow up imaging indicated gradual reduction of thickness and extension of the longitudinal direction of cervical OPLL after surgery (**Fig. 8.2b**).

WFNS Spine Committee Recommendations

Several important clinical studies have provided evidence-based recommendations to

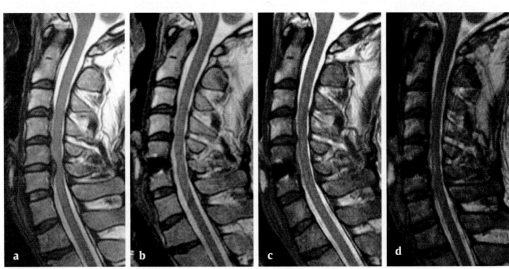

Fig. 8.1 Illustrative case 1. MR images obtained before and after surgery demonstrating successful decompression of the spinal cord and stable condition after surgery. (**a**) Before surgery, (**b**) 3 years after surgery, (**c**) 10 years after surgery, (**d**) 15 years after surgery.

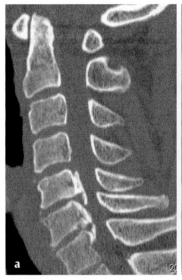
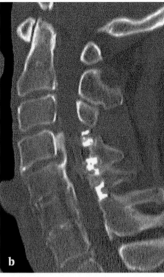

Fig. 8.2 Illustrative case 2. CT images obtained before and after surgery demonstrating gradual resolution of ossification of the posterior longitudinal ligament (OPLL). (**a**) Before surgery, (**b**) 17 years after surgery.

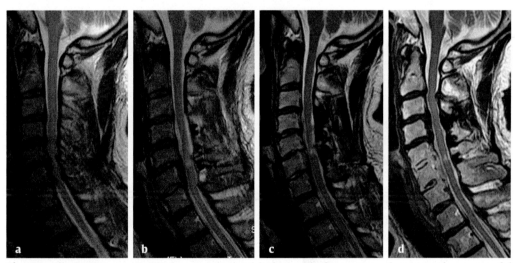

Fig. 8.3 Illustrative case 2. MR images obtained before and after surgery demonstrating successful decompression of the spinal cord and stable condition after surgery. (**a**) Before surgery, (**b**) 3 months after surgery, (**c**) 5 years after surgery, (**d**) 17 years after surgery.

manage patients with CSM. Nikolaidis et al performed a systematic review of a database to explore whether surgery for CSM was associated with improved outcomes compared to conservative nonoperative treatment.[38] They suggested that there is low-quality evidence that surgery might provide faster pain relief than conservative nonoperative treatment in patients with cervical radiculopathy; however, there is little or no difference in the long-term. There is also low-quality evidence that patients with mild myelopathy feel subjectively better shortly after surgery, but there is little or no difference in the long term. Kadanka et al conducted a 3-year prospective randomized study focusing on the results of conservative versus surgical treatment for CSM.[39] Their study did not show that surgery is superior to conservative treatment for mild-to-moderate CSM. Rhee et al reviewed the role of conservative nonoperative treatment for CSM through a systematic search in PubMed and the Cochrane Collaboration Library for articles published between 1956 and 2012.[40] Conservative nonoperative treatments included physical therapy, medications, injections, orthoses, and traction. They noted a paucity of evidence regarding the effectiveness of conservative nonoperative treatment for CSM. They suggested that conservative nonoperative treatment cannot be routinely recommended. In the largest prospective evaluation and first global assessment of surgical outcomes in patients with CSM, Fehlings et al noted that surgery results in improved clinical outcomes, functional status, and QOL, as evaluated by the mJOA scale.[41] Four hundred seventy-nine symptomatic patients with CSM were evaluated in this prospective, multicenter study from 16 global sites. They suggested that surgical decompression for CSM is safe and effective in improving the functional status and QOL of patients with CSM, irrespective of differences in medical systems and sociocultural determinants of health.

The AOSpine North America and the Cervical Spine Research Society developed clinical practice guidelines for the management of CSM.[42] They recommended surgical intervention for moderate-to-severe CSM. They also recommended surgical intervention for mild CSM when there is neurological deterioration with conservative nonoperative treatment. They did not recommend prophylactic surgery for nonmyelopathic patients, with evidence of cervical cord compression without signs or symptoms of radiculopathy. These patients should be followed clinically. Their guidelines promote standardization of clinical care for CSM, recommend decrease in the heterogeneity of management strategies and, finally, encourage surgeons to make evidence-based informed decisions. The WFNS Spine committee followed the GRADE-ADOLOPMENT approach for development of guideline recommendations to develop adapted recommendations

(**Table 8.1**).[43] Parthiban et al conducted a review of the literature on conservative nonoperative treatment and surgery for CSM, and explored the general consensus regarding its applicability in various clinical situations across the world.[12] They reported that surgical intervention is generally recommended for moderate-to-severe CSM, and either surgical intervention or rehabilitation should be prescribed for mild CSM, with nonoperative management being considered for slowly progressive mild CSM, and surgical intervention when rapid progression is noted. Prophylactic surgery should not be performed for nonmyelopathic patients with evidence of cervical cord compression without signs or symptoms of radiculopathy. On the other hand, nonmyelopathic patients with cord compression and clinical evidence of radiculopathy with or without electrophysiological confirmation are potential candidates for deterioration, thus carrying a high risk and, hence, need to be counselled. These patients are recommended to undergo surgery or close observation with rehabilitation if the patient refuses surgery.

Conclusion

Although there is no definite consensus on the surgical indications for mild CSM, symptoms of pain or walking disability might be key factors suggesting the surgical indications, because those symptoms considerably affect not only the functional condition but also mental condition. Surgeons need to consider the surgical indication for mild CSM using both evidence-based and narrative-based medicine. To make surgery for CSM much more reliable and convincing, spine surgeons are now facing the great challenge of contributing to the realization of a society of good health and longevity. Recent technical innovations, including imaging technology, application of artificial intelligence to spine surgery, computer-based navigation systems, and robotic technologies, are worthy of note and appear very promising.

Table 8.1 WFNS Spine Committee Recommendations for the Management of Patients with CSM as proposed by Parthiban et al[12]

Grade	Recommendations
Moderate-to-severe CSM (mJOA < 15)	Surgical intervention is recommended.
Mild CSM (mJOA 15–17)	Suggest offering surgical intervention or rehabilitation for patients with mild CSM.
	If at the beginning nonoperative management was followed, we recommend operative intervention when rapid progression of symptoms appear.
	Nonoperative conservative management may be considered for slowly progressive disease.
Nonmyelopathic patients with evidence of cervical cord compression without signs or symptoms of radiculopathy	Should not be offered a prophylactic surgery.
	These patients should be counselled about the potential risk of worsening, educated about the signs and symptoms of progression, and followed-up regularly.
	An informed consent should be obtained about neurological deficits that may follow trivial injury.
Nonmyelopathic patients with cord compression and clinical evidence of radiculopathy with or without electrophysiological confirmation	Patients are potential candidates who may deteriorate thus carrying high risk and hence need to be counselled about it. These patients are recommended to undergo surgery or close observation with rehabilitation if the patient refuses to undergo surgery.
	In the event of developing myelopathic signs, they are advised to go for surgery at the earliest.
	An informed consent should be obtained about neurological deficits that may follow trivial injury.

Abbreviations: CSM: cervical spondylotic myelopathy; mJOA: modified Japanese Orthopaedic Association scale.

Take-home Points

- Approximately 20% of patients with mild CSM who received initial conservative treatment might need surgical treatment during follow-up. The following factors are possible predictors of deterioration during nonoperative management: circumferential compression in axial MRI, angular-edged deformity, high-signal intensity on T2-weighted MRI/low-signal intensity on T1-weighted MRI of the spinal cord, hypermobility/instability of the spinal segment, kyphosis, and presence of OPLL and cervical stenosis.

- Surgical intervention should be offered for mild CSM when neurological deterioration or rapid progression is noted with conservative nonoperative treatment.

- Prophylactic surgery should not be offered for nonmyelopathic patients with evidence of cervical cord compression without signs or symptoms of radiculopathy.

References

1. Yonenobu K, Abumi K, Nagata K, Taketomi E, Ueyama K. Interobserver and intraobserver reliability of the japanese orthopaedic association scoring system for evaluation of cervical compression myelopathy. Spine 2001;26(17):1890–1894, discussion 1895

2. Tetreault L, Kopjar B, Nouri A, et al. The modified Japanese Orthopaedic Association scale: establishing criteria for mild, moderate and severe impairment in patients with degenerative cervical myelopathy. Eur Spine J 2017;26(1):78–84

3. Bednarik J, Kadanka Z, Dusek L, et al. Presymptomatic spondylotic cervical cord compression. Spine 2004;29(20):2260–2269

4. Wilson JR, Barry S, Fischer DJ, et al. Frequency, timing, and predictors of neurological dysfunction in the nonmyelopathic patient with cervical spinal cord compression, canal stenosis, and/or ossification of the posterior longitudinal ligament. Spine 2013; 38(22, Suppl 1):S37–S54

5. Kovalova I, Kerkovsky M, Kadanka Z, et al. Prevalence and imaging characteristics of nonmyelopathic and myelopathic spondylotic cervical cord compression. Spine 2016; 41(24):1908–1916

6. Matsumoto M, Chiba K, Ishikawa M, Maruiwa H, Fujimura Y, Toyama Y. Relationships between outcomes of conservative treatment and magnetic resonance imaging findings in patients with mild cervical myelopathy caused by soft disc herniations. Spine 2001;26(14):1592–1598

7. Yoshimatsu H, Nagata K, Goto H, et al. Conservative treatment for cervical spondylotic myelopathy. prediction of treatment effects by multivariate analysis. Spine J 2001;1(4):269–273

8. Naito K, Yamagata T, Ohata K, Takami T. Management of the patient with cervical cord compression but no evidence of myelopathy: what should we do? Neurosurg Clin N Am 2018;29(1):145–152

9. Zileli M, Borkar SA, Sinha S, et al. Cervical Spondylotic Myelopathy: Natural Course and the Value of Diagnostic Techniques -WFNS Spine Committee Recommendations. Neurospine 2019;16(3):386–402

10. Zileli M, Maheshwari S, Kale SS, Garg K, Menon SK, Parthiban J. Outcome Measures and Variables Affecting Prognosis of Cervical Spondylotic Myelopathy: WFNS Spine Committee Recommendations. Neurospine 2019;16(3):435–447

11. Zileli M. Recommendations of WFNS Spine Committee. Neurospine 2019;16(3):383–385

12. Parthiban J, Alves OL, Chandrachari KP, Ramani P, Zileli M. Value of surgery and nonsurgical approaches for cervical spondylotic myelopathy: WFNS Spine Committee recommendations. Neurospine 2019;16(3):403–407

13. Shimomura T, Sumi M, Nishida K, et al. Prognostic factors for deterioration of patients with cervical spondylotic myelopathy after nonsurgical treatment. Spine 2007;32(22):2474–2479

14. Sumi M, Miyamoto H, Suzuki T, Kaneyama S, Kanatani T, Uno K. Prospective cohort study of mild cervical spondylotic myelopathy without surgical treatment. J Neurosurg Spine 2012;16(1):8–14

15. Al-Mefty O, Harkey LH, Middleton TH, Smith RR, Fox JL. Myelopathic cervical spondylotic lesions demonstrated by magnetic resonance imaging. J Neurosurg 1988;68(2):217–222

16. Ohshio I, Hatayama A, Kaneda K, Takahara M, Nagashima K. Correlation between histopathologic features and magnetic resonance images of spinal cord lesions. Spine 1993; 18(9):1140–1149

17. Takahashi M, Yamashita Y, Sakamoto Y, Kojima R. Chronic cervical cord compression: clinical significance of increased signal intensity on MR images. Radiology 1989; 173(1):219–224

18. Bednarik J, Kadanka Z, Dusek L, et al. Presymptomatic spondylotic cervical myelopathy: an updated predictive model. Eur Spine J 2008;17(3):421–431

19. Matsumoto M, Toyama Y, Ishikawa M, Chiba K, Suzuki N, Fujimura Y. Increased signal intensity of the spinal cord on magnetic resonance images in cervical compressive myelopathy. Does it predict the outcome of conservative treatment? Spine 2000;25(6):677–682

20. Salem HM, Salem KM, Burget F, Bommireddy R, Klezl Z. Cervical spondylotic myelopathy: the prediction of outcome following surgical intervention in 93 patients using T1- and T2-weighted MRI scans. Eur Spine J 2015;24(12):2930–2935

21. Tetreault LA, Dettori JR, Wilson JR, et al. Systematic review of magnetic resonance imaging characteristics that affect treatment decision making and predict clinical outcome in patients with cervical spondylotic myelopathy. Spine 2013; 38(22, Suppl 1):S89–S110

22. Oshima Y, Seichi A, Takeshita K, et al. Natural course and prognostic factors in patients with mild cervical spondylotic myelopathy with increased signal intensity on T2-weighted magnetic resonance imaging. Spine 2012;37(22):1909–1913

23. Kong LD, Meng LC, Wang LF, Shen Y, Wang P, Shang ZK. Evaluation of conservative treatment and timing of surgical intervention for mild forms of cervical spondylotic myelopathy. Exp Ther Med 2013;6(3): 852–856

24. Matsunaga S, Sakou T, Taketomi E, Komiya S. Clinical course of patients with ossification of the posterior longitudinal ligament: a minimum 10-year cohort study. J Neurosurg 2004; 100(3, Suppl Spine):245–248

25. Facon D, Ozanne A, Fillard P, Lepeintre JF, Tournoux-Facon C, Ducreux D. MR diffusion tensor imaging and fiber tracking in spinal cord compression. AJNR Am J Neuroradiol 2005;26(6):1587–1594

26. Mamata H, Jolesz FA, Maier SE. Apparent diffusion coefficient and fractional anisotropy in spinal cord: age and cervical spondylosis-related changes. J Magn Reson Imaging 2005;22(1):38–43

27. Hori M, Okubo T, Aoki S, Kumagai H, Araki T. Line scan diffusion tensor MRI at low magnetic field strength: feasibility study of cervical spondylotic myelopathy in an early clinical stage. J Magn Reson Imaging 2006;23(2):183–188

28. Ellingson BM, Ulmer JL, Kurpad SN, Schmit BD. Diffusion tensor MR imaging in chronic spinal cord injury. AJNR Am J Neuroradiol 2008;29(10):1976–1982

29. Uda T, Takami T, Tsuyuguchi N, et al. Assessment of cervical spondylotic myelopathy using diffusion tensor magnetic resonance imaging parameter at 3.0 tesla. Spine 2013;38(5):407–414

30. Guan X, Fan G, Wu X, et al. Diffusion tensor imaging studies of cervical spondylotic myelopathy: a systemic review and meta-analysis. PLoS One 2015;10(2):e0117707

31. Banaszek A, Bladowska J, Podgórski P, Sąsiadek MJ. Role of diffusion tensor mr imaging in degenerative cervical spine disease: a review of the literature. Clin Neuroradiol 2016;26(3):265–276

32. Zheng W, Chen H, Wang N, et al. Application of diffusion tensor imaging cutoff value to evaluate the severity and postoperative neurologic recovery of cervical spondylotic myelopathy. World Neurosurg 2018;118:e849–e855

33. Neo M, Fujibayashi S, Takemoto M, Nakamura T. Clinical results of and patient satisfaction with cervical laminoplasty for considerable cord compression with only slight myelopathy. Eur Spine J 2012;21(2):340–346

34. Stoffman MR, Roberts MS, King JT Jr. Cervical spondylotic myelopathy, depression, and anxiety: a cohort analysis of 89 patients. Neurosurgery 2005;57(2):307–313, discussion 307–313

35. Fehlings MG, Wilson JR, Kopjar B, et al. Efficacy and safety of surgical decompression in patients with cervical spondylotic myelopathy: results of the AOSpine North America prospective multi-center study. J Bone Joint Surg Am 2013;95(18):1651–1658

36. Tetreault L, Nagoshi N, Nakashima H, et al. Impact of depression and bipolar disorders on functional and quality of life outcomes in patients undergoing surgery for degenerative cervical myelopathy: analysis of a combined prospective dataset. Spine 2017;42(6):372–378

37. Badhiwala JH, Witiw CD, Nassiri F, et al. Efficacy and safety of surgery for mild Degenerative cervical myelopathy: result of the AOSpine north America and international prospective multicenter studies. Neurosurgery 2019;84(4):890–897

38. Nikolaidis I, Fouyas IP, Sandercock PA, Statham PF. Surgery for cervical radiculopathy or myelopathy. Cochrane Database Syst Rev 2010; (1):CD001466

39. Kadanka Z, Mares M, Bednaník J, et al. Approaches to spondylotic cervical myelopathy: conservative versus surgical results in a 3-year follow-up study. Spine 2002; 27(20):2205–2210, discussion 2210–2211

40. Rhee JM, Shamji MF, Erwin WM, et al. Nonoperative management of cervical myelopathy: a systematic review. Spine 2013; 38(22, Suppl 1):S55–S67

41. Fehlings MG, Ibrahim A, Tetreault L, et al. A global perspective on the outcomes of surgical decompression in patients with cervical spondylotic myelopathy: results from the prospective multicenter AOSpine international study on 479 patients. Spine 2015;40(17):1322–1328

42. Fehlings MG, Tetreault LA, Riew KD, et al. A clinical practice guideline for the management of patients with degenerative cervical myelopathy: recommendations for patients with mild, moderate, and severe disease and nonmyelopathic patients with evidence of cord compression. Global Spine J 2017; **7**(3, Suppl)70S–83S

43. Schünemann HJ, Wiercioch W, Brozek J, et al. GRADE Evidence to Decision (EtD) frameworks for adoption, adaptation, and de novo development of trustworthy recommendations: GRADE-ADOLOPMENT. J Clin Epidemiol 2017;81:101–110

09 Surgical Indications and Preferences for Cervical Spondylotic Myelopathy and OPLL

Salman Sharif, Sandeep Vaishya, Syed Maroof Ali, and Yousuf Shaikh

Introduction

Cervical spondylotic myelopathy (CSM) is an important cause of spinal cord dysfunction globally and is triggered by the degeneration of the cervical column.[1] This chapter has been divided into two parts. In the first part, authors will explain the causes of cervical myelopathy with the exclusion of ossified posterior longitudinal ligament (OPLL), and in the second part, myelopathy caused by OPLL. Each section has its own indications and surgical preferences.

Cervical Spondylotic Myelopathy

The typical CSM symptoms are instability of gait, loss of fine motor control of the upper limbs, weakness, and neck pain with a reduced range of motion along with urinary urgency at times. In advanced stages of the disease, it can lead to significant neurological deficits. Patients with minor symptoms usually do not require surgery and can be managed with physical therapy and medicines, depending on the symptoms, while patients with progressively worsening neurological symptoms and cord compression (with or without cord changes) usually require surgery.

Sometimes patients may present in an emergency. They may have had a pre-existing compression but either had mild or no symptoms, but a trivial trauma may precipitate a cord injury. This fact has to be kept in mind while deciding whether to operate or conservatively manage a patient.

Indications of Surgery

The indications of surgery can be summarized as below:
- Progressively worsening neurological deficits
- Significant pain and numbness in the upper extremities
- Sudden worsening after a trivial trauma
- Fixed neurological deficit not improving with time
- Failure of conservative management

Type of Surgery

There has been a perennial debate about the anterior versus posterior surgery. Even in anterior surgery, the debate is between multilevel anterior cervical discectomy and fusion (ACDF) versus corpectomy (and variations of it, such as oblique corpectomy), while in posterior surgery, it is between laminectomy versus laminoplasty. There are pros and cons to all procedures, and although in some cases the approach and procedure might be well-defined, in other cases, there is no single approach superior to another, and that is where the debate starts. In this chapter, authors have given an overview of all available procedures, their indications, results, and the complications associated with them. The available surgical procedures are mentioned below:
- Anterior surgery
  - ACDF
  - Anterior cervical corpectomy
  - Oblique corpectomy

- Hybrid procedures combining corpectomy with ACDF or cervical disk arthroplasty (CDA) with ACDF
- Posterior surgery
  - Cervical laminectomy (with or without fusion)
  - Cervical laminoplasty (and many variations of the procedure)
  - Posterior minimally invasive decompression
- Combined anterior and posterior procedures

This is done either in a single stage or as a second procedure in which a patient has been operated before, either anteriorly or posteriorly.

Anterior Approach

In the 1950s, surgeons started from posterior and then moved to anterior procedures. The anterior approach to the cervical spine was developed in the 1950s by Robinson and Smith, Smith and Robinson, and Cloward.[1–3] Robinson and Smith's original paper reported their first eight patients and suggested that disk degeneration leads to osteophyte formation, subluxation, and instability, while Cloward developed instrumentation for interbody fusion by creating bone dowels.

ACDF can decompress the anterior spinal cord, preserve the spinal column's stability, and is associated with a low prevalence of graft extrusion or migration. For many years, standard ACDF techniques were popular with autograft and later with artificial grafts like titanium or polyetheretherketone (PEEK) cages or allografts. Since the 1990s, most authors prefer a locking cervical plate, in order to supplement fusion and prevent graft migration. On the other hand, several authors have mentioned a higher risk of complications where cervical plate is used. In a series of more than 2200 cases, Xie et al reviewed their complications in relation to the cervical plate and found 10.7% incidence of complications related to the plate, including loosening or breaking of the screw and the plate and its malpositioning.[4]

Interestingly, they had not looked at dysphagia in that series, which is the most common complication of anterior cervical surgery and more so after plating. In the last few years, several studies have been conducted where a graft or cage alone was used, obviating the need for a cervical plate to reduce the plate-related complications. Shenghua et al in a randomized prospective study compared 104 patients of multilevel CSM operated with either zero-profile PEEK cage with a screw or a cervical plate. They found that the incidence of dysphagia was significantly higher in the group with plating.[5]

ACDF could result in greater improvements in cervical lordosis and segmental height and less blood loss than anterior cervical corpectomy and fusion (ACCF). At the same time, it was suggested that ACCF could provide improved visualization compared to ACDF in removing the osteophytes and ossified ligament.[6,7]

In a meta-analysis, Guan et al could find no difference in efficacy while comparing ACCF with ACDF, but the latter was superior to operation time, blood loss, and hospital stay.[8]

In another meta-analysis, Han et al found similar data; in addition, they also found that ACDF was superior to ACCF in complication rates.[9]

Anterior Cervical Discectomy and Fusion

ACDF is the most standard and commonly used procedure for CSM. It allows the removal of the disk, uncovertebral joints, and osteophytes. If there is focal OPLL, then that can also be taken care of at the same time. The disks which have migrated significantly cranial or caudal may need a corpectomy instead of a discectomy. When performed at multiple levels, ACDF provides a better kyphosis correction as the distraction is over multiple segments.[10] Several authors have reported a higher rate of pseudoarthrosis as the number of fused segments increase.

However, some authors argue that ACDF may not be the optimal surgical approach for

CSM due to the risk of incomplete decompression, limited visual exposure, and a high rate of nonunion due to graft-host interfaces.[11,12] The most commonly used technique is to perform a discectomy and insert a graft. For the first few decades, an autograft from the iliac crest was the only source of graft. But in the last two decades, the availability of other materials has made it possible to make different types of grafts. The commonly used ones are made of PEEK, titanium, or porous tantalum apart from allografts. These are usually supplemented with a locking plate. Cervical locking plates have also evolved over a period of time, as the initial plates required a bicortical purchase, leading to a risk of dural penetration. With the availability of locking screw-plate design since the mid-1990s, it became much easier to use. Various types of screw plate systems are available today— rigid, dynamic, and translational. Zero profile PEEK cages with screws have become popular in recent years and obviate the use of a plate. They are also useful in the fusion of adjacent segment disease where a plate is already in place; thus, obviating the need to remove it. Another advantage of these is that it could be used for a nonadjacent segment disk disease, sparing the intervening motion segment. An alternate means of improving the fusion rate after multilevel decompression is the use of ACCF. In addition to improving the fusion rate, ACCF also provides for a more extensive decompression and, at the same time, provides enough bone to be used as an autograft.

Disk arthroplasty can be an option in very selected patients. Generally speaking, it is not recommended for people with myelopathy, as many surgeons believe that arthrodesis is required to prevent motion at the involved segment. Buchowski et al conducted a multicentric randomized control trial in single-level cervical disk disease with myelopathy and enrolled 199 patients. They found that the results were equally good in both fusion and arthroplasty groups, and preservation of motion did not have any negative impact on myelopathy.[13]

Cervical Corpectomy and Fusion

When the compression extends beyond the disk level, or there are significant osteophytes behind the vertebral body, then performing a corpectomy is a better option than carrying out a discectomy alone. As a corpectomy gives more space, one can directly attack the pathology and perform a more extensive decompression. A corpectomy makes it easier to remove the osteophytes from behind the intact cranial and caudal vertebral bodies, as the surgeon is working at an angle rather than the straight trajectory as in a discectomy. In 1969, Boni and Denaro, developed a technique which they termed multiple subtotal corpectomies.[14,15] The technique was called "multiple" because it is performed at multiple levels, "subtotal" because the lateral walls of the vertebral body were preserved, and "corpectomy" because the central part of the vertebral body was entirely removed. The original technique, as described by Boni and Denaro, required modified Cloward instrumentation at multiple levels and then widening of the holes at multiple levels, and deepening of the bony trench with the removal of the posterior walls of the vertebral bodies (up to the posterior longitudinal ligament) and removal of any element of conflict with the spinal cord.[16] After a corpectomy, either a strut graft or a metal cage can be used. Some settling of the graft or subsidence of the cage is expected, but in the osteoporotic spine, it can be significant, sometimes requiring a refixation or supplementation by posterior fusion. Expandable cages are a good option and easier to use but provide less space for the bone graft to be filled. Fusion rates after corpectomy are reported to be better than ACDF.[11,12]

George et al suggested a technique of oblique corpectomy without fusion for elderly patients in whom the involved segments were already fused.[17] Other groups were following this technique.[18] Tykocki et al reviewed all published literature on oblique corpectomy and found nearly 800 cases.[19] In the cases of CSM and OPLL, they found an improvement rate of about 70%. Although this technique does not require the use of an implant, it still did not become very popular amongst surgeons due to technical challenges and higher complication rates, particularly Horner's syndrome. Other possible complications are the risk of injury to the vertebral artery and the inability to correct kyphosis.

Hybrid Procedures

In the last decade, hybrid procedures have also become popular, possibly involving a corpectomy at one or two levels along with discectomy at another. This provides an advantage of 3-point fixation of the plate, thus providing more stability. Ryu et al.[20] reported that a combination of a single-level corpectomy with discectomy was superior to two-level corpectomy and provided higher fusion rates, better lordosis, and lesser complications related to the implant. Another example of a hybrid procedure for multilevel discectomy can be discectomy and fusion at one level and CDA at another. This will help in retaining some movement of the neck, particularly in 3- or 4-level discectomies.[21]

Posterior Approach

Posterior procedures like laminectomy and hemilaminectomy started much before the anterior procedures. The usual procedure was a C3–C7 laminectomy but it became less common after anterior surgeries became popular. There were two reasons for this—first, the anterior surgery could directly attack the pathology; second, the long-term side effects, such as the development of kyphosis and axial neck pain. Then in the 1970s, laminoplasty started becoming popular and removed some of the disadvantages of laminectomy. Much later, posterior fixation techniques were developed and, along with laminectomy, became a popular alternative. There is a lot of debate over the superiority of one technique over the other, and ample literature is available to support all views, although there are recommended guidelines for certain situations.

Posterior procedures can be grossly divided into a laminectomy alone, laminectomy with fusion, and laminoplasty.

Laminectomy

Laminectomy involves removal of the lamina at the involved levels, and according to published literature, it is a safe and effective procedure with success ranging from 62 to 70%. It provides good long-term relief from symptoms. For more than four decades, laminectomy alone was the standard treatment for long-segment compressive myelopathy. But laminectomy alone may compromise the flexibility of the spine and can also lead to instability.[22] Many cervical laminectomy patients develop a deformity called swan neck deformity, which may need corrective surgery.

Cervical Laminoplasty

In 1973 in Japan, Oyama and Hattori introduced the laminoplasty to prevent post-laminectomy invasion of the laminectomy membrane.[23] This procedure was popularized by Japanese surgeons in the 1970s and 1980s. Over the years, different techniques were devised to perform the procedure. Unilateral open-door laminoplasty was introduced by Hirabayashi and coworkers in 1977, and it continues to be one of the standard techniques for posterior decompression of the cervical spine.[24,25] Gutters are created with high-speed drills at the junction between the articular processes and the laminae. The gutters on the dominant side of the symptoms are cut completely to achieve laminotomy. The spinous processes and the laminae are laterally displaced to the gutters' hinges on the opposite side. The spinal canal is enlarged by opening the posterior bony elements, and the laminae are kept open with three or four sutures on the facet capsule on the hinge side.[26]

As compared to the original technique, the spinal canal was kept open by suture on the facet capsule on the hinge side, but it was difficult to maintain the increased canal diameter; hence, currently various implants of titanium/ceramic or hydroxyapatite are used on the laminotomy side to keep it open.

The purpose of the development of laminoplasty was to preserve the posterior muscular structures, in order to prevent kyphosis and instability and prevent the formation of the postlaminectomy membrane.

The other most popular technique was described by Kurokawa et al.[27] In this technique, the spinous process was split in between, and then lateral gutters were drilled in the lamina on either side, and the gap in the spinous process was kept open by either bone graft or metal implant.

General complications of laminoplasty are axial neck pain, C5 root palsy, kyphosis, and, rarely, epidural hematoma.

Complications of unilateral single door laminoplasty—if lamina is fixed with lateral mass with miniplates, then wider dissection is required, leading to increased muscle atrophy and increased complications associated with the implant. If bone chips are used for fusion, there may be excess bone growth, leading to restriction of neck movements.

Cervical Laminectomy and Fusion

The modern era of cervical spine surgery in the treatment of cervical instability began with the reports of Roy-Camille, who treated spinal instability with plates and screws inserted in the lateral masses.[28,29] He designed cervical lateral mass plates with 13-mm distance holes and different lengths. The technique became more popular in the last 20 years when cervical polyaxial screws became widely available. Laminectomy provides a more extensive decompression as compared to laminoplasty and prevents the development of kyphosis. The incidence of axial neck pain is also less as compared to laminoplasty, although the range of motion is less.

Cervical Minimally Invasive Decompression

In certain cases, with predominantly posterior compression by hypertrophic ligamentum flavum, a minimally invasive decompression can be performed either by a tubular retractor or an endoscope. It can be performed at multiple levels. The advantage of a minimally invasive procedure would be the preservation of posterior elements, including spinous processes and interspinous ligament, thus providing a full range of movement and preventing future instability. But if there is any preexisting instability, then laminectomy and lateral mass fusion is a better option.

In a recent meta-analysis between laminoplasty and laminectomy and fusion, Lin et al found that the incidence of C5 root palsy was significantly higher in fusion patients.[30] Other authors have explained this fact by theorizing that wider decompression in fusion patients makes the tethering effect of C5 root worse.[31,32]

As compared to OPLL, where the guidelines and decisions are better defined, in CSM, anterior versus posterior debate has ambiguous answers. There are numerous publications in favor of both techniques. Even in some nonrandomized studies, there was an equal improvement in both groups with no clear superiority of one technique over the other. Goghawala et al are conducting a randomized control trial and a nonrandomized arm (eligible patients but decline randomization).[33] There will be 250 patients enrolled in the study and will be studying the anterior (multilevel discectomy and fusion and single-level corpectomy and fusion) and posterior (both laminectomy and lateral mass fusion and laminoplasty). The results of the above study should be out by 2021 and hopefully answer some controversies.

Combined Anterior and Posterior Approaches

When the compression is both ventral and dorsal and over a long segment, a combined approach can be chosen if the surgeon feels that either approach alone will not solve it. It can be performed as a single-stage procedure or sometimes at different times. In patients with severe osteoporosis, it may be useful to combine anterior surgery with posterior fixation, because the risk of graft subsidence is high. Occasionally, it may be a supplement to a previously performed anterior or posterior procedure.

To summarize, anterior surgery should be applied in the following cases: (1) if the compression is predominantly anterior, (2) in presence of cervical kyphosis, and (3) up to three levels of disease.

More than three levels is not a contraindication to anterior surgery, and many surgeons prefer it, but it may increase the risk of complications like dysphagia and pseudoarthrosis.

Posterior surgery should be applied in the following cases: (1) in multilevel compression—usually more than three levels, (2) if the neck pain is a significant feature, then fusion is a better option than laminoplasty, and (3) if the compression extends to extremes of the cervical spine—C2–3 and C7 levels.

Relative indications for posterior surgery are: (1) previous anterior surgery, (2) osteoporotic bone, (3) old age with comorbidities.

In a lordotic or straight spine, both anterior and posterior surgeries can be done, depending on the compression site. In equivocal situations, many times it is the surgeon's experience and preference which will decide whether it should be anterior or posterior surgery. The surgeons should consider the technique they are most comfortable with and which can ensure a good outcome in patients.

Surgical Outcomes of Cervical Spondylotic Myelopathy

Most authors report good outcomes as far as neurological recovery is concerned with a low incidence of complications, whether surgery is anterior or posterior. **Table 9.1** shows the outcome after anterior surgery and compares ACDF with ACCF. **Table 9.2** shows the outcome after posterior surgery and compares laminoplasty with laminectomy and fusion, while **Table 9.3** compares anterior with posterior surgery. As is evident from the tables, enough data compares various anterior techniques and different posterior techniques. Data for anterior versus posterior surgery is very scant, and there are no significant randomized studies.

In a recent publication, Montano et al, in a meta-analysis, suggested that for multilevel cervical myelopathy, ACDF should be the preferred option to laminoplasty.[54]

We can see from the above tables that there is a reasonable amount of data comparing various anterior techniques and different posterior techniques. However, data is scanty where anterior versus posterior is concerned.

Complications

Anterior Surgery Complications

Dysphagia: One of the most common complications after anterior surgery is dysphagia. Although it resolves in most patients over a few days to weeks, in a few cases, it can persist for a long time. It is more commonly seen in the older age groups and reoperations. Shriver et al, in a meta-analysis, reported an overall dysphagia rate of 8.5% and the rate of moderate or severe dysphagia to be 4.4%.[55]

Cerebrospinal fluid (CSF) leak: It is an unusual complication, although more commonly seen in cases of OPLL rather than CSM, seen in about 1% of patients.[56,57] Even if it happens, it can be managed easily by repairing it with sutures and glue and dural substitutes. Some patients with a bad tear that does not allow a watertight closure may require lumbar CSF drainage for a few days.

Injury to the recurrent laryngeal nerve: This is a dreaded complication, although its incidence is very low, ranging between 1 and 2%. The injury is generally transient and recovers over a period of 4 to 6 weeks. In rare cases, it can be a permanent injury leading to hoarseness of voice. Sometimes, particularly in old patients, it can lead to respiratory complications too. It is more commonly seen in reoperations than first-time surgery.[56–58]

Esophageal injury: This is another rare but dreaded complication. If it can be identified during surgery, then it should be repaired there and then. Halani et al reviewed the literature and found 153 published cases after

Table 9.1 Outcome after anterior surgery comparing ACDF and ACCF

Study	Sample size		Mean age (years)		Sex (male/female)		Follow-up (months, years)		Graft		Outcome	Complications
	ACDF	ACCF	ACDF	ACCF	ACDF	ACCF	ACDF	ACCF	ACDF	ACCF	ACDF vs. ACCF	
Li et al[34]	47	42	51.3 ± 6.5		58M/31F		79.6 ± 20.5M		Autograft, cage	Autograft, cage	JOA^a (0.10 [−0.97, 0.77]) Odom criteria (NE) Fusion rate (NE) Cobb angles C2–C7 (0.01 [−2.24, 2.24])	–
Liu et al[35]	69	39	46.1 ± 6.8	47.8 ± 6.4	39M/30F	26M/13F	26.8M (12–29M)	26.4M (12–37)	Cage, Atlantis plate	Titanium mesh cage, Atlantis plate	JOA (−0.49 [−1.08, 0.28]) NDI (−0.4 [−1.52, 0.72]) Odom criteria^b (1.36 [0.50, 3.73]) Fusion rate (26.97 [1.48, 493.03]) Segmental angle 2.93 (0.23,5.63) Cobb angles C2–C7 (8.64 [4.07, 13.21])	Dysphagia, hoarseness, C5 palsy, infection, CSF leak, epidural hematoma
Kyung et al[36]	25	15	50.3 ± 7.5	54.1 ± 9.8	19M/6F	11M/4F	87.3 ± 21.7 M	94.3 ±25.3	Autograft, cage	Autograft	JOA (0.3 [−1.4, 2.00]) VAS^a (0.8 [−0.98, 2.58]) Fusion rate (0.52 [0.05, 5.55]) Cobb angles C2–C7 (3.28 [0.47, 7.03])	Dysphagia, hoarseness, donor site pain, CSF leak, epidural hematoma

(Continued)

Table 9.1 (*Continued*) Outcome after anterior surgery comparing ACDF and ACCF

Study	Sample size		Mean age (years)		Sex (male/female)		Follow-up (months, years)		Graft		Outcome	Complications
Lin et al[10]	57	63	58.7 ± 9.7	57.9 ± 9.0	38M/19F	43M/20F	24 M	24M	Autograft, cage, semi-constrained plating system	Autograft, TMC, semi-constrained plating systems	JOA (0.59, −0.02, 1.02 [CI]) NDI (−2.24 [−3.02, −1.46]) Odom criteria (1.62 [0.70, 3.73]) Fusion rate (NE) Segmental angle (3.26 [2.35, 4.17])	Dysphagia, hoarseness, C5 palsy, CSF leak, epidural hematoma
Guo et al[37]	43	24	52.7 ± 9.4	55.2 ± 10.1	24M/19F	13M/11F	37.7 ± 7.2	37.3 ± 7.3	Autograft and PEEK cage	Autograft and titanium cage	JOA (0.79–1.08, 0.28 [CI]) Fusion rate (1.83 [0.11, 30.58]) Cobb angles ([3.50 [−0.19, 7.19]]) Segmental angles (5.8 [2.41, 9.19])	CSF leak, epidural hematoma
Park et al[38]	45	52	49.3 ± 9.7	49.4 ± 8.7	28M/17F	22M/30F	25.7 ± 6.2	23.3 ± 6.6	Allograft	Allograft	Cobb angles C2–C7 (1.60 [−1.91, 5.11])	-

Abbreviations: ACCF, anterior cervical corpectomy and fusion; ACDF, anterior cervical discectomy and fusion; CSF, cerebrospinal fluid; JOA, Japanese Orthopaedic Association; NDI, neck disability index; NE, not estimable; PEEK, polyetheretherketone; TMC, titanium mesh cages; VAS, visual analogue scale.

[a] JOA, VAS, NDI, Cobb angles, segmental angles scores comparison given as mean difference independent variable (fixed, CI).

[b] Fusion rate comparison given as Mantel–Haenszel statistical method independent variable (fixed variable, CI).

Table 9.2 Interventions and their outcomes in laminoplasty

Reference	Procedure (n, sample size)	Follow-up	Surgical complications	Clinical outcome	Radiographic outcome
Woods et al[39]	Laminoplasty using Mitek suture another fixation (39)	Average of 24 months	LAMP: chronic pain 2, recurrent stenosis 1, persistent radiculopathy 1, revision surgery 2	Gait pain postoperatively better in LAMP, $p < 0.05$	Sagittal alignment postoperatively better in LAMP, $p < 0.05$
	Laminectomy and fusion (82)		LAMT: chronic pain 2, dysphagia1, infection 1, junctional stenosis 1, kyphosis 1, revision surgery 2	Neck pain $p > 0.05$	Junctional kyphosis $p > 0.05$
Highsmith et al[40]	Instrumented open-door laminoplasty (30)	Laminoplasty 42.3 months (13–69 months)	LAMP: infection 2, sterile seromas 2, C5 paresis 1, urinary retention 1, revision surgery 4	Nurick score or JOA score $p > 0.05$ VAS score improvement LAMP 02 (pain scores increased slightly postoperatively)	Radiographic outcomes were similar between the groups
	Laminectomy and fusion (26)	Laminectomy 41.3 months (12–85 months)	LAMT: infection 4, sterile seromas 2, C5 paresis 1, revision surgery 2	LAMT 2.8, $p < 0.05$	
Manzano et al[41]	Open-door expansile laminoplasty (9)	> 12 months	No complications in the two groups	Nurick grade SF-36 score, NDI, self-reported outcome measures were improved only in LAMP, $p < 0.05$	ROM was decreased only in LAMT, $p > 0.05$ Percent of change in the area of spinal canal LAMP 34% LAMT 76%, $p < 0.05$
	Laminectomy and fusion (7)				

(Continued)

Table 9.2   (*Continued*) Interventions and their outcomes in laminoplasty

Reference	Procedure (*n*, sample size)	Follow-up	Surgical complications	Clinical outcome	Radiographic outcome
Nurboja et al[42]	Standard laminoplasty (154)	Laminoplasty 96 months	N/A	LAMP was associated with more neck pain and worse quality of life (4 or more levels involved); there was no difference (3 or fewer levels) VAS score $p > 0.05$ EQ-5D questionnaire improve significantly in LAMT	A greater extent of decompression in LAMP, $p < 0.05$
	Laminotomy (114)	Laminotomy 58 months			Sagittal alignment $p > 0.05$
Du et al[43]	Open-door laminoplasty (36)	Laminoplasty 92 months (7–11 months)	N/A	Final follow-up JOA score and neurological recovery rate $p > 0.05$	Loss of curvature Index LAMP 2.60 ± 1.01 LAMT 1.22 ± 0.72, $p < 0.05$
	Laminectomy and fusion (32)	Laminectomy and fusion 89 months (7-12 months)		Axial symptom incidence LAMP 66.7% (24/36) LAMT 37.5% (12/32), $p < 0.05$	
Yang et al[44]	Plate-only open door laminoplasty (75)	> 24 months	LAMP C5 paresis 3, CSF leakage 1, kyphosis 3, restenosis 1, axial pain 9	JOA score and Nurick score $p > 0.05$ NDI scores and VAS scores better improvement in LAMP, $p < 0.05$ Better neck function recovery in LAMP	Increase of dural sac area LAMP 31.99% LAMT 52.7% $p < 0.001$ Spinal cord shift LAMP 1.2 mm LAMT 2.4 mm $p < 0.001$ Curvature index $p > 0.05$ Greater loss of ROM in LAMT
	Laminectomy and fusion (66)		LAMT C5 paresis 11, CSF leakage 3, kyphosis 2, infection 1, axial pain 23		

Abbreviations: CSF, cerebrospinal fluid; JOA, Japanese Orthopaedic Association; LAMP, laminoplasty; LAMT, laminectomy; NDI, neck disability index; ROM, range of motion; SF-36, short form-36; VAS, visual analogue scale.

Table 9.3 Comparing anterior with posterior surgery for CSM

	Anterior vs. posterior–pseudoarthrosis	Anterior vs. posterior–C5 palsy	Anterior vs. posterior–infection	Anterior vs. posterior–dysphagia	Anterior vs. posterior–pain
Liu et al[45]	1/25 (4.0%) – 0/27 (0%)	0/25 (0%) – 2/27 (7.4%)	NR – NR	2/25 (8.0%) – 0.27 (0%)	0/25 (0%) – 1.27 (3.7)
Edwards et al[47]	1/13 (7.7%) – 0/13 (0%)	NR – NR	NR – NR	4/13 (30.8%) – 0/13 (0%)	8/13 (61.5%) – 8/13 (61.5%)
Hosono[48]	NR – NR	NR – NR	NR – NR	NR – NR	5/26 (19.2) – 43/72 (59.7%)
Shibuya et al[49]	6/34 (17.6%) – 0/49 (0%)	3/34 (8.8%) – 5/49 (10.2%)	NR – NR	NR – NR	10/20 (50%) – 32/41 (78%)
Yonenobu et al[50]	NR – NR	4/41 (9.8%) – 3/42 (7.1%)	NR – NR	NR – NR	NR – NR
Kristof et al[51]	NR – NR	NR – NR	1/42 (2.3%) – 4/61 (6.5%)	3/42 (7.1%) – 0/61 (0%)	NR – NR
Benzel et al[52]	NR – NR	NR- NR	1/17 (5.9%) – NR	NR – NR	NR – NR
Hirai et al[53]	2.5% – NR	2.5% (1/39) vs. 6.38% (3/47)	NA	NA	0 vs. 1/13(7.6%)

Abbreviations: CSM, cervical spondylotic myelopathy; NR, not responded; NA, not available.

anterior cervical surgery.[59] The most common cause was implant failure or erosion by the implant, while intraoperative injury was a less common cause. The repair was usually done either primarily or using a modified muscle flap.

Implant failure: There can be implant failure in 1 to 3% of patients after anterior surgery. It can result in graft fracture, graft subsidence, pullout or break in screws, fracture of the plate and, rarely, fracture of vertebral body and pseudoarthrosis. Subsidence of the cage after a corpectomy can lead to kyphosis and an increased load on the screws leading to screw fracture. It may require an additional posterior stabilization.

Yee et al.[56] did a meta-analysis of 240 articles to look for complications in anterior cervical spine surgery and found the following complications: dysphagia 5.3%, recurrent laryngeal nerve palsy 1.3%, infection 1.2%, esophageal perforation 0.2%, adjacent segment disease 8.1%, pseudarthrosis 2.0%, graft or hardware failure 2.1%, CSF leak 0.5%, hematoma 1.0%, Horner's syndrome 0.4%, C5 palsy 3.0%, vertebral artery injury 0.4%, and new or worsening neurological deficit 0.5%.

C5 root palsy: C5 root palsy is a known complication of surgery for CSM.[31,32] This complication is known in both anterior and posterior surgeries, although the incidence is slightly more in posterior surgery. Most of them are temporary and resolve over a period of a few months. The incidence ranges from 3 to 8%. Most patients improve spontaneously over 1 to 3 months after regular physiotherapy.

Surgical site hematoma: Hematoma and infection also are rare complications, but occur more often in posterior surgeries.

Posterior Surgery Complications

Complications specific to posterior surgeries include the formation of laminectomy membrane, which can cause a delayed compression. Suppose the laminectomy is performed only in limited segments and not extended a level above, in that case, the cord may not migrate posteriorly properly, and the adjacent level may cause compression of the migrated cord. Similarly, if laminectomy is done in a kyphotic spine, then the posterior cord migration may not occur, and anterior compression will continue to compress the cord.

In open-door laminoplasty, if the lamina is not fixed properly, whether with a spacer or bone, there is a chance that it can fall back and cause compression as before. This is known as spring back closure, and it was reported only with suture fixation and not when plate fixation of lamina has been done.[60]

Ossification of Posterior Longitudinal Ligament

OPLL is a pathological process characterized by progressive calcification of the ligament, with subsequent narrowing of the cervical canal. This may lead to spinal cord compression and neurological sequelae. OPLL was first described in the Japanese and East Asian populations, where it is a common cause of cervical myelopathy. In Japan, the incidence of OPLL has been estimated at 1.9 to 4.3%. In other Asian countries, that incidence is as high as 3%. Recent research has shown that OPLL has an incidence rate of 0.1 to 1.7% among the North Americans and Europeans with cervical spine disorders.[61,62] Lee and Turner historically described the natural history of cervical myelopathy.[63] They described exacerbation of symptoms, followed by often long periods of static or worsening function or, in rare instances, improvement. Very few patients had steady progressive deterioration. Although surgery is often necessary for patients with symptomatic neurological deterioration caused by OPLL, controversy remains regarding the optimal timing of surgery and surgical indications. Surgical decompression and stabilization via cervical fusion are widely accepted as the optimal treatment for patients with cervical radiculopathy or myelopathy caused by OPLL.

Patients with symptomatic OPLL present with various myelopathic symptoms and usually require surgery rather than conservative treatment. Although the spinal cord can be decompressed directly and successfully via an anterior approach, indirect decompression by a posterior approach has been widely used to treat OPLL. Compared to the anterior approach, the posterior approach is technically less demanding and seldom associated with severe complications such as intraoperative neural injury, symptomatic CSF leakage, graft dislodgement, and adjacent segment disease. It is generally preferred for multisegmental lesions, which is often the case in OPLL patients.

Types of OPLL

The commonly applied classification for OPLL is from the Japanese Ministry of Health and Welfare's investigation committee on OPLL. A sagittal view of the spine is required to classify OPLL into four classic subtypes: continuous, segmental, mixed, and localized (**Fig. 9.1**). The continuous type spreads across the vertebral bodies and their intervening

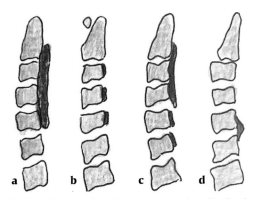

Fig. 9.1 Types of ossified posterior longitudinal ligament (OPLL): continuous (**a**), segmental (**b**), mixed (**c**), localized (**d**).

disk spaces. The segmental type only affects each vertebral body. The mixed type has features of both the segmental and continuous types. The localized type is defined as the ossification involving the intervening disk spaces, only affecting the vertebral body. The mixed and continuous types are mostly found in patients with progression to myelopathy.[64]

Parameters for OPLL Surgery Indications and Postoperative Recovery

K-line

Fujiyoshi described the K-line, which connects the midpoints of the spinal canal at C2 and C7 on a neutral lateral radiograph. OPLL did not exceed the K-line in the K-line (+) type and exceeded in the K-line (–) type.[65] Fujiyoshi suggested that the surgical approach was decided based on the K-line. They suggested posterior decompression and fusion in patients with K-line (–) OPLL. Twenty-one patients underwent this intervention and had an excellent postoperative recovery following the intervention. The author also emphasizes that cervical lordotic alignment should be maintained to get better neurological outcomes postoperatively. Katsumi et al studied 38 patients who underwent posterior decompression and fusion (PDF) surgery. His results showed better neurological outcomes among patients who had an OPLL with K-line (–).[66]

Takeuchi et al divided 41 patients into K-line +/– group. They concluded that patients with K-line (–) OPLL in flexed neck positions have no improvement in motor function, especially OPLL with beak-shaped ossification tends to have a poor outcome after laminoplasty compared to those with K-line (+) OPLL. They also showed progression of OPLL with laminoplasty after 5 years follow-up compared to fusion cases. They recommended fusion in these cases.[67] Similar findings were reported by Koda et al, who concluded that laminoplasty should not be done in patients with K-line (–) OPLL. Anterior decompression and fusion (ADF) should be considered in these cases. However, PDF can also be done in these patients as a possible alternative for this kind of OPLL.[68]

The role of sagittal vertical axis (SVA) remains controversial to date. One of the studies conducted by Chang Lee et al did not find any clinical impact on the outcome of patients undergoing laminoplasty.[69] Another study has quoted that smaller SVA correlates with higher chances of postoperative kyphosis.[70] In another study, patients who had a laminectomy done for OPLL had worsening of symptoms compared with either laminoplasty or fusion. The author has also mentioned that in patients with SVA < 40 mm or significant lordosis, posterior fusion, or laminoplasty are preferable.[71] Overall, the clinical significance of SVA remains controversial (**Fig. 9.2** and **Flowchart 9.1**).

Japanese Orthopedic Association (JOA) Score

Considering the fact that pathological changes that occur in neurons are largely irreversible, it becomes difficult to quantify the degree of improvement beforehand. CSM is a dynamic process where the disease tends to progress over time. A lot of studies initially advocated superior results of surgical intervention but suffered from a major flaw. There was no universal tool to define the degree of neurological deterioration accurately. The problem was solved in 1975 when the JOA score was introduced.[72] The score subsequently underwent modification to be known as mJOA in 1994.[73] The score was validated by a large-scale prospective trial involving 479 patients.[74] As a result, patients were grouped in to mild (mJOA > 14), a moderate (mJOA 12–14) and a severe form (mJOA < 12). This classification now represents the basic layout for further decisions about conservative or operative options for CSM.

In 2011, Kalb proposed a recovery rate based on JOA:

- Recovery rate = (postoperative JOA score – preoperative JOA score) / (17 – preoperative JOA score) × 100.
- The highest attainable JOA score is 17.

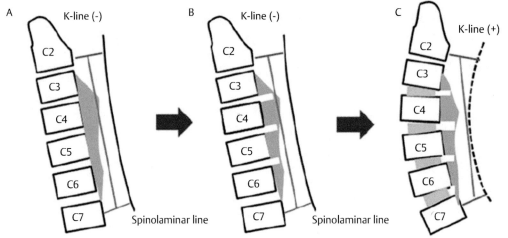

Fig. 9.2 Showing K-line negative as well positive ossified posterior longitudinal ligament (OPLL). Sagittal vertical axis (SVA) < 40 mm.

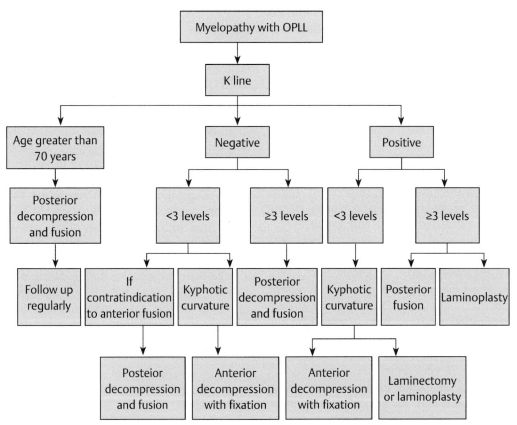

Flowchart 9.1 Algorithm explaining the approach towards ossified posterior longitudinal ligament (OPLL) management.

- A recovery rate > 75% is considered an excellent outcome.
- A recovery rate of 50 to 75% is regarded as a good outcome.
- A recovery rate of 25 to 49% is considered to be a fair outcome.
- A recovery rate < 25% is considered to be a poor outcome.[75]

Fehlings et al published CSM management guidelines for surgery in cervical degenerative myelopathy.[76] Five systematic reviews were incorporated to establish these guidelines, taking into consideration efficacy and effectiveness, safety of nonoperative and surgical management, the impact of preoperative duration of symptoms, myelopathy severity, and treatment outcomes. According to their guideline recommendations, all patients should go under surgical intervention with moderate-to-severe OPLL. Patients with longer duration of symptoms that is greater than 12 months with severe JOA tend to have less improvement of JOA after 1 year follow-up compared to those who have shorter duration of symptoms.

Anterior Approaches

Indications for Anterior Approach

Following are the indications of anterior approach procedures for OPLL:

- Persistent or recurrent radiculopathy nonresponsive to conservative treatment (3 years)
- Progressive neurological deficit
- The static neurological deficit with severe radicular pain when associated with confirmatory imaging (CT, MRI) and clinical–radiological correlation
- Straightened spine or kyphotic spine with three or less compression levels
- Focal OPLL or localized to small segment < 3 vertebrae
- Comorbidities and age < 60 years. Studies have shown that elderly patients with multiple comorbid conditions and age > 60 years may have

longer hospital stay and higher chances of untoward complications.[77]

- Carotid screening with minimal atherosclerotic plaque. The actual reported incidence of stroke following ACDF is very low and estimated to be 1/1000.[78] However, there is no proven evidence of an association between the degree of plaque and risk of stroke. A handful of case reports suggest the duration of retraction on the carotid artery as a risk factor for postoperative stroke.[79]

Types of Anterior Cervical Approaches

Anterior Cervical Corpectomy and Fusion

Three papers were related to the ACCF, and all of them were retrospective. The first article published in 2018 had 353 patients who had undergone an uninstrumented corpectomy. The functional gain was achieved in most of these patients postoperatively after long-follow-up when the duration of their symptoms was less than 1 year, age less than 50 years, and Nurick grade less than 4.[80] Chen et al published data on 229 patients who had undergone ACF for multilevel OPLL, had good JOA recovery, and maintained their cervical lordosis and sagittal balance. It is limited to retrospective studies and surgeries by two surgeons.[81] Wang presented 32 patients who underwent ACCF with a microscope for cervical myelopathy secondary to OPLL. They claimed that the use of a microscope might reduce intraoperative bleeding and postoperative complications.[82]

Anterior Cervical Discectomy and Fusion

Two studies were related to ACDF for cervical OPLL. Nakajima showed that increasing the transverse area of the cord at the level of the largest spinal cord compression is an independent and significant factor for long-term recovery in 80 patients of mixed type OPLL. The remnants of OPLL progressed postoperatively, especially in the mixed type of OPLL. The problem with this study was that the number of involved segments was not mentioned.[83] Lei performed a large cervical discectomy to remove localized OPLL in 24 patients. The benefit of this approach was that corpectomy was avoided, and postoperative recovery was good with a satisfactory radiographic outcome.[84]

Anterior Cervical Antedisplacement and Fusion (ACAF)

Yang, in 2019, performed ACAF in 63 patients to treat OPLL and degenerative kyphotic spine (DKS). They proposed that dura act as a suspensory tent when the vertebrae, along with its ossified ligament, is brought forward. This may protect the spinal cord with excellent JOA recovery.[85] Similarly, Sun et al recruited 31 patients who also underwent ACAF for cervical OPLL. They reported good neurological recovery and a reduction in the complications.[86] One of the benefits proposed by Yang et al is the ability to deal with multilevel OPLL with anterior approach.[86] In this retrospective study, the authors compared ACAF with ACCF, as the anterior approach is relatively contraindicated in multilevel OPLL. With the advent of ACAF, it can be done safely without causing many complications postoperatively. As these studies have a small sample size, further validation with a prospective randomized study is required.[86–88]

Complications of Anterior Approach

A long list of complications has been attributed to the anterior approach to the cervical spine. However, in experienced hands, they usually tend to be minimal or temporary. Certain factors should be taken into consideration while planning an anterior approach. These particularly include the number of levels being addressed, the age of the patient, comorbidities, and degree of carotid stenosis. As stated above, increasing age, comorbidities, and significant carotid stenosis may complicate an anterior approach. However, they do not represent an acute contraindication to approach. This merely requires an increased understanding of possible complications and appropriate measures being taken to reduce them.

Posterior Approaches

Indications for Posterior Approach

Generally, these include:

- Location of the compressive pathology (particularly when OPLL is associated with ossification of the yellow ligament [OYL]).
- The number of levels involved, generally more than three-level disease.
- Patient's comorbidities: Age more than 60 years and multiple comorbidities are an indication for the posterior approach.
- Additional factors affecting the choice of the anterior versus posterior approach include the extent of ventral compression (K-line +/−) and radiculopathy pain, numbness, or weakness.

Posterior approaches consist of laminectomy alone, laminectomy with fusion, and laminoplasty.

Types of Posterior Cervical Approaches

Surgeons have a choice of standard laminectomy alone or skip laminectomy (which involves the preservation of key posterior muscle attachments and the selective removal of partial laminae), laminoplasty and its multiple variations, and laminectomy with fusion and stabilization. The comparative efficacy of the most common approaches, that is, posterior laminoplasty versus laminectomy with posterior spinal fusion remains unclear. A good prospective study that includes 479 patients from 5 different regions compared OPLL to other forms of degenerative myelopathy. Patients with OPLL were at higher risk of perioperative complications than patients with other form of degenerative cervical myelopathy.[89]

Laminectomy

Laminectomy is the most common surgical procedure for managing the CSM. Several recent studies have reported that laminectomy can improve postoperative JOA scores and lead to a cure rate of more than 50%.[90] In a retrospective study, 82 patients had

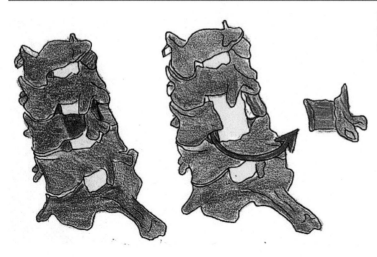

Fig. 9.3 Shows complete laminectomy in the cervical spine.

undergone extensive laminectomy, that is, laminectomy with ¼ of facet joint to expose nerve roots in patients with cervical OPLL and shoulder pain. Most patients have excellent recovery; only two patients had C5 palsy (**Fig. 9.3**).[91]

Laminectomy with Fusion

Laminectomy with fusion is performed to stabilize the residual structure, in order to prevent complications of standalone laminectomies such as kyphosis. Fusion can be done between vertebral bodies (known as interbody or anterior fusion) to the bone lamina (posterior fusion), to the transverse process (posterolateral fusion), or using a combination of these fusion techniques. In a meta-analysis of different articles, fusion surgery is preferred over laminoplasty if there is a high-canal occupying ratio of OPLL or long-term effectiveness and relief from symptoms. Therefore, the articles used in this were mostly retrospective, and only two studies were prospective.[92] Chen et al, in a retrospective study published in 2014, included 83 patients with OPLL, who were operated by two surgeons. It showed that patients with laminoplasty have more progression of OPLL than the laminectomy and fusion group. This study needs to be validated with prospective and randomized trials, so that intervention for OPLL can be further optimized.[81]

A meta-analysis states that decompression and fusion are better in faster recovery, lead to improvement in neurological function, and result in decrease in incidence for OPLL progression. In contrast, complication rates were similar in both groups, given that PDF is preferred over decompression alone for long-term effectiveness. Since the meta-analysis is primarily comprised of retrospective studies with a handful of prospective studies, it poses an inherent bias and results cannot be generalized.[93]

Laminoplasty

Laminoplasty also helps reach the spinal cord in tumors, vascular problems, and functional surgery, in which procedures such as laminectomy are difficult. However, laminoplasty should be avoided in patients with cervical kyphosis and significant preoperative axial neck pain. Neck pain itself could be a common complication of laminoplasty.

Many laminoplasty techniques and variations have been described, but they all share the principle of expanding the cervical canal and protecting part or all of the posterior elements. Modifications have been made to the cutting site of the lamina or spinous process. More recently, proposed techniques include using ceramic spacers and titanium miniplates, which can reduce surgical time and improve the procedure's safety. These newly developed procedures are intended to maintain the musculature attachments in the paraspinal muscles and the posterior tension band. Two of the most common methods for laminoplasty are open-door and French door techniques. Although various surgical modifications have been suggested, the basic concepts are the same. According to an author, indications for open-door laminoplasty (also referred to as tension-band laminoplasty) were CSM and one-sided radiculopathy, severe ossification of OPLL, and patients who have a small spinous process and cannot undergo double-door Laminoplasty.[94] Double-door laminoplasty indications are small-sized prominent OPLL, CSM with bilateral radiculopathy, and canal stenosis with instability requiring fusion. Precise minimum expansion ratio to attain adequate decompression of the spinal cord is not known, but the eventual decision depends upon the surgeon and level of expertise.

In the open-door technique, the hinge is created unilaterally; in the French door modification, the hinge is created bilaterally. In the open-door procedure, the opening is made on the opposite lateral mass-laminar junction, while the French door is performed at the midline, providing enough space for the spinal cord (**Figs. 9.4 and 9.5**).

Four good articles were related to laminoplasty intervention in OPLL patients. The first is a prospective study of 31 patients with 5 years follow-up after laminoplasty. The patients did not develop neurological deterioration even after the progression of OPLL. After 5 years, sagittal cervical lordosis was lost in some patients, but no neurological decline was seen. Preservation of muscle attachment from the C2–C7 spinous process also leads to a decrease in axial neck pain in these patients.[95] Another review article has described the benefit of laminoplasty in contrast to fusion surgeries. Their indications for laminoplasty were developmentally narrow spinal canal or canal compromise < 60%, multisegmented OPLL, and absence of kyphotic spine. They also showed that both types of laminoplasty had similar outcomes and were considered cost-effective.[96] A study by Qian et al included 137 patients with CSM or OPLL who underwent laminoplasty due to cervical myelopathy. Patients with cervical lordosis or mild cervical kyphosis have better clinical outcomes than marked cervical kyphosis. The author also contraindicates laminoplasty in patients with large range of motion (ROM)

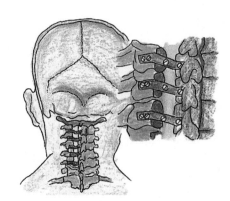

Fig. 9.4 Open-door multilevel laminoplasty.

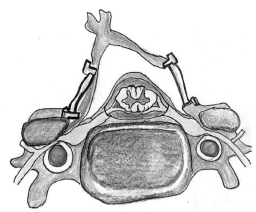

Fig. 9.5 Open-door laminoplasty of a single segment.

preoperatively.[82] The last article mainly outlines the complications after laminoplasty. This was a multi-institutional retrospective study analyzing 581 patients who developed complications following different types of laminoplasty. In their analysis, only 18 patients suffered from lower extremity dysfunction and the cause was epidural hematoma, spinal cord herniation through injured dura, and vertebral artery injury during the intervention.[71,97]

Suture Anchor in Lateral Mass for Open-Door Laminoplasty

In one study, the suture anchor system made it possible to reliably anchor the lateral mass and enable faster fixation of the hydroxyapatite spacers in the open-door-laminoplasty.[98] The anchor is inserted in the pedicle part of the vertebral arch with an insertion angle at a cross-section of around 30° superiorly. Postoperatively, these patients had no long-term axial pain, their visual analogue scale (VAS) score improved, and no serious complication was observed in OPLL group.[98]

Anterior versus Posterior Approaches

Seventy-five patients were included in this study. It concludes that ADF should be considered in multilevel OPLL, as it directly decompresses the affected level by removing the OPLL. Enhanced surgical skill and expertise are required to reduce the operative complications. In contrast, PDF helps restore cervical lordosis and indirect decompression of the affected levels. Both methods produce comparable long-term results in terms of JOA recovery. Finally, laminoplasty is not suitable with multilevel OPLL, as this leads to instability in the spine and causes progression of OPLL in the long term.[99] In another retrospective study, both ADF and PDF interventions were compared in patients with massive OPLL > 50% canal-occupying ratio. In patients with kyphotic deformity, ADF was preferred. ADF was associated with less blood loss, more operative time and complications compared to PDF, which was associated with more blood loss, postoperative axial pain, and less complications. Postoperative JOA recovery was similar in both cases as there was no difference seen in both groups.[100] In a meta-analysis, Wu et al concluded that there is an inverse correlation in preoperative JOA score and postoperative JOA score improvement.[101] The author also mentioned that an anterior approach leads to a better JOA improvement compared to posterior approaches.

ACF/ADF versus Laminoplasty Based on Canal Diameter

Chen et al published a meta-analysis in 2020, based on 818 patients from nonrandomized control trial articles. Their analysis preferred for an anterior approach if the canal diameter was ≥ 60% compromised or the kyphotic alignment of the spine. Otherwise, if the occupying ratio was less than 60%, laminoplasty was considered a safe and effective option. This meta-analysis did not consider the number of segments involved for either approach.[102] Similar findings were reported by Qin et al in a systematic review with meta-analysis of 10 nonrandomized studies.[103] Two groups were analyzed: one with canal diameter < 60% and one with > 60%. The initial group has no significant difference in postoperative JOA recovery with either intervention, in contrast to the second group where JOA recovery is seen in ACCF patients compared to laminoplasty patients. In another nonrandomized control trial, patients were selected based on their MRI findings and curvature. The surgeon preferred an anterior approach if the canal stenosis was >50% or with poor cervical curvature, otherwise laminoplasty could be considered an alternative option.[104] Another meta-analysis compared anterior approach versus laminoplasty while considering the number of segments involved with OPLL. The author stated that if involved segments are less than three, the anterior approach is recommended; otherwise, laminoplasty is preferred. However, the quality of evidence is low and more validating studies are required to suggest intervention, according to the number of segments affected.[105] Further prospective studies have validated the advantage of the anterior approach in cases of severe canal stenosis. In a prospective study, ADF was superior in patients with kyphotic deformity and canal compromise more than 50%; otherwise, laminoplasty and ADF have no significant difference. However, ADF was also associated with long operative time and complications compared to laminoplasty alone.[103]

Special Circumstances

C2 Level OPLL and Preferred Approach
Posterior surgery is recommended in patients with C2 level OPLL, as this is much safer and easier to perform compared to the anterior approach. Surgery is indicated in patients with the narrowest diameter at the C2 level and high-intensity MRI signals at C2.[106]

Revision Surgery
According to this retrospective study, patients who initially underwent a posterior approach or underwent an anterior procedure based on progressive neurological deterioration. There was no mention of cervical curvature changes in this study as patients were subjected to revision surgery solely based on neurology.[73] Similarly, three articles related to ACAF as revision surgery for OPLL were identified. All these articles were retrospective with small numbers, and their results concluded that they had improvement in JOA recovery as well as a change in K-line from negative to positive.[64,84,107]

Combined Approaches and Other Studies

Hybrid Procedures
The patients included in this study had multilevel OPLL and degenerative disk disease, and hybrid surgery with ACCF and CDA showed satisfactory clinical and radiological outcomes. This study's limitations were that as this was a retrospective study, the patient sample was small, and there was no control group to compare these findings with. The only way to prove its significance is to carry out a clinical trial or a case-control study to prove its benefits.[108] Another article showed 540-degree cervical fusion provides safe decompression, cervical realignment, and favorable outcomes for extensive cervical OPLL with kyphotic deformity. As this is a combined procedure, it avoids the shortcomings of both anterior and posterior approaches for extensive OPLL. This prospective cohort was based on 18 patients only.[109]

Conclusion

CSM requires surgery in patients with progressive neurological deficits or persistent radiculopathy, provides an improvement in 70 to 80% of patients, and stabilizes the disease in others. Both anterior and posterior procedures are safe, with almost the same rate of complications in both groups. In many cases, it is still uncertain whether anterior or posterior surgery is a better option, and to answer this question, it will require more extensive multicentric double-blind trials. The neurosurgical data lacks prospective quality trials to ascertain the benefit of one approach over another. Most of the literature is primarily composed of retrospective data or small prospective cohorts, which naturally poses a bias in the study methodology. Based on the available literature, the indications cited above provide a good framework to follow until further studies validate the results. One of the aspects worth mentioning is the promising results of ACAF in the treatment of OPLL.

Take-home Points

- Anterior surgery is ideal for decompression in cervical myelopathy and OPLL when the compression is mainly anterior, with kyphosis, or when the disease segments are less than or equal to three.

- Going beyond three levels via anterior approach is not a contraindication to surgery, but the risk of complication may increase with the number of segments involved.

- Posterior approach is preferred in multilevel compression involving more than three levels. In the presence of neck pain, laminectomy/laminoplasty alone is avoided and fusion may be considered. However, in case of compression involving the upper or lower segments of cervical spine, posterior approach may be a safer option.

- Other possible indications for posterior surgery include previous anterior surgery, osteoporotic bone, and old age with comorbidities

- In cases of lordotic or straight spine, both anterior and posterior surgeries can be done with comparable outcomes. To ensure a good outcome, surgeons should proceed with the approach that they are most comfortable with.

References

1. Robinson RA, Smith GW. Anterolateral cervical disc removal and interbody fusion for cervical disc syndrome. Bull Johns Hopkins Hosp 1955;96:223–224

2. Smith GW, Robinson RA. The treatment of certain cervical-spine disorders by anterior removal of the intervertebral disc and interbody fusion. J Bone Joint Surg Am 1958;40-A(3):607–624

3. Cloward RB. The anterior approach for removal of ruptured cervical disks. J Neurosurg 1958;15(6):602–617

4. Ning X, Wen Y, Xiao-Jian Y, et al. Anterior cervical locking plate-related complications; prevention and treatment recommendations. Int Orthop 2008;32(5):649–655

5. He S, Feng H, Lan Z, et al. A randomized trial comparing clinical outcomes between zero-profile and traditional multilevel anterior cervical discectomy and fusion surgery for cervical myelopathy. Spine 2017 (e-pub ahead of print). doi:10.1097/BRS.0000000000002323

6. Burkhardt JK, Mannion AF, Marbacher S, et al. A comparative effectiveness study of patient-rated and radiographic outcome after 2 types of decompression with fusion for spondylotic myelopathy: anterior cervical discectomy versus corpectomy. Neurosurg Focus 2013;35(1):E4

7. Gore DR. The arthrodesis rate in multilevel anterior cervical fusions using autogenous fibula. Spine 2001;26(11):1259–1263

8. Guan L, Hai Y, Yang J-C, Zhou L-J, Chen X-L. Anterior cervical discectomy and fusion may be more effective than anterior cervical corpectomy and fusion for the treatment of cervical spondylotic myelopathy. BMC Musculoskelet Disord 2015;16:29

9. Han Y-C, Liu Z-Q, Wang S-J, Li L-J, Tan J. Is anterior cervical discectomy and fusion superior to corpectomy and fusion for treatment of multilevel cervical spondylotic myelopathy? A systemic review and meta-analysis. PLoS One 2014;9(1):e87191

10. Lin Q, Zhou X, Wang X, Cao P, Tsai N, Yuan W. A comparison of anterior cervical discectomy and corpectomy in patients with multilevel cervical spondylotic myelopathy. Eur Spine J 2012;21(3):474–481

11. Oh MC, Zhang HY, Park JY, Kim KS. Two-level anterior cervical discectomy versus one-level corpectomy in cervical spondylotic myelopathy. Spine 2009;34(7):692–696

12. Fountas KN, Kapsalaki EZ, Nikolakakos LG, et al. Anterior cervical discectomy and fusion associated complications. Spine 2007; 32(21):2310–2317

13. Buchowski JM, Anderson PA, Sekhon L, Riew KD. Cervical disc arthroplasty compared with arthrodesis for the treatment of myelopathy. Surgical technique. J Bone Joint Surg Am 2009;91(Suppl 2):223–232

14. Boni M, Cherubino P, Denaro V, Benazzo F. Multiple subtotal somatectomy. Technique and evaluation of a series of 39 cases. Spine 1984;9(4):358–362

15. Boni M, Denaro V. [Surgical treatment of cervical arthrosis. Follow-up review (2–13 years) of the 1st 100 cases operated on by anterior approach]. [in French] Rev Chir Orthop Repar Appar Mot 1982;68(4):269–280

16. Denaro V, Di Martino A. Cervical spine surgery: an historical perspective. Clin Orthop Relat Res 2011;469(3):639–648

17. George B, Zerah M, Lot G, Hurth M. Oblique transcorporeal approach to anteriorly located lesions in the cervical spinal canal. Acta Neurochir (Wien) 1993;121(3-4):187–190

18. Chacko AG, Turel MK, Sarkar S, Prabhu K, Daniel RT. Clinical and radiological outcomes in 153 patients undergoing oblique corpectomy for cervical spondylotic myelopathy. Br J Neurosurg 2014;28(1):49–55

19. Tykocki T, Poniatowski LA, Czyz M, Wynne-Jones G. Oblique corpectomy in the cervical spine. Spinal Cord 2018;56(5):426–435

20. Ryu WHA, Platt A, Deutsch H. Hybrid decompression and reconstruction technique for cervical spondylotic myelopathy: case series and review of the literature. J Spine Surg 2020;6(1):181–195

21. Zhu Y, Fang J, Xu G, Ye X, Zhang Y. A hybrid technique for treating multilevel cervical myelopathy: cervical artificial disc replacement combined with fusion. Oncol Lett 2019;17(1):360–364

22. Geck MJ, Eismont FJ. Surgical options for the treatment of cervical spondylotic myelopathy. Orthop Clin North Am 2002; 33(2):329–348

23. Oyama M, Hattori S. A new method of cervical laminectomy. Chubu Seisaishi. 1973;16:792–794

24. Hirabayashi K. Expansive open-door laminoplasty for cervical spondylotic myelopathy. Jpn J Surg 1978;32:1159–1163 [in Japanese]

25. Hirabayashi K, Miyakawa J, Satomi K, Maruyama T, Wakano K. Operative results and postoperative progression of ossification among patients with ossification of cervical posterior longitudinal ligament. Spine 1981; 6(4):354–364

26. Hirabayashi K, Watanabe K, Wakano K, Suzuki N, Satomi K, Ishii Y. Expansive open-door laminoplasty for cervical spinal stenotic myelopathy. Spine 1983;8(7):693–699

27. Kurokawa T, Tsuyama N, Tanaka H, et al. Enlargement of spinal canal by sagittal splitting of spinous processes. Bessatsu Seikeigeka 1982;2:234–240 [in Japanese]

28. Roy-Camille R, Saillant G, Mazel C, et al. Rachis cervical traumatique non neurologique. In: Roy-Camille R, et al., eds. 1eres Journees d'orthopedie de la Pitie. Paris, France: Masson; 1979

29. Roy-Camille R, Saillant G. [Surgery of the cervical spine. 3. Complex fractures of the lower cervical spine. Tetraplegia]. Nouv Presse Med 1972;1(40):2707–2709 [in French]

30. Lin X, Cai J, Qin C, Yang Q, Xiao Z. Comparison of clinical outcomes and safety between laminectomy with instrumented fusion versus laminoplasty for the treatment of multilevel cervical spondylotic myelopathy. Medicine (Baltimore) 2019;98(8):e14651

31. Shou F, Li Z, Wang H, Yan C, Liu Q, Xiao C. Prevalence of C5 nerve root palsy after cervical decompressive surgery: a meta-analysis. Eur Spine J 2015;24(12):2724–2734

32. Wang T, Wang H, Liu S, Ding WY. Incidence of C5 nerve root palsy after cervical surgery: a meta-analysis for last decade. Medicine (Baltimore) 2017;96(45):e8560

33. Ghogawala Z, Benzel EC, Heary RF, et al. Cervical spondylotic myelopathy surgical trial: randomized, controlled trial design and rationale. Neurosurgery 2014;75(4):334–346

34. Li J, Zheng Q, Guo X, et al. Anterior surgical options for the treatment of cervical spondylotic myelopathy in a long-term follow-up study. Arch Orthop Trauma Surg 2013;133(6):745–751

35. Liu Y, Qi M, Chen H, et al. Comparative analysis of complications of different reconstructive techniques following anterior decompression for multilevel cervical spondylotic myelopathy. Eur Spine J 2012; 21(12):2428–2435

36. Song KJ, Lee KB, Song JH, Song JH. Efficacy of multilevel anterior cervical discectomy and fusion versus corpectomy and fusion for multilevel cervical spondylotic myelopathy: a minimum 5-year follow-up study. Eur Spine J 2012;21(8):1551–1557

37. Guo Q, Bi X, Ni B, et al. Outcomes of three anterior decompression and fusion techniques in the treatment of three-level cervical spondylosis. Eur Spine J 2011;20(9): 1539–1544

38. Park Y, Maeda T, Cho W, Riew KD. Comparison of anterior cervical fusion after two-level discectomy or single-level corpectomy: sagittal alignment, cervical lordosis, graft collapse, and adjacent-level ossification. Spine J 2010;10(3):193–199

39. Woods BI, Hohl J, Lee J, Donaldson W III, Kang J. Laminoplasty versus laminectomy and fusion for multilevel cervical spondylotic myelopathy. Clin Orthop Relat Res 2011; 469(3):688–695

40. Highsmith JM, Dhall SS, Haid RW Jr, Rodts GE Jr, Mummaneni PV. Treatment of cervical stenotic myelopathy: a cost and outcome comparison of laminoplasty versus laminectomy and lateral mass fusion. J Neurosurg Spine 2011;14(5):619–625

41. Manzano GR, Casella G, Wang MY, Vanni S, Levi AD. A prospective, randomized trial comparing expansile cervical laminoplasty and cervical laminectomy and fusion for multilevel cervical myelopathy. Neurosurgery 2012;70(2):264–277

42. Nurboja B, Kachramanoglou C, Choi D. Cervical laminectomy vs laminoplasty: is there a difference in outcome and postoperative pain? Neurosurgery 2012;70(4):965–970, discussion 970

43. Du W, Wang L, Shen Y, Zhang Y, Ding W, Ren L. Long-term impacts of different posterior operations on curvature, neurological recovery and axial symptoms for multilevel cervical degenerative myelopathy. Eur Spine J 2013;22(7):1594–1602

44. Yang L, Gu Y, Shi J, et al. Modified plate-only open-door laminoplasty versus laminectomy and fusion for the treatment of cervical stenotic myelopathy. Orthopedics 2013;36(1):e79–e87

45. Liu T, Yang HL, Xu YZ, Qi RF, Guan HQ. ACDF with the PCB cage-plate system versus laminoplasty for multilevel cervical spondylotic myelopathy. J Spinal Disord Tech 2011;24(4):213–220

46. Yoshida M, Tamaki T, Kawakami M, Hayashi N, Ando M. Indication and clinical results of laminoplasty for cervical myelopathy caused by disc herniation with developmental canal stenosis. Spine 1998;23(22):2391–2397

47. Edwards CC II, Heller JG, Murakami H. Corpectomy versus laminoplasty for multi-level cervical myelopathy: an independent matched-cohort analysis. Spine 2002;27(11): 1168–1175

48. Hosono N, Yonenobu K, Ono K. Neck and shoulder pain after laminoplasty. A noticeable complication. Spine 1996;21(17): 1969–1973

49. Shibuya S, Komatsubara S, Oka S, Kanda Y, Arima N, Yamamoto T. Differences between subtotal corpectomy and laminoplasty for cervical spondylotic myelopathy. Spinal Cord 2010;48(3):214–220

50. Yonenobu K, Hosono N, Iwasaki M, Asano M, Ono K. Laminoplasty versus subtotal corpectomy. A comparative study of results in multisegmental cervical spondylotic myelopathy. Spine 1992;17(11):1281–1284

51. Kristof RA, Kiefer T, Thudium M, et al. Comparison of ventral corpectomy and plate-screw-instrumented fusion with dorsal laminectomy and rod-screw-instrumented fusion for treatment of at least two vertebral-level spondylotic cervical myelopathy. Eur Spine J 2009;18(12):1951–1956

52. Benzel EC, Lancon J, Kesterson L, Hadden T. Cervical laminectomy and dentate ligament section for cervical spondylotic myelopathy. J Spinal Disord 1991;4(3):286–295

53. Hirai T, Yoshii T, Sakai K, et al. Long-term results of a prospective study of anterior decompression with fusion and posterior decompression with laminoplasty for treatment of cervical spondylotic myelopathy. J Orthop Sci 2018;23(1):32–38

54. Montano N, Ricciardi L, Olivi A. Comparison of anterior cervical decompression and fusion versus laminoplasty in the treatment of multilevel cervical spondylotic myelopathy: a meta-analysis of clinical and radiological outcomes. World Neurosurg 2019;130: 530–536.e2

55. Shriver MF, Lewis DJ, Kshettry VR, Rosenbaum BP, Benzel EC, Mroz TE. Dysphagia rates after anterior cervical diskectomy and fusion: a systematic review and meta-analysis. Global Spine J 2017;7(1):95–103

56. Yee TJ, Swong K, Park P. Complications of anterior cervical spine surgery: a systematic

review of the literature. J Spine Surg 2020; 6(1):302–322

57. Tasiou A, Giannis T, Brotis AG, et al. Anterior cervical spine surgery-associated complications in a retrospective case-control study. J Spine Surg 2017;3(3):444–459

58. Erwood MS, Hadley MN, Gordon AS, Carroll WR, Agee BS, Walters BC. Recurrent laryngeal nerve injury following reoperative anterior cervical discectomy and fusion: a meta-analysis. J Neurosurg Spine 2016; 25(2):198–204

59. Halani SH, Baum GR, Riley JP, et al. Esophageal perforation after anterior cervical spine surgery: a systematic review of the literature. J Neurosurg Spine 2016;25(3):285–291

60. Mochida J, Nomura T, Chiba M, Nishimura K, Toh E. Modified expansive open-door laminoplasty in cervical myelopathy. J Spinal Disord 1999;12(5):386–391

61. Stapleton CJ, Pham MH, Attenello FJ, Hsieh PC. Ossification of the posterior longitudinal ligament: genetics and pathophysiology. Neurosurg Focus 2011;30(3):E6

62. Yoshimura N, Nagata K, Muraki S, et al. Prevalence and progression of radiographic ossification of the posterior longitudinal ligament and associated factors in the Japanese population: a 3-year follow-up of the ROAD study. Osteoporos Int 2014; 25(3):1089–1098

63. Sadasivan KK, Reddy RP, Albright JA. The natural history of cervical spondylotic myelopathy. Yale J Biol Med 1993;66(3): 235–242

64. Abiola R, Rubery P, Mesfin A. Ossification of the posterior longitudinal ligament: etiology, diagnosis, and outcomes of nonoperative and operative management. Global Spine J 2016;6(2):195–204

65. Fujiyoshi T, Yamazaki M, Kawabe J, et al. A new concept for making decisions regarding the surgical approach for cervical ossification of the posterior longitudinal ligament: the K-line. Spine 2008;33(26):E990–E993

66. Katsumi K, Hirano T, Watanabe K, et al. Perioperative factors associated with favorable outcomes of posterior decompression and instrumented fusion for cervical ossification of the posterior longitudinal ligament: a retrospective multicenter study. J Clin Neurosci 2018;57:74–78

67. Takeuchi K, Yokoyama T, Numasawa T, et al. K-line (-) in the neck-flexed position in patients with ossification of the posterior longitudinal ligament is a risk factor for poor clinical outcome after cervical laminoplasty. Spine 2016;41(24):1891–1895

68. Koda M, Mochizuki M, Konishi H, et al. Comparison of clinical outcomes between laminoplasty, posterior decompression with instrumented fusion, and anterior decompression with fusion for K-line (-) cervical ossification of the posterior longitudinal ligament. Eur Spine J 2016;25(7):2294–2301

69. Lee CK, Shin DA, Yi S, et al. Correlation between cervical spine sagittal alignment and clinical outcome after cervical laminoplasty for ossification of the posterior longitudinal ligament. J Neurosurg Spine 2016;24(1):100–107

70. Matsuoka Y, Endo K, Nishimura H, et al. Cervical kyphotic deformity after laminoplasty in patients with cervical ossification of posterior longitudinal ligament with normal sagittal spinal alignment. Spine Surgery and Related Research 2018 (e-pub ahead of print). doi:https://doi.org/10.22603/ ssrr.2017-0078

71. Lee CH, Jahng TA, Hyun SJ, Kim KJ, Kim HJ. Expansive laminoplasty versus laminectomy alone versus laminectomy and fusion for cervical ossification of the posterior longitudinal ligament: is there a difference in the clinical outcome and sagittal alignment? Clin Spine Surg 2016;29(1):E9–E15

72. Zhu MP, Tetreault LA, Sorefan-Mangou F, Garwood P, Wilson JR. Efficacy, safety, and economics of bracing after spine surgery: a systematic review of the literature. Spine J 2018;18(9):1513–1525

73. Kato S, Oshima Y, Oka H, et al. Comparison of the Japanese Orthopaedic Association (JOA) score and modified JOA (mJOA) score for the assessment of cervical myelopathy: a multicenter observational study. PLoS One 2015;10(4):e0123022

74. Tetreault L, Kopjar B, Nouri A, et al. The modified Japanese Orthopaedic Association scale: establishing criteria for mild, moderate and severe impairment in patients with degenerative cervical myelopathy. Eur Spine J 2017;26(1):78–84

75. Kalb S, Martirosyan NL, Perez-Orribo L, Kalani MY, Theodore N. Analysis of demographics, risk factors, clinical presentation, and surgical treatment modalities for the ossified posterior longitudinal ligament. Neurosurg Focus 2011;30(3):E11

76. Fehlings MG, Tetreault LA, Riew KD, et al. A clinical practice guideline for the management of patients with degenerative cervical myelopathy: recommendations for patients with mild, moderate, and severe disease and nonmyelopathic patients with evidence of cord compression. Global Spine J 2017; 7(3, Suppl)70S–83S

77. Di Capua J, Somani S, Kim JS, et al. Elderly age as a risk factor for 30-day postoperative outcomes following elective anterior cervical discectomy and fusion. Global Spine J 2017; 7(5):425–431

78. Härtl R, Alimi M, Abdelatif Boukebir M, et al. Carotid artery injury in anterior cervical spine surgery: multicenter cohort study and literature review. Global Spine J 2017; 7(1, Suppl)71S–75S

79. Du YQ, Duan WR, Chen Z, Wu H, Jian FZ. Carotid artery-related perioperative stroke following anterior cervical spine surgery: a series of 3 cases and literature review. J Stroke Cerebrovasc Dis 2019;28(2):458–463

80. Sarkar S, Rajshekhar V. Long-term sustainability of functional improvement following central corpectomy for cervical spondylotic myelopathy and ossification of posterior longitudinal ligament. Spine 2018;43(12):E703–E711

81. Chen Y, Yang L, Liu Y, Yang H, Wang X, Chen D. Surgical results and prognostic factors of anterior cervical corpectomy and fusion for ossification of the posterior longitudinal ligament. PLoS One 2014;9(7):e102008

82. Qian S, Wang Z, Jiang G, Xu Z, Chen W. Efficacy of laminoplasty in patients with cervical kyphosis. Med Sci Monit 2018;24:1188–1195

83. Nakajima H, Watanabe S, Honjoh K, Kitade I, Sugita D, Matsumine A. Long-term outcome of anterior cervical decompression with fusion for cervical ossification of posterior longitudinal ligament including postsurgical remnant ossified spinal lesion. Spine 2019; 44(24):E1452–E1460

84. Lei T, Wang H, Tong T, Ma Q, Wang L, Shen Y. Enlarged anterior cervical diskectomy and fusion in the treatment of severe localised ossification of the posterior longitudinal ligament. J Orthop Surg Res 2016;11(1):129

85. Zhang B, Sun J, Xu X, et al. Skip corpectomy and fusion (SCF) versus anterior controllable antedisplacement and fusion (ACAF): which is better for patients with multilevel cervical OPLL? Arch Orthop Trauma Surg 2019;139(11):1533–1541

86. Yang H, Sun J, Shi J, Shi G, Guo Y, Yang Y. Anterior controllable antedisplacement fusion (ACAF) for severe cervical ossification of the posterior longitudinal ligament: comparison with anterior cervical corpectomy with fusion (ACCF). World Neurosurgery 2018;115:e428–e436

87. Wang H, Sun J, Tan Y, et al. Anterior controllable antedisplacement and fusion as revision surgery after posterior decompression surgery in patients with ossification of the posterior longitudinal ligament. World Neurosurg 2019;123:e310–e317

88. Yang H, Guo Y, Shi J, et al. Surgical results and complications of anterior controllable antedisplacement fusion as a revision surgery after initial posterior surgery for cervical myelopathy due to ossification of the posterior longitudinal ligament. J Clin Neurosci 2018;56:21–27

89. Nakashima H, Tetreault L, Nagoshi N, et al. Comparison of outcomes of surgical treatment for ossification of the posterior longitudinal ligament versus other forms of degenerative cervical myelopathy: results from the prospective, multicenter AOSpine CSM-International Study of 479 patients. J Bone Joint Surg Am 2016;98(5):370–378

90. Jain SK, Salunke PS, Vyas KH, Behari SS, Banerji D, Jain VK. Multisegmental cervical ossification of the posterior longitudinal ligament: anterior vs posterior approach. Neurol India 2005;53(3):283–285, discussion 286

91. Zhao X, Xue Y, Pan F, et al. Extensive laminectomy for the treatment of ossification of the posterior longitudinal ligament in the cervical spine. Arch Orthop Trauma Surg 2012;132(2):203–209

92. Lee CH, Sohn MJ, Lee CH, Choi CY, Han SR, Choi BW. Are there differences in the progression of ossification of the posterior longitudinal ligament following laminoplasty versus fusion?: a meta-analysis. Spine 2017; 42(12):887–894

93. Mehdi SK, Alentado VJ, Lee BS, Mroz TE, Benzel EC, Steinmetz MP. Comparison of clinical outcomes in decompression and fusion versus decompression only in patients with ossification of the posterior longitudinal ligament: a meta-analysis. Neurosurg Focus 2016;40(6):E9

94. Hirabayashi S, Matsushita T. Two types of laminoplasty for cervical spondylotic myelopathy at multiple levels. ISRN Orthop 2011;2011:637185

95. Sakaura H, Hosono N, Mukai Y, Iwasaki M, Yoshikawa H. Medium-term outcomes of C3-6 laminoplasty for cervical myelopathy: a prospective study with a minimum 5-year follow-up. Eur Spine J 2011;20(6):928–933

96. Matsumoto M, Chiba K, Toyama Y. Surgical treatment of ossification of the posterior longitudinal ligament and its outcomes: posterior surgery by laminoplasty. Spine 2012;37(5):E303–E308

97. Seichi A, Hoshino Y, Kimura A, et al. Neurological complications of cervical laminoplasty for patients with ossification of the posterior longitudinal ligament-a multi-institutional retrospective study. Spine 2011;36(15):E998–E1003

98. Ozawa T, Toyone T, Shiboi R, et al. Modified open-door laminoplasty using a ceramic spacer and suture fixation for cervical myelopathy. Yonsei Med J 2015; 56(6):1651–1655

99. Chen Y, Guo Y, Lu X, et al. Surgical strategy for multilevel severe ossification of posterior longitudinal ligament in the cervical spine. J Spinal Disord Tech 2011;24(1):24–30

100. Yoshii T, Sakai K, Hirai T, et al. Anterior decompression with fusion versus posterior decompression with fusion for massive cervical ossification of the posterior longitudinal ligament with a ≥50% canal occupying ratio: a multicenter retrospective study. Spine J 2016;16(11):1351–1357

101. Wu D, Liu C-Z, Yang H, Li H, Chen N. Surgical interventions for cervical spondylosis due to ossification of posterior longitudinal ligament: a meta-analysis. Medicine (Baltimore) 2017;96(33):e7590

102. Chen Z, Liu B, Dong J, et al. Comparison of anterior corpectomy and fusion versus laminoplasty for the treatment of cervical ossification of posterior longitudinal ligament: a meta-analysis. Neurosurg Focus 2016;40(6):E8

103. Sakai K, Okawa A, Takahashi M, et al. Five-year follow-up evaluation of surgical treatment for cervical myelopathy caused by ossification of the posterior longitudinal ligament: a prospective comparative study of anterior decompression and fusion with floating method versus laminoplasty. Spine 2012;37(5):367–376

104. Hou Y, Liang L, Shi GD, et al. Comparing effects of cervical anterior approach and laminoplasty in surgical management of cervical ossification of posterior longitudinal ligament by a prospective nonrandomized controlled study. Orthop Traumatol Surg Res 2017;103(5):733–740

105. Liu X, Min S, Zhang H, Zhou Z, Wang H, Jin A. Anterior corpectomy versus posterior laminoplasty for multilevel cervical myelopathy: a systematic review and meta-analysis. Eur Spine J 2014;23(2):362–372

106. Lee SE, Jahng T-A, Kim H-J. Surgical outcomes of the ossification of the posterior longitudinal ligament according to the involvement of the C2 segment. World Neurosurg 2016;90:51–57

107. Kawaguchi Y, Nakano M, Yasuda T, Seki S, Hori T, Kimura T. Anterior decompressive surgery after cervical laminoplasty in patients with ossification of the posterior longitudinal ligament. Spine J 2014;14(6):955–963

108. Chang H-C, Tu T-H, Chang H-K, et al. Hybrid corpectomy and disc arthroplasty for cervical spondylotic myelopathy caused by ossification of posterior longitudinal ligament and disc herniation. World Neurosurg 2016;95:22–30

109. Lee SH, Kim KT, Lee JH, et al. 540° cervical realignment procedure for extensive cervical OPLL with kyphotic deformity. Spine 2016;41(24):1876–1883

10 Cervical Anterior Decompression and Fusion Techniques

Ibet Marie Y. Sih, Karlo M. Pedro, Scott C. Robertson, and Salman Sharif

Introduction

Cervical spondylosis generally pertains to degenerative condition of the cervical spine, which includes the spectrum of findings from disc protrusion, ossification of the posterior longitudinal ligament (OPLL), facet joint hypertrophy, hypertrophied or ossified ligament flavum, central and foraminal stenosis, and kyphotic deformity of the spine. Clinical manifestations include radiculopathy, axial pain syndromes, and myelopathy.

Surgery for cervical spondylosis is suggested with failure of medical management. The main goals of surgery are: to provide neural decompression to address myelopathy, radiculopathy, or pain, restore or maintain the stability of the cervical spine, and prevent progression of deformity.

While these goals can be achieved either by anterior, posterior or combined approaches, anterior surgery offers the advantage of being able to address ventral pathologies like OPLL, herniated disc, and disc-osteophyte complex, which are otherwise difficult to visualize through a posterior corridor. In addition, the anterior approach may be very beneficial for patients with focal cervical kyphosis, large herniated disc compressing on the ventral spine, and significant anterior neural foraminal stenosis.

The following chapter will elucidate the different techniques of anterior cervical decompression and fusion.

Indications and Patient Selection

The indications of cervical spine surgery mainly include treatment of degenerative spine conditions such as cervical spondylosis secondary to disc pathology (protrusion), cervical spondylotic myelopathy (CSM) secondary to spinal stenosis, and cervical radiculopathy secondary to foraminal stenosis. Significant improvement after surgery may be expected with the above conditions after failure of trial medical management.

Overall, cervical spine surgery mainly aims to provide neural decompression to address myelopathy, radiculopathy, or pain. Other objectives are to: (1) restore or maintain the stability of the cervical spine; (2) maintain sagittal and coronal balance; and (3) prevent progression of deformity.

When surgery is indicated, the cervical spine can be approached by either anterior, posterior, or combined surgical approaches.

Anterior surgery offers the advantage of being able to address ventral pathologies like OPLL, herniated disc, and disc-osteophyte complex, which are otherwise difficult to visualize through a posterior corridor. Anterior approaches also provide an unobstructed view of the disc space, facilitating more complete discectomies and thereby promoting overall better rates of fusion. In addition, the anterior approach may be very beneficial for patients with focal cervical kyphosis, large herniated disc compressing on the ventral spine, and significant anterior neural foraminal stenosis.

The history of anterior cervical decompression started when this procedure was introduced by Smith and Robinson for cervical degenerative disease.[1] Through the years, several modifications have been made, with the goal of addressing ventral pathologies of the cervical spine.

The commonly performed anterior procedures include the following: anterior cervical discectomy without fusion, anterior cervical discectomy and fusion (ACDF), anterior cervical corpectomy and fusion (ACCF), and several modifications—oblique corpectomy, skip corpectomy and hybrid surgery. Anterior cervical discectomy without fusion is limited to treat ventral compression secondary to soft disc protrusion without significant disc height collapse, usually seen in young patients with maintained cervical lordosis, and no advanced degenerative spine condition (wherein there may be concomitant pathologies like facet joint disease or multilevel disc disease).[2] As an option, total disc replacement may be done in young patients with soft disc protrusion but there is no available high-quality data yet to support its efficacy.

ACDF is opted for one- to three-level central and paracentral disc protrusion with compression of the cord and respective nerve root. Aside from being able to remove osteophytic compression, ACDF is able to improve the curvature of the cervical spine and provide distraction and further decompression of foramina.

The addition of vertebral body removal or corpectomy (ACCF) to discectomy is made on the basis of the presence of significant retrovertebral compression from either a ligamentous or bony element pathology. Anterior cervical corpectomy is therefore a better option in patients with long-segment stenosis from OPLL, traumatic vertebral body disruption, osteomyelitis or neoplasm.[3] Advantages of corpectomy include greater surface available for fusion, lower pseudoarthrosis rate (due to lesser number of bone–graft interface needed to heal as compared to ACDF), and improved visualization of anterior thecal sac.

A study by Fraser and Hartl looked into the difference in the fusion rates between ACDF and ACCF. In this meta-analysis, it has been shown that the fusion rate between ACDF and ACCF for two-level disc disease with plate is statistically similar, but for three-level disc problems, ACCF with plate offers higher fusion rate (96.2%), although with more intraoperative blood loss compared to simple discectomy with plate system (82.5%).[4]

Preoperative Planning

Appropriate planning for surgery requires adequate imaging to supplement the physical examination findings of cervical spondylosis. A good resolution (at least 1.5 Tesla) cervical MRI provides the best modality in imaging the spinal canal and soft-tissue details including the disc, ligaments, the spinal cord and nerve roots. T2-weighted hyperintense signal changes within the spinal cord may signify edema or myelopathic changes.[5] Complementary imaging with cervical CT and X-rays (AP, lateral, oblique views and dynamic views) provide additional information to evaluate the extent of OPLL, facet joint disease, foraminal stenosis, and potential instability. Other important details to determine from imaging studies include the course of the vertebral artery, presence of nerve root compression, and length and quality of vertebral body segments (for the size of plates to be used). For patients with prior anterior decompression surgeries, preoperative evaluation with laryngoscopy can help guide in the decision which side will be approached for revision surgeries. If extensive anterior surgery was done in the past, option of decompression via the posterior approach may be chosen to decrease the risk of injury to anterior structures. Patients who are on corticosteroids or nonsteroidal anti-inflammatory drugs (NSAIDs) are advised to stop these medications 10 days before surgery, if possible. Smoking is known to negatively impact fusion rates; hence, it is discouraged at least 2 months prior and 3 to 6 months after surgery.[6]

Neuroanesthetic Considerations

Patients with CSM are at a very high risk for spinal cord injuries even with minor neck manipulation due to compromised spinal canal diameter. Even small degrees of flexion or extension may lead to additional neurologic deficits during the process of induction. Although routine orotracheal intubation using standard laryngoscopy may be done to patients with stable neck and nonseverely stenotic spinal canals, fiberoptic intubation is preferred, especially in patients with instability and with severe spinal stenosis. Induction is carried out using intravenous propofol, and neuromuscular blocking agent is administered to relax the neck muscles. If neuromonitoring using somatosensory-evoked potentials (SSEPs) is planned, the combination of sevoflurane or isoflurane, fentanyl and nondepolarizing muscle relaxant (e.g., Rocuronium) is used to optimize potentials. Preoperative antibiotics are generally institution-based, depending on local antibiogram results, but is recommended to be administered generally 30 minutes prior to skin incision to coincide with its peak concentration. The use of preoperative steroids during cervical anterior decompressive surgeries has been shown in a randomized study to decrease airway edema and improve swallowing function but can significantly affect fusion rate in short term.[7] Hence, the use of dexamethasone as preoperative medication remains at the discretion of the surgeon.

The routine use of intraoperative neuromonitoring remains to be proven by high-quality randomized studies.[8,9] In institutions where this is routinely utilized, typically a combination of electromyography (EMG), SSEPs, and motor-evoked potentials (MEPs) are used. Baseline preoperative determination of signals is performed after intubation and before the patient is positioned. Any change in these baseline values are used to alert surgeons intraoperatively to signify potential neurologic injury.

Positioning and Skin Marking

The patient is positioned supine on a radiolucent bed to facilitate intraoperative fluoroscopy. The neck is maintained in midline and in slightly extended position to maximize exposure to the anterior cervical spine. A shoulder roll is placed under the scapula and another one is placed under the lordosis of the neck to maintain the neck in slightly extended position and to provide support to the neck. Taping of the shoulders and the chin, with proper support of soft tissues (i.e., the nose), to prevent skin and pressure sores may be done to improve exposure of the neck. For unstable spine with listhesis, the use of Gardner–Wells tongs and weight traction of a factor of 5 to 10 to the level of listhesis or intended reduction may be helpful. The arms are pulled down and tucked to the side to reduce soft-tissue preclusion in X-ray visualization of the vertebral bodies **(Figs. 10.1a, b)**.

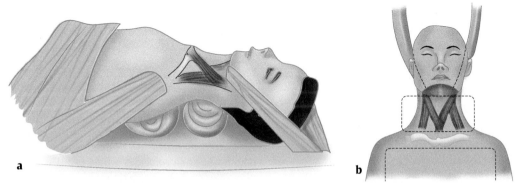

a b

Fig. 10.1 Patient positioning (lateral view) during anterior cervical surgery **(a)**. The cervical spine is extended for maximal exposure with the chin and mandible, and shoulders strapped down to the operating table. The head is supported with a doughnut headrest and the neck and shoulders are supported with rolls. Patient positioning (top view) during anterior cervical surgery **(b)**. Chin and mandible and shoulder straps are shown in blue lines, while the doughnut head rest and neck and shoulder rolls are shown in dotted lines.

Useful estimates for localization in the cervical spine are provided by several anatomic landmarks as outlined in **Table 10.1**. Identification of the desired anatomic level may be more precisely identified by using an intraoperative image intensifier prior to incision.

A transverse skin incision spanning from midline of the neck to the medial border of the sternocleidomastoid muscle (SCM) is generally sufficient in most cases, even in surgeries that require multilevel discectomies. In some situations, this transverse incision can be extended beyond the midline and laterally across the SCM to provide adequate exposure. The key to adequate exposure is proper dissection of fascial planes superior, inferior, and lateral to the skin incision to allow and maximize sliding of the skin over the deeper layers of the neck. Some surgeons may however prefer a longitudinal incision along the medial border of the SCM for surgeries involving more than three-level corpectomies or for extremely obese patients **(Fig. 10.2)**.

Choice of Laterality of Approach

The choice whether to approach the cervical spine from the right or left is based on several factors. In general, a right-sided approach is preferred by right-handed surgeons because of comfort and ergonomic consideration. Theoretically, a left-sided approach has the advantage of avoiding damage to the right recurrent laryngeal nerve (RLN), which has a more variable and superficial course compared to the left. This must however be weighed against the potential for a thoracic duct injury which is reported to be more frequent in left-sided approaches.[10] A prior surgery to either side may also affect the choice of laterality during second surgery. A current review on the rate of occurrence of RLN injury after anterior cervical surgery however showed no correlation of side of approach in the incidence of RLN injury.[11] Several methods were proposed to decrease the incidence of RLN injury, including reduction of endotracheal tube (ETT) cuff pressure below 20 mm Hg, use of methylprednisolone,

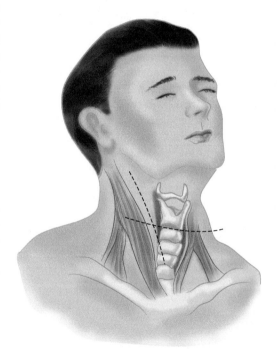

Table 10.1   Anatomic landmarks for cervical localization

Anatomic structure	Corresponding cervical level
Hyoid bone	C2–C3 disc space
Thyroid cartilage (inferior border)	C4 vertebral body
Cricoid cartilage	C6 vertebral body [a]

[a] In some patients, the anterior tubercle of C6 (also known as Chassaignac's tubercle) can be palpated.

Fig. 10.2   Skin incision and anatomic landmarks. Useful estimates for localization in the cervical spine are provided by several anatomic landmarks. The hyoid bone coincides with C2–3 disc space, the inferior border of thyroid cartilage with C4–5 disc space, and the cricoid cartilage with C6 vertebral body. Dashed lines approximate a transverse incision for a C4–C5 discectomy, while the solid line shows a longitudinal incision along the medial border of the sternocleidomastoid muscle (SCM).

and use of EMG monitoring, but none of these are proven and duplicated in randomized studies.[12–14]

Exposure of the Vertebral Column

After skin incision, the platysma may be cut across using electrocautery or split vertically using sharp Metzenbaum scissors. Blunt dissection is then employed using finger dissection or rolled sponge ("cherry sponge") to develop an avascular plane between the SCM and the tracheoesophageal bundle. This blunt dissection is continued with a medial trajectory until the underlying vertebral column is palpable **(Fig. 10.3)**. Attention must be given to the superior and inferior thyroid arteries, which extend from the carotid artery to the midline (thyroid gland), in order to avoid inadvertent injury to these important arteries. Should there be a need for extensive exposure, sacrifice of one artery with careful ligation may be done. The prevertebral

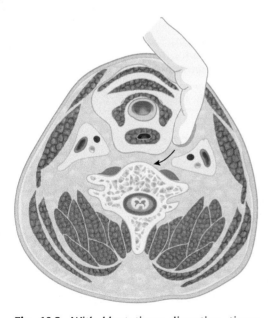

Fig. 10.3 With blunt tissue dissection, tissue planes can be separated to reach the prevertebral plane, with the carotid sheath lateral and the trachea-esophageal complex medial to the exposed working area.

fascia is exposed and dissected in the midline to expose the anterior borders of the vertebral bodies and the anterior longitudinal ligament (ALL). At this point, a lateral view using an intraoperative image intensifier is obtained to confirm the appropriate cervical level. This is facilitated using a needle bent in bayonet fashion and inserted into the desired intervertebral disc level.

Once the appropriate level is confirmed, the medial insertions of the longus colli muscles on both sides which run within the anterolateral surface of the vertebral bodies are dissected using mild electrocautery. It is important that during this part of the procedure, dissection is only limited to the medial attachment of the muscles, as the sympathetic chain of cervical plexus runs underneath this muscle and its injury may lead to Horner's syndrome. Laterally directed sharp retractor blades may be docked at the dissected region of the longus colli muscles and locked in place using the corresponding retractor system to give the final surgical working window. Two laterally directed retractor blades on each side attached to retractor systems may be used for long construct surgeries (two-level corpectomies), in order to provide physical shield or barrier, protecting the esophagus and the carotid sheath from potential harm of drilling. Once properly positioned, the anterior longitudinal ligament is dissected off from the ventral surface of vertebral body before commencing the discectomy.

A pin retractor system to distract disc spaces may be assembled by inserting pins into the rostral and caudal vertebral bodies **(Fig. 10.4)**. If corpectomy is to be done, the pins may be placed on the rostral and caudal vertebral bodies to the corpectomy region. Additional segmental pin placement within the construct region may not be necessary, and as a rule, distraction of 1 to 2 mm per disc level may be allowed by the pin distractor system to maximize exposure. It is important to consciously not overdistract the cervical spine, because this may cause undue strain and stretching of the nerve roots and

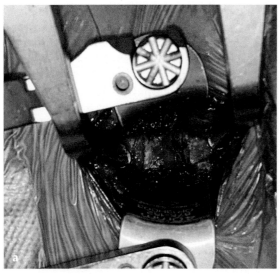

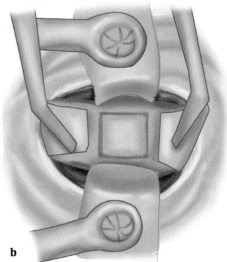

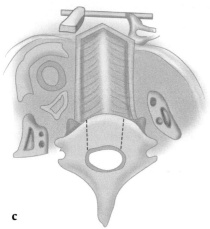

Fig. 10.4 Intraoperative picture showing the retractor blades docked at the dissected medial borders of the longus colli muscles and the vertebral body pins superior and inferior to the intended corpectomy level (**a**). Corresponding illustration of Fig. 10.4 a (**b**). Axial view illustration (**c**) showing where the retractor blades are docked to provide adequate exposure and shield off the carotid sheath (lateral) and the trachea-esophageal complex (medial).

the spinal cord and may lead to postoperative pain syndromes (including intrascapular pain). For other surgeons who prefer not to use the pin distractor system, vertically or longitudinally directed blunt retractor blades properly assembled perpendicular to the initial retractor system may be used to provide a good surgical window and circumferential barrier to drilling. At this point, the operating microscope is brought to the surgical field to carry on with the subsequent steps of the surgery. The use of magnifying loupes and headlight may be done but is suboptimal if the operating microscope is not available.

Discectomy and Corpectomy Technique

Using a blade 15 knife, a rectangular incision (annulotomy) outlining the borders of the disc space (at least 15 mm in lateral width to approximate the region of the uncovertebral joint) is done at the index disc level. For corpectomies, all the disc spaces may be scored with the knife to facilitate discectomies and improve the corrective distraction of the cervical spine by the pin retractor system. If the disc spaces are completely covered by osteophytes, drilling off the anterior osteophytes to expose the disc space may be done. The anterior osteophytic overgrowth at the anterior border of the vertebral bodies may be drilled off also to flatten the anterior border and optimize the placement of plates later on.

Discectomy is done using serial dissection and removal of disc elements with curettes, disc rongeurs and coarse diamond burr drill. It is important to work in a lateral-to-medial fashion and to maintain the tip of curettes or burr within the disc space at all times. Next, the posterior longitudinal ligament (PLL) is carefully opened with a blunt hook inferolateral to the posterior border of the vertebral body and carefully incised with a reverse Karlin knife or blade 11 knife. The PLL may then be resected using fine Kerrison rongeurs (1–2 mm, preferably with thin foot plate, 130 degrees up bite). Special care is done to avoid pushing on the central thecal sac and compression of the cord during discectomy and removal of PLL. "Undercutting" of the PLL and the posterior osteophyte may provide additional decompression to the central thecal sac of the cord. A right-angled nerve hook is then carefully inserted within the neural foramina to ensure that the paramedian gutter is free of any disc-osteophyte and ligamentous compression. The offending osteophyte or ligament is then removed via anterior foraminotomy using a fine round diamond drill or 1-mm Kerrison rongeur. The lateral extent of discectomy is achieved by palpation of the pedicle on each side with a blunt hook and frequently with the appearance of venous epidural bleeding, which should be properly controlled with a gentle hemostatic agent such as Surgicel.

If corpectomy is to be done, after superficial or partial discectomies providing spaces superior and inferior to the vertebral body to be removed, the anterior portion of the vertebral body may be removed using Leksell rongeur or automated ultrasonic bone cutters to save bone for autologous bone graft material. Deeper resection is carried out and completed with high-speed coarse diamond drill.

The posterior cortical bone (posterior vertebral body border) and the PLL or OPLL may further be softened with drilling. Either a nerve hook or fine curette to dissect the PLL or OPLL from the thecal sac is carefully done. Serial removal of the PLL or OPLL and posterior osteophytes may be done with Kerrison rongeurs and nerve hook. Sometimes, it may be prudent to leave thin islands of floating OPLL, which are intimately adherent to the thecal sac to avoid incidental durotomies.[15] The goal of leaving thinner islands is to achieve decompression of the cord and to allow for an adequate space for construct placement (without causing unnecessary compression later on). A safe and sufficient decompression is generally achieved when a 15 to 20 mm wide trough is created after discectomies or corpectomies. It is important to always be oriented midline to avoid iatrogenic vascular injuries at the same time, in order to be able to maximize decompression with adequate trough diameters, and this can be supported with identification of the uncovertebral joint.

Endplate Preparation

A key step in successful bone fusion is preparation of the graft site with adequate end plate preparation to achieve intimate contact with the graft. End plate preparation involves drilling enough to expose raw endplate but not too far extensive to cause endplate disruption, which may lead to telescoping of graft material or subsidence. In addition, to achieve intimate contact, a rectangular space is created with parallel decorticated surface. Other surgeons prefer to make a central cutout in the endplate, with a matching surface on the graft in order to increase stability. It is essential that the anterior lips of the superior and inferior endplate are drilled in order to get an unobstructed view of posterior disc space, allow smooth passage of bone graft, and provide a flushed surface for the placement of cervical plate.

Graft Selection and Harvesting

Size Selection and Placement

For both discectomy and corpectomy procedures, graft size can be predicted based on preoperative assessment of lateral radiographs. A safe estimate of graft size is generally 1 to 2 mm greater than what is measured and a depth about 60 to 80% of the measured AP dimension of the vertebral body to take the magnification factor into account.

One method used to optimize fusion is based on application of Wolff's Law, which states that fusion is optimal when construct is maintained under compressive loading. To apply this concept, autologous grafts are placed in between vertebral bodies, which are separated in tension using distraction pins. This way, once distraction pins are released, the graft in situ are compressed under pressure. Caution, however, must be observed with the use of cervical distractors, as excess tension may cause undue strain and stretching of the nerve roots and the spinal cord. Use of pins in osteoporotic bone may also lead to fracture, as pins may toggle within the vertebral body.

For discectomy procedures, commercial sizers may be used as guide in the selection of properly matched allograft. Grafts are inserted carefully and never forced into position to avoid potential nerve injury and iatrogenic fracture (**Fig. 10.5**). In multilevel ACDF, the smallest disc level is grafted first before proceeding to a larger disc level. Once in place, the graft must have adequate clearance from the decompressed thecal sac and must be recessed at least 2 to 3 mm from the anterior border of the vertebral body.

For corpectomy procedures, calipers may be used to determine the size of the graft. Resected bone during corpectomy can be used to fill the central marrow cavity of structural graft or the hollow center of cage allograft. Other surgeons use demineralized bone matrix as a supplement or add-on to autologous bone chips.

Graft Choice: Allograft versus Autograft

Three options are available to achieve fusion in anterior cervical surgery: allogenic bone graft (allograft), autologous bone graft (autograft), or synthetic cages.

When cervical plating is used, studies have shown that using allograft versus

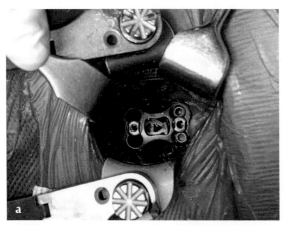
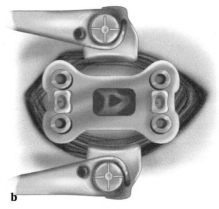

Fig. 10.5   Intraoperative picture of the corpectomy construct set in place (**a**), consisting of titanium cage (with bone graft) with slightly recessed anterior margin, and titanium cervical plate with screws locked at the superior and inferior vertebral bodies. The graft is under compressive loading to optimize fusion (Wolff's law). Corresponding illustration of Fig. 10.5 a (**b**).

autograft makes no difference in rate of nonunion in up to two to three-level ACDF. Samartzis and colleagues have shown fusion rates of up to 97.5% for multilevel ACDF with either autograft or allograft.[16] A recent systematic review of 13 studies on this topic have similarly shown that autologous bone graft and allograft have similar effectiveness in terms of fusion rates, pain scores, and functional outcomes.[17] A similar study comparing autologous bone graft with polyethylene ether ketone (PEEK) showed that PEEK has a comparable fusion rate with autologous bone graft.[18]

Bone Graft Harvesting

Autologous bone graft is most commonly harvested from the anterior iliac crest. To do this, a 4 to 5 cm oblique incision is made just inferior to the iliac crest, at 2 to 3-finger breadths lateral to the anterior superior iliac spine (ASIS), to avoid the lateral femoral cutaneous nerve injury (**Fig. 10.6**). A combination of electrocautery and Cobbs elevator is used to sharply dissect muscles subperiosteally and expose both the outer and inner table of the iliac crest. The surgeon must be wary of the peritoneal cavity medially. An oscillating saw, or an osteotome, is used to harvest a tricortical bone graft. The bone graft donor site should then be sealed with bone wax or Floseal. Reconstruction of the bony defect may be considered using bone void fillers.

An alternative to iliac crest bone graft is an autologous fibular graft, which can be used for longer reconstruction such as multilevel corpectomy (**Fig. 10.7**). To harvest the fibula, the leg must be properly positioned even prior to draping to facilitate easy harvesting during the surgery. A bolster is placed underneath the calf muscle and the donor leg is flexed at the knee and internally rotated to expose the outer lateral aspect of the leg. A longitudinal incision is made along the mid-portion of the fibula. A plane of dissection is made in between peroneus longus muscle anteriorly and gastrocnemius muscle posteriorly. To avoid instability of the ankle joint, an

8-cm portion of fibula proximal to the malleolus should be left intact. A total of 18 cm of fibular bone can be harvested for use as graft.

Cervical Plating

Anterior Cervical Plating Options

Anterior cervical plating offers several advantages over nonplated constructs, especially in two or more level surgeries. Plates are believed to provide rigid fixation and higher fusion rates, resist graft settling and eventual development of segmental kyphosis, and reduce the incidence of graft displacement or extrusion. This must however be weighed against several detrimental effects including additional operative time and cost, complications associated with plate loosening, as well as making revision surgeries more complicated and cumbersome.

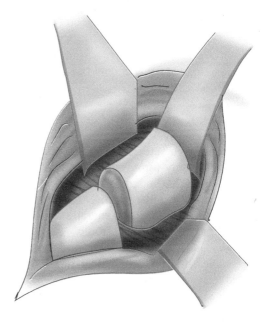

Fig. 10.6 Bone graft is harvested from the iliac crest with an oblique incision lateral to the anterior superior iliac spine. An osteotomy saw or an osteotome is used to obtain a tricortical graft. Careful placement of this incision is essential to avoid injury to the lateral femoral cutaneous nerve.

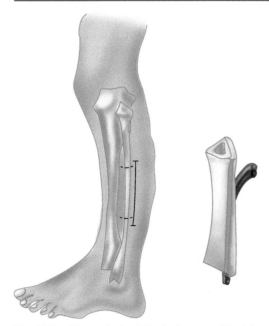

Fig. 10.7 A "vascularized fibular bone graft" with muscle cuff and vascular pedicle can be harvested when long struts are needed. The longitudinal line approximates the skin incision, while the horizontal dotted lines outline the borders of the graft site.

A systematic review and meta-analysis on the topic whether anterior plate is necessary after cervical discectomy showed that the addition of cervical plates after single, two-level, or even three-level discectomy leads to increased fusion rate, decreased subsidence rate, and slightly improved visual analogue scale (VAS) neck pain scores at follow-up.[19]

Compared to discectomy, the use of anterior cervical plate is generally a standard of practice after corpectomy. A one- to two-level ACDF with anterior plate leads to acceptable fusion rates compared to non-plated constructs. However, as proven by several studies, a three-level corpectomy, even if supplemented by anterior plate construct, leads to extremely high rate of graft failure, so that a combination of anterior and posterior surgery is often recommended in these cases.[20] Graft failure can be improved biomechanically by adding one or two screws

in the middle portion of the graft to bring the graft close to the plate.

The use of standalone cages has also been studied in a meta-analysis by Cheung and colleagues.[21] Compared to conventional ACDF with plating, the use of standalone interbody cage is associated with lower dysphagia rate and adjacent segment disease, although this procedure is associated with higher rates of subsidence and cervical kyphosis.[21]

Anterior Cervical Plating Techniques

A plate of adequate size must be used to complement fusion after discectomy or corpectomy. A properly fitted anterior plate must not exceed the span of the desired level to be fused nor should it be short to avoid the dangerous complications of improper screw placement. An ideal plate should have screw holes adjacent to their respective endplates. The plate should be centered by checking if it is within the boundaries of the uncinate processes. The screw length to be used is usually preselected, based on measurement of vertebral body depth on a lateral radiograph or is determined intraoperatively using bayoneted needles inserted into the disc space as marker. The screws are inserted at a medial angulation, aiming toward the center of the vertebral body (triangulation technique) and away from the plate (superior screws oriented superiorly and inferior screws oriented inferiorly). Aside from providing more strength (creating a double lock system) with this type of screw purchase, this technique avoids potential damage to the vertebral artery. Tapping of screws may or may not be needed during screw placement. Unicortical purchase is usually sufficient, especially with modern locking plates. Bicortical purchase is recommended for osteopenic patients or those with highly unstable spine. Once all screws are driven in place, a lateral radiograph is requested to confirm proper screw placement.

The use of newer systems including mini-plates and interbody constructs may be an option, as this may provide a customized fit at each level of fusion and also potentially provide easier revision surgeries when needed in the future.

Closure

Once screw placement is confirmed, retractors are removed carefully and bleeding points are meticulously searched and controlled using bipolar cautery. Soft tissues are allowed to assume their final midline position and their surfaces are inspected repeatedly for any signs of bleeding from scratch or abrasion brought about by contact with the retractor system or newly implanted instrumentation. Once hemostasis is achieved, the wound is irrigated and bony defect from the distraction pins are filled with bone wax or Surgicel. A drain (JP or cigar-shaped Penrose drain) may be placed. Platysma is reapproximated with inverted absorbable sutures (Vicryl 3-0). Skin is closed in subcuticular fashion.

Contemporary Issues

Postoperative Neck Stabilization

A rigid cervical collar is fitted in the operating room prior to awakening. In general, cervical orthosis is recommended to be worn 2 to 4 weeks postoperatively in order to relieve muscle spasm and avoid instability during the period by which the bony construct is allowed to fuse.

Outpatient Surgery

An increasing number of patients had been subjected to day surgery for ACDF. Reported as early as 1996, proponents to this procedure mainly cite the advantage of this strategy in terms of cost savings compared to inpatient surgery.[22,23] Furthermore, outpatient ACDF is found to be safe with overall complications rates not significantly different from inpatient surgery.[24] While this practice will most likely continue in some centers, it must be noted that there is no strong level I or II evidence in the literature supporting this strategy.

Some surgeons however have raised concerns over the delicate nature of cervical surgery, in that complications like airway compromise from cervical edema and hematoma may develop in delayed fashion during when these patients may already have been discharged from the clinic. It should be considered also that for simple single discectomy and decompression, day surgeries may be an option, and for the more complex surgeries of multilevel discectomies and corpectomies with CSM and OPLL, inpatient surgery is still the mainstay of treatment.

Radiographic Monitoring

No consensus exists with regard to the ideal timing of radiographic assessment of cervical fusion after surgery. In fact, many surgeons will recommend different follow-up regimens as well as different modalities to document evidence of fusion after ACDF or ACCF. In one study which looked into the common practice of spine surgeons, approximately 96% will request an AP and lateral radiographic views during follow-up and only 46% will request for dynamic X-rays.[25] A systematic literature review has shown that approximately 90% of patients undergoing ACDF will have fusion documented on radiograph at 1 year post surgery.[26] In clinical practice, the four most common criteria used to document fusion include the following: (1) presence of bridging trabecular bone between endplates; (2) absence of a radiolucent gap between the graft and endplate (defined as radiolucency occupying < 50% of the graft vertebral interface); (3) absence of or minimal motion (< 4° of angulation or < 3mm translation) between adjacent vertebral bodies on flexion-extension radiographs; and (4) absence of or < 2 mm motion between the spinous processes on flexion-extension radiographs.[27] Among these four, the last criterion is one that is highly recommended, as it avoids subjectivity in assessment and has a low false positivity rate.

The following radiographic monitoring may be adopted to evaluate fusion and stability of the construct: (1) cervical AP and lateral X-rays at 2 weeks, 1, 3, 6 and 12 months postoperatively; (2) cervical flexion and extension lateral X-rays at 6 and 12 months postoperatively.

Take-home Points

- Anterior approaches to the cervical spine include anterior cervical discectomy without fusion, ACDF, ACCF, and several modifications—oblique corpectomy, skip corpectomy, and hybrid surgery.

- Anterior surgery for CSM offers the advantage of decompressing the spinal cord from any anterior disc, osteophyte, or ligamentous pathologies while at the same time restoring the natural lordosis of the cervical spine.

- Proper patient screening and selection and perioperative planning are important in the evaluation and treatment of patients with CSM. Clinical and radiological assessment including the number of levels to be treated should be taken into consideration.

- Key procedural steps in anterior cervical decompression and fusion include adequate discectomy/corpectomy, meticulous endplate preparation, proper graft selection, and careful fitting of cervical plate, which should be strictly followed to ensure improvement of signs and symptoms, and at the same time decrease the risks of failure of constructs.

References

1. Smith GW, Robinson RA. The treatment of certain cervical-spine disorders by anterior removal of the intervertebral disc and interbody fusion. J Bone Joint Surg Am 1958; 40-A(3):607–624

2. Hadley MN, Sonntag VK. Cervical disc herniations. The anterior approach to symptomatic interspace pathology. Neurosurg Clin N Am 1993;4(1):45–52

3. Gillis CC, O'Toole J, Traynelis VC. Cervical interbody strut techniques. In: Benzel's Spine Surgery: Techniques, Complication Avoidance, and Management. Philadelphia: Elsevier; 2017:532–539

4. Fraser JF, Härtl R. Anterior approaches to fusion of the cervical spine: a metaanalysis of fusion rates. J Neurosurg Spine 2007; 6(4):298–303

5. Al-Mefty O, Harkey LH, Middleton TH, Smith RR, Fox JL. Myelopathic cervical spondylotic lesions demonstrated by magnetic resonance imaging. J Neurosurg 1988;68(2):217–222

6. Theodore N, Soriano-Baron H, Sonntag VK. Anterior cervical instrumentation. In: Youmans and Winn Neurological Surgery. Philadelphia: Elsevier; 2017:2656–2667

7. Jeyamohan SB, Kenning TJ, Petronis KA, Feustel PJ, Drazin D, DiRisio DJ. Effect of steroid use in anterior cervical discectomy and fusion: a randomized controlled trial. J Neurosurg Spine 2015;23(2):137–143

8. Di Martino A, Papalia R, Caldaria A, Torre G, Denaro L, Denaro V. Should evoked potential monitoring be used in degenerative cervical spine surgery? A systematic review. J Orthop Traumatol 2019;20(1):19

9. Ajiboye RM, D'Oro A, Ashana AO, et al. Routine use of intraoperative neuromonitoring during ACDFs for the treatment of spondylotic myelopathy and radiculopathy is questionable: a review of 15,395 cases. Spine 2017;42(1):14–19

10. Derakhshan A, Lubelski D, Steinmetz MP, et al. Thoracic duct injury following cervical spine surgery: a multicenter retrospective review. Global Spine J 2017; **7**(1, Suppl)115S–119S

11. Beutler WJ, Sweeney CA, Connolly PJ. Recurrent laryngeal nerve injury with anterior cervical spine surgery risk with laterality of surgical approach. Spine 2001; 26(12):1337–1342

12. Jung A, Schramm J. How to reduce recurrent laryngeal nerve palsy in anterior cervical spine surgery: a prospective observational study. Neurosurgery 2010;67(1):10–15, discussion 15

13. Pedram M, Castagnera L, Carat X, Macouillard G, Vital JM. Pharyngolaryngeal lesions in patients undergoing cervical spine surgery through the anterior approach: contribution

of methylprednisolone. Eur Spine J 2003; 12(1):84–90

14. Dimopoulos VG, Chung I, Lee GP, et al. Quantitative estimation of the recurrent laryngeal nerve irritation by employing spontaneous intraoperative electromyographic monitoring during anterior cervical discectomy and fusion. J Spinal Disord Tech 2009;22(1):1–7

15. Mizuno J, Nakagawa H, Song J, Matsuo N. Surgery for dural ossification in association with cervical ossification of the posterior longitudinal ligament via an anterior approach. Neurol India 2005;53(3):354–357

16. Samartzis D, Shen FH, Matthews DK, Yoon ST, Goldberg EJ, An HS. Comparison of allograft to autograft in multilevel anterior cervical discectomy and fusion with rigid plate fixation. Spine J 2003;3(6):451–459

17. Tuchman A, Brodke DS, Youssef JA, et al. Autogenous versus allograft for cervical spinal fusion. Global Spine J 2017;7(1):59–70

18. Chou YC, Chen DC, Hsieh WA, et al. Efficacy of anterior cervical fusion: comparison of titanium cages, polyetheretherketone (PEEK) cages and autogenous bone grafts. J Clin Neurosci 2008;15(11):1240–1245

19. Oliver JD, Goncalves S, Kerezoudis P, et al. Comparison of outcomes for anterior cervical discectomy and fusion with and without anterior plate fixation: a systematic review and meta-analysis. Spine 2018;43(7): E413–E422

20. Vaccaro AR, Falatyn SP, Scuderi GJ, et al. Early failure of long segment anterior cervical plate fixation. J Spinal Disord 1998; 11(5):410–415

21. Cheung ZB, Gidumal S, White S, et al. Comparison of anterior cervical discectomy and fusion with a stand-alone interbody cage versus a conventional cage-plate technique: a systematic review and meta-analysis. Global Spine J 2019;9(4):446–455

22. Silvers HR, Lewis PJ, Suddaby LS, Asch HL, Clabeaux DE, Blumenson LE. Day surgery for cervical microdiscectomy: is it safe and effective? J Spinal Disord 1996;9(4): 287–293

23. Ban D, Liu Y, Cao T, Feng S. Safety of outpatient anterior cervical discectomy and fusion: a systematic review and meta-analysis. Eur J Med Res 2016;21(1):34

24. Yerneni K, Burke JF, Chunduru P, et al. Safety of outpatient anterior cervical discectomy and fusion: a systematic review and meta-analysis. Neurosurgery 2020;86(1):30–45

25. Bohl DD, Hustedt JW, Blizzard DJ, Badrinath R, Grauer JN. Routine imaging for anterior cervical decompression and fusion procedures: a survey study establishing current practice patterns. Orthopedics 2012;35(7):e1068–e1072

26. Noordhoek I, Koning MT, Vleggeert-Lankamp CLA. Evaluation of bony fusion after anterior cervical discectomy: a systematic literature review. Eur Spine J 2019;28(2):386–399

27. Oshina M, Oshima Y, Tanaka S, Riew KD. Radiological fusion criteria of postoperative anterior cervical discectomy and fusion: a systematic review. Global Spine J 2018; 8(7):739–750

Anterior Cervical Body Replacement with Expandable Cylindrical Cages for Cervical Spondylotic Myelopathy and OPLL

Joachim M.K. Oertel and Anna Prajsnar-Borak

Introduction

Cervical spondylotic myelopathy (CSM) is a common cause of atraumatic spinal cord dysfunction. It was described in 1952 by Brain and colleagues.[1] Although a significant effort has been made to understand the pathophysiological mechanisms, static and dynamic factors contribute to the clinical syndrome, the underlying mechanism is still not fully understood. Ischemic damage, cerebrospinal fluid (CSF) pulsations as well as mechanical compression of the spinal cord have all been discussed as an underlying cause.

Concerning the clinical course, a large number of patients remain asymptomatic despite a clear myelopathic signal alteration on the MRI. Once clinically symptomatic, the disease might progress, improve, or remain stable. Thus, natural history and clinical course are highly variable.[2]

MRI is the diagnostic modality of choice, providing crucial information regarding intrinsic spinal cord abnormalities, number of level involvement, spinal cord atrophy, and surrounding structures. CT provides information regarding bony structure and presence of ossification of the posterior longitudinal ligament (OPLL).

If the decision for surgery is made, the treatment of choice is anterior decompression and fusion. The first ventral cervical stabilization was introduced by Bailey and Badgley in 1952.[3] Robinson and colleagues and, shortly afterward, Cloward described the anterior cervical discectomy and fusion (ACDF) techniques for various indications in the 50s.[4,5] Since then, the concept of surgery has remained more or less unchanged. The advantageous and excellent results of ACDF have been presented in numerous studies.[6]

Background

In case of multi-level spinal cord compression, there is an ongoing debate whether to decompress from anterior or posterior, or anterior and posterior with 360° stabilization. While many authors prefer a posterior decompression because of the easy access to the spinal canal and the easy extension to multiple levels, others are in favor of an anterior approach because of the superior stability and the easy restoration of the physiological cervical lordosis. Multilevel anterior cervical decompression and fusion applied in treatment of CSM, however, poses several technical challenges.[7] Looking through the literature, the discussion regarding which type of cervical decompression (anterior vs. posterior, multilevel discectomy vs. corpectomy) provides best results is still ongoing.[6,8–11]

Decision regarding primary treatment strategy for patients with CSM remains based on patient-specific variables and surgeon preferences. Once the decision for an anterior corpectomy is made, the surgeon can choose between bone graft rigid mesh cages and expandable cylindrical cages. The anterior cervical corpectomy and fusion (ACCF) with implantation of expandable cages combined with an anterior plating system for sufficient decompression and fusion is a relatively new concept. Among various anterior approaches, ACCF is one of the most reliable procedures for treating multilevel CSM with satisfactory results.[12,13] The benefits of this operative intervention have been well established and include an excellent and direct ventral spinal cord decompression without interrupting and demanding of posterior neck muscles, maintaining cervical lordosis, and restoring of pre-existing postsurgical (postlaminectomy) kyphosis. High-fusion rate correlates with high success rate, which is reported in 70 to 80% of patients. Reduction of graft subsidence rate, which was a commonly observed phenomenon after ACCF, is another important advantage of anterior cervical body replacement with expandable cylindrical cage followed by anterior plating technique.

However, the incidence of nonunion for ACCF is higher than in ACDF. The reported implant-associated complications with ACCF, including implant dislodgement, and failed bony fusion with pseudoarthrosis, ranging from 2 to 20%, cannot be overlooked. The incidence of pseudoarthrosis and nonunion correlates with the number of instrumented levels. Additionally, ACCF is associated with more intraoperative blood loss in comparison to ACDF.

In terms of diagnostics, postoperative MRI features, certain artifacts in MRI after ACCF may remarkably confuse the obtained image, particularly in patients with additional underlying pathology, reducing the quality of examination, negatively influencing MR images, and limiting the ability of adequate interpretation of the obtained image.

In this chapter, the authors focus on the technical nuances of anterior cervical body replacement with expandable cylindrical cages followed by anterior plating for CSM and OPLL.

Indications for Anterior Corpectomy and Cage Implantation

Probably the most difficult aspect of anterior corpectomy and cage fusion is to select the ideal patient. On one hand, the biomechanics with multilevel discectomy are better compared with corpectomy, and on the other hand, the complication rate is higher with corpectomy and vertebral body replacement than with discectomy and cage implantation alone.[14,15] Thus, the indication for anterior corpectomy, cage implantation, and subsequent anterior plating is rather rare.

The clinical symptoms, the location of spinal cord compression, the individual condition of the patient, and the personal preference of the surgeon are all aspects that have to be taken into account. The selection criteria for an anterior corpectomy differ significantly between surgeons. Some do not hesitate to remove the vertebral body, while others try to avoid the anterior corpectomy at almost all costs. The authors of the chapter favor the anterior corpectomy in all cases when there is an anterior stenosis and spinal cord compression, which cannot be resolved sufficiently via discectomy alone. A grading of the various aspects to favor an anterior corpectomy is shown in **Table 11.1**.

Exclusion Criteria and Contraindications

The anterior corpectomy and plating can be performed almost always. However, the individual risk has to be taken into account. Thus, earlier anterior surgery, earlier radiation, individual deformity, other local factors such as scars, and so on might all influence the decision for the ideal surgical strategy.

Table 11.1 Decision-making for anterior corpectomy

Criteria	Strength of recommendation in favor of anterior corpectomy
Mainly posterior stenosis	–
Short anterior stenosis	+
Long anterior stenosis including the spinal canal behind the body of the vertebra	++
Personal preference of the surgeon	++
Long anterior spinal cord compression / OPLL	+++
Restoration of lordosis required	+++
Symptoms from anterior spinal cord like paresis	++++

Table 11.2 Compilation of preoperative findings

Criteria	Strength of recommendation in favor of surgery
Spinal canal stenosis, no myelopathy	(+)
Spinal canal stenosis, myelopathic changes on MRI, no clinical symptoms	+
Spinal canal stenosis, myelopathic changes on MRI, gait ataxia	++
Spinal canal stenosis, myelopathic changes on MRI, sensory changes or severe ataxia	+++
Spinal canal stenosis, myelopathic changes on MRI, motor weakness	++++

Preoperative Workup

First, the decision for surgery has to be based on the neurological symptoms and signs. Since cervical myelopathy might not improve, despite surgical decompression, early surgery is recommended. A compilation of preoperative findings is shown in **Table 11.2**. Sometimes, there are significant neurological deficits without obvious myelopathic changes on MRI. In these cases, the authors recommend a detailed neurological workup. If no other causes than a spinal canal stenosis is found, surgery is recommended. However, these patients do not benefit as much from surgery in the experience of the authors.

Once the decision for surgery is made, the preoperative workup includes an MRI, a CT as well as flexion extension X-ray (**Table 11.3**). Based on these data, the number of involved levels and extent of compression are determined.

When to add a posterior osteosynthesis is another dispute without unequivocal answer. The authors of this chapter do only anterior corpectomy and plating in single corpectomy. As soon as two or more vertebrae are involved, a posterior osteosynthesis with screw rod system is added.

Surgical Technique

Preoperative Planning

Best the day before surgery, latest the morning before surgery, a detailed planning of the procedure should be done. The authors

Table 11.3 Preoperative diagnostic workup

Investigating modality	Quality of imaging
MRI	Ligamentum flavum hypertrophy Soft disc prolapse Soft tissue foraminal stenosis Myelopathic changes of spinal cord Vertebral artery course
CT	Bony stenosis Calcification of disc prolapses OPLL Quality of bone for spondylodesis and osteosynthesis
Flexion extension X-ray	To rule out instability in adjacent levels

Abbreviation: OPLL, ossification of the posterior longitudinal ligament.

Table 11.4 Preoperative checklist

Criteria	Yes	No
Patient written consent obtained?		
Preoperative workup complete (MRI, CT, X-ray, anesthesia consultation)		
Recurrent laryngeal nerve palsy ruled out?		
Head fixation system and retractor system available?		
Mayfield clamp available?		
Vertebral body replacement implant available?		
What is the expected size?	Diameter? Height? Angulation of endplates?	
Ventral plating and screw system available?		
What is the expected size?	Plate length? Plate shape? Length of screws?	

recommend using a standard checklist to evaluate the requirements for the planned procedure **(Table 11.4)**.

The procedure is performed under the status of general endotracheal anesthesia. In patients with severe spinal cord compression or instability, fiberoptic intubation is recommended. Perioperative antibiotics are administered. The patient is placed on the operating table in the supine position. Pressure points are appropriately padded and protected. For vertebral body replacement, three-pin head holder fixation is recommended. If a carbon clamp is available, it should be used to allow anterior posterior X-ray imaging. If no carbon clamp is available, the head can be fixed in an oblique position of the Mayfield clamp to allow AP X-ray imaging. The head is fixed in a slightly retroflexed extended position. In severe spinal cord compression, sensory-evoked potential monitoring is recommended **(Figs. 11.1a, b)**.

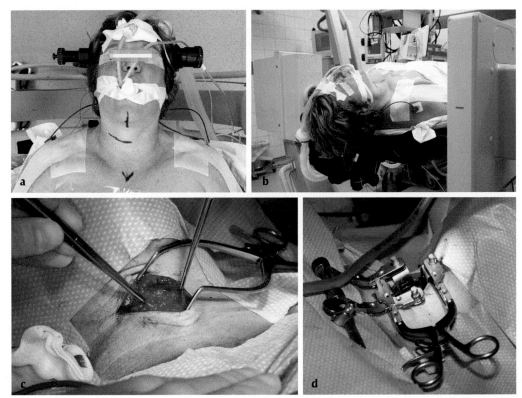

Fig. 11.1 Positioning and approach. The patient is placed in supine position. The head is fixed using a carbon Mayfield clamp in extension and slight retroflexion. C-arm is positioned for intraoperative fluoroscopy control (**a**). Here, a right-sided approach is planned (**b**). After skin incision, the platysma muscle is dissected (**c**). After reaching the anterior vertebral column, a retractor system for craniocaudal and lateral retraction is inserted (**d**).

Procedure

The level of skin incision is determined by lateral fluoroscopy using a clamp or K-wire. The skin incision can be done horizontal and vertical on the right or on the left side. Up to two-level corpectomy, a horizontal skin incision is sufficient. On more levels, a vertical skin incision can be considered. The side of surgery depends on the personal preference of the surgeon. In general, it is easier to decompress the contralateral structures from the opposite direction (the right-side compression from the left-side, and vice versa.)

After dissection of platysma muscle (**Fig. 11.1c**), the carotid artery and the jugular vein are left lateral, the esophagus and trachea medial, and the prevertebral fascia is localized. It is dissected; the longus colli

muscle exposed on both sides, coagulated, cut, and pushed aside. Fluoroscopically, the correct level is confirmed. A retractor system is inserted for lateral tissue retraction. If available, another retractor system for craniocaudal retraction is inserted (**Fig. 11.1d**). The latter facilitates spondylectomy, cage implantation, and subsequent plating. Without second retractor system, Caspar screws are inserted into the adjacent vertebrae and gentle retraction is applied.

Under microscopic view, the evacuation of the adjacent disc spaces follows (**Figs. 11.2a, b**). For a firm position of the vertebral body replacement, it is important to preserve the integrity of the endplates of the adjacent vertebral bodies. The complete annulus should be removed. Complete discectomy prior to

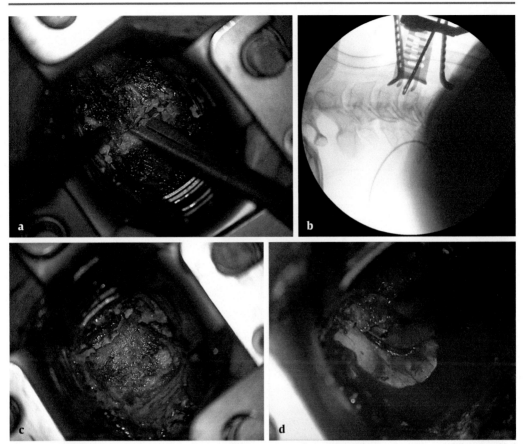

Fig. 11.2 Anterior decompression. Sequential intraoperative photographs showing anterior cervical discectomy C4–5 and C5–6 as well as corpectomy C5. First, the disc spaces are evacuated (**a, b**). Once discectomies above and below the vertebral body are completed, the corpectomy with high-speed drill is continued until a thin layer of bone is remaining (**c**). The last layer of bone is stepwise resected, and the dura decompressed (**d**).

removal of the vertebral body also facilitates evaluation of the depth of the vertebral body as well as the location of the spinal canal. Sufficient lateral decompression of neuroforamen, particularly in patients with concomitant radiculopathy, is performed first. Turning to the vertebral body removal, a high-speed drill is highly recommended, until a thin layer of posterior cortical bone is remaining (**Fig. 11.2c**), which is then approached using small Kerrison rongeurs (**Fig. 11.2d**). Mostly, the posterior longitudinal ligament is simultaneously resected. Sometimes, particularly with OPLL, the dura is very adherent to the ligament, so a dural tear is not rarely seen.

In this case, the duraplasty should be applied using dural substitute as usual.[16,17]

Once the decompression is completed, the expandable cage is selected. Particular attention is paid to the selection of angulation, in order to achieve good endplate alignment. Overdistraction should be avoided, but an appropriate size of the expandable cage is mandatory to avoid screw loosening and kyphotic deformity development. After insertion of the cage (**Figs. 11.3a, b**), the position should be confirmed in lateral and AP X-ray (**Figs. 11.3c, d**). The expansion of the cylindrical cage should be performed under fluoroscopy control to avoid overdistraction.

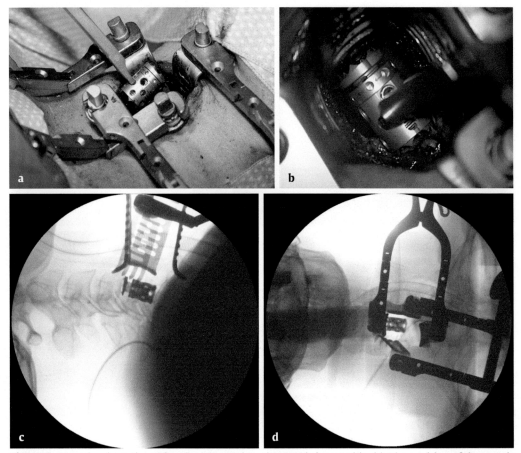

Fig. 11.3   Cage implantation. After decompression, the cage is inserted (**a, b**). The position of the cage is controlled by lateral and AP fluoroscopy to achieve optimal positioning (**c, d**).

Before the application of the plate, the anterior osteophytes are removed and an ideal plane for the plating is reconstructed. The size of the plate is determined, and the plate is inserted (**Fig. 11.4a**). Again, lateral X-ray is performed to confirm the plate position; then, the screws are inserted (**Figs. 11.4b, c**). After removal of the retractor systems, hemostasis is obtained, and a drain inserted (**Fig. 11.4d**).

Postoperative Management

The risk for postoperative infection and hemorrhage is similar to other ACDF cases. However, in severe OPLL, there is a significantly higher risk of postoperative deficits;

thus, a close neurological observation is recommended. In cases with poor bone quality or a planned posterior osteosynthesis in a second surgery later on, a stiff neck immobilization is mandatory, in order to prevent instability and relieve nuchal muscle spasm.

Outcome

The authors performed more the 200 cervical vertebral body replacements since 2010. Between 2011 and 2016, 135 consecutive patients were evaluated. Their mean age was 63 years with a range of 15 to 88 years. The mean follow-up scored 6.5 months. Sixty cases received an expandable cylindrical cage with separate anterior plate, and 75 patients

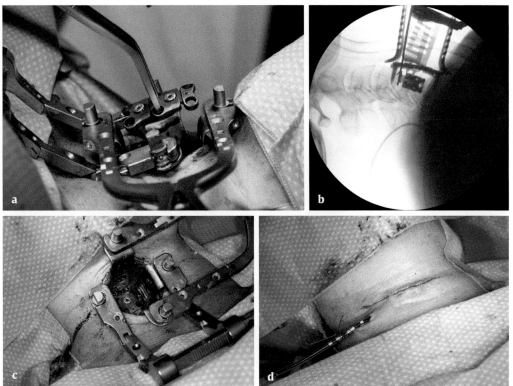

Fig. 11.4 Anterior plating and wound closure. The size of the plate is determined, and the plate is inserted (**a**). Lateral X-ray is performed to confirm the plate position; then, the screws are inserted (**b, c**). After removal of the retractor systems, hemostasis is obtained, and a drain inserted followed by wound closure (**d**).

received an expandable cylindrical cage with integrated anterior plate. Sixty patients were subjected to a single corpectomy, 63 to a two-body corpectomy, 11 to a three-body corpectomy, and 1 to a four-body corpectomy. In 72 of the cases, a posterior fixation was additionally performed.

Neck pain improved in 75%, sensory deficits improved in 71%, motor deficits improved in 85%, and gait ataxia improved in 70%.

Complications

Common complications include:

- Transient dysphagia in 50 to 60% of patients; in 5%, it may persist.
- Failed bony fusion with pseudoarthrosis in 2 to 20%.
- Injury of recurrent laryngeal nerve (permanent 4%, transient 11%).
- Horner's syndrome (rare).
- Injury to carotid artery, vertebral artery, jugular vein, or thoracic duct (rare).
- Perforation of esophagus, trachea, or pharynx (rare).

The authors themselves experienced in their series of 135 cases, 14 complications (10.3%). These consisted of 1 epidural bleeding requiring revision surgery, 2 wound infections, and 11 revision due to implant failure.

Illustrative Case Presentation

An 83-year-old man suffering from progressed clumsiness and gait ataxia for 1 year. In the neurological examination, hyperreflexia and spasticity in lower extremities were seen. MRI showed an advanced multilevel CSM with stenosis in C3–4, C4–5,

C5–6 (**Figs. 11.5a–c**). The indication for microsurgical C3–C6 decompression, ventral corpectomy C4 and C5, anterior cervical body replacement with expandable cylindrical cage was made (**Fig. 11.5d**). In further course, because of the number of segments decompressed, supplemental posterior decompression with instrumentation with lateral mass screws from C3 to C6 was done. In the postoperative course, the patient improved remarkably.

Conclusion

The anterior cervical corpectomy with subsequent vertebral body replacement and plating provides good results and stable fusion rates with an acceptable number of complications.

Take-home Points

- Excellent decompression of the spinal cord and nerve roots with high fusion rate can be achieved by using anterior cervical body replacement with expandable cylindrical cages.

- Identification of both sides uncovertebral joints are the most reliable reference in determining the extent of lateral exposure and decompression.

- There is a higher risk of complications including implant failure.

- Thus, the indication for corpectomy and vertebral body replacement with subsequent plating should be seen as a subgroup of patients with severe spinal cord compression.

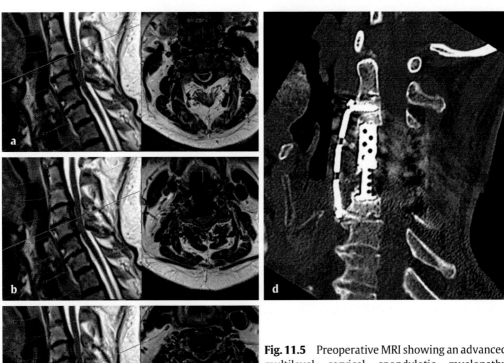

Fig. 11.5 Preoperative MRI showing an advanced multilevel cervical spondylotic myelopathy (CSM) with stenosis in C3–4, C4–5, C5–6 (**a–c**). Postoperative CT sagittal reconstruction showing the status postcorpectomy C4 and C5, vertebral body replacement C4 and C5, and anterior plating C3 to C6 (**d**).

References

1. Lavelle WF, Bell GR. Cervical myelopathy: history and physical examination. Spine Surgery 2007;19:6–11
2. Matz PG, Anderson PA, Holly LT, et al; Joint Section on Disorders of the Spine and Peripheral Nerves of the American Association of Neurological Surgeons and Congress of Neurological Surgeons. The natural history of cervical spondylotic myelopathy. J Neurosurg Spine 2009;11(2):104–111
3. Bailey RW, Badgley CE. Stabilization of the cervical spine by anterior fusion. J Bone Joint Surg Am 1960;42-A:565–594
4. Robinson RA, Smith GW. Anterolateral cervical disc removal an interbody fusion for cervical disc syndrome. Bull Johns Hopkins Hosp 1955;96:223–224
5. Cloward RB. The anterior approach for removal of ruptured cervical disks. J Neurosurg 1958;15(6):602–617
6. Hillard VH, Apfelbaum RI. Surgical management of cervical myelopathy: indications and techniques for multilevel cervical discectomy. Spine J 2006; 6(6, Suppl):242S–251S
7. Sasso RC, Ruggiero RA Jr, Reilly TM, Hall PV. Early reconstruction failures after multilevel cervical corpectomy. Spine 2003;28(2):140–142
8. Hussain M, Nassr A, Natarajan RN, An HS, Andersson GB. Corpectomy versus discectomy for the treatment of multilevel cervical spine pathology: a finite element model analysis. Spine J 2012;12(5):401–408
9. Ikenaga M, Shikata J, Tanaka C. Long-term results over 10 years of anterior corpectomy and fusion for multilevel cervical myelopathy. Spine 2006;31(14):1568–1574, discussion 1575
10. Konya D, Ozgen S, Gercek A, Pamir MN. Outcomes for combined anterior and posterior surgical approaches for patients with multisegmental cervical spondylotic myelopathy. J Clin Neurosci 2009;16(3):404–409
11. Kawakami M, Tamaki T, Iwasaki H, Yoshida M, Ando M, Yamada H. A comparative study of surgical approaches for cervical compressive myelopathy. Clin Orthop Relat Res 2000; (381):129–136
12. Andaluz N, Zuccarello M, Kuntz C. Long-term follow-up of cervical radiographic sagittal spinal alignment after 1- and 2-level cervical corpectomy for the treatment of spondylosis of the subaxial cervical spine causing radiculomyelopathy or myelopathy: a retrospective study. J Neurosurg Spine 2012;16(1):2–7
13. Gao R, Yang L, Chen H, Liu Y, Liang L, Yuan W. Long term results of anterior corpectomy and fusion for cervical spondylotic myelopathy. PLoS One 2012;7(4):e34811
14. Benzel E, ed. The Cervical Spine. Philadelphia: Lippincott Williams & Wilkins; 2012
15. Benzel E. Biomechanics of the Spine Stabilization. Rolling Meadows: Thieme; 2001
16. Müller SJ, Burkhardt BW, Oertel JM. Management of dura ltears in endoscopic lumbar spinal surgery: a review of the literature. World Neurosurg 2018;119:494–499
17. Oertel JM, Burkhardt BW. Full endoscopic treatment of dural tears in lumbar spine surgery. Eur Spine J 2017;26(10):2496–2503

12 Cervical Oblique Corpectomy

Oscar L. Alves and D'jamel Kitumba

Introduction

Cervical spondylosis is the most common cause of myelopathy in adults worldwide. Degenerative cervical stenosis, caused by osteophytes, disc herniation or ossified posterior longitudinal ligament (OPLL), gradually develops and compromises the spinal cord. Surgical decompression for symptomatic cervical myelopathic stenosis is often required.[1] Depending on the location of the compression, on the number of the involved levels, and on sagittal alignment of the cervical spine, different approaches have been postulated.[2] Among the anterior approaches, whenever the compression extends behind the vertebral body, a cervical corpectomy is considered the procedure of choice.[3] As a significant part of the vertebral body is removed during the decompressive corpectomy, there is a need for later reconstruction with a cylinder and stabilization with plates and screws. Besides their own cost, these implants are associated with complications such as migration, subsidence, screw and plate breakage, fusion failure, dysphagia, and persistent low-grade infection.

In order to circumvent these problems, in 1993, George et al proposed the oblique corpectomy (OC) as an alternative to the anterior cervical corpectomy to effectively decompress the neural elements without the need for bone grafting and plating.[4] In this chapter, we review all the major issues related to this rather recent technique to treat spondylotic cervical myelopathy.

Selection Criteria for Oblique Corpectomy

To achieve good outcomes, both clinical and functional, the selection criteria must be respected. In 1999, George et al treated a total of 101 cervical spondylotic patients, 66 with myelopathy and 35 with radiculopathy, through oblique corpectomy without interbody stabilization. Oblique corpectomy was performed on one to five levels and from C2–C3 to C7–T1.[5] Indications for this approach was the presence of a predominantly anterior compression of the spinal cord, which could be associated with unilateral radiculopathy.[5–7] Patients should preferentially have hard collapsed discs, straight or kyphotic spine curvature, and a high risk for pseudarthrosis. Patients are less amenable to oblique corpectomy if they have a lordotic curvature, soft discs on the pathological or adjacent levels (herniated or not), or instability (defined as > 2 mm translatory motion on lateral dynamic radiographs). All these features pose a greater risk for postoperative instability that would require arthrodesis.[6]

Moreover, the basic surgical principles of oblique corpectomy have been used to successfully access intradural lesions such as tumors, vascular anomalies, as well as spinal epidural abscess.[8–12]

Surgical Technique of Oblique Corpectomy

Surgery is done under general anesthesia and endotracheal intubation. It is never enough to stress the importance of neuromonitoring and fiberoptic intubation on these patients to prevent inadvertent neurological injury during the intubation or surgical procedure. Patient is positioned supine with slight ipsilateral shoulder elevation, slight rotation, and extension of the head to the contralateral side. Pathological levels are confirmed with fluoroscopy before sterilization and draping.

The anterolateral approach to cervical spine has been widely described in the literature.[4,6,13] A vertical skin incision is done along the medial border of the sternocleidomastoid (SCM) muscle and extended approximately 2 cm above and below the operating level (s), until the mastoid tip for C2–C3 level or to the suprasternal notch if C7–T1 level has to be approached. Platysma is divided in the same orientation as the skin incision, then the approach progresses in depth through a natural plane without crossing neural structures or blood vessels, between the SCM, laterally, and the trachea, esophagus, internal jugular vein, vagus, and internal carotid artery, medially, exposing deeply the anterolateral aspect of the cervical spine, which is partially covered by the longus colli and longus capitis (LC) muscles (**Fig. 12.1**).

At this point, the lateral border of the classical anterior approach is no more than the medial border of the anterolateral approach (**Fig. 12.2**). The stellate ganglion and cervical sympathetic trunk (CST) run under the LC

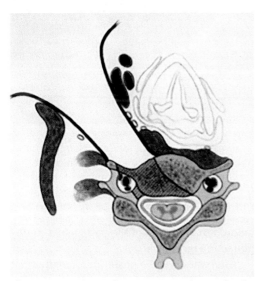

Fig. 12.1 Schematic representation of the anterolateral approach to the cervical spine through a natural corridor between the sternocleidomastoid (SCM) muscle, laterally, and internal jugular vein (IJV), internal carotid artery (ICA), esophagus and trachea, medially, exposing the entry zone for the oblique corpectomy.

muscle fascia, and in order to avoid injury to these structures, this fascia has to be incised medially to the CST, held with stitches, and then smoothly retracted laterally, respecting the connections with cervical nerve roots. The other option is to dissect it medial to lateral and then put a blade retractor, but this technique has been associated with a greater incidence of postoperative Horner's syndrome (HS).

Once the transversarium foramen is identified above and below the surgical levels of interest, the LC muscles are incised horizontally along the transverse process and excised en bloc, exposing the entire course of the vertebral artery (VA). At this stage, a key maneuver to effectively control the VA is the subperiosteal dissection of the VA inside the transversarium foramen. This leaves the periosteal sheath covering the VA and the surrounding venous plexus to avoid excessive bleeding and damage of the VA. It is mandatory, in every case, to identify on the preoperative cervical spine MRI or CT the location and course of the VA, especially its entry point in the transversarium foramen, in order to avoid major vascular complications. The VA can then be mobilized, depending on the need to expose the entire length of the foramen and the nerve root. Moreover, the VA does not need to be mobilized in every single case, especially when only myelopathy is present.

The next step is to identify the uncovertebral joint, since drilling is owed to begin 3 mm medial from it to avoid VA injury. An important concept to preserve stability is to leave intact the anterior longitudinal ligament, as well as the intervertebral discs adjacent to the untouched part of the vertebral bodies intact (**Fig. 12.3**). Drilling is done with a 4 mm cutting-drill from the aforementioned entry point straight backward to the posterior cortical bone. Once the posterior cortical bone has been reached, the surgeon must change the orientation of the microscope to a more oblique view and direct the bone drilling to the opposite side. This should be done with care not to violate neither the

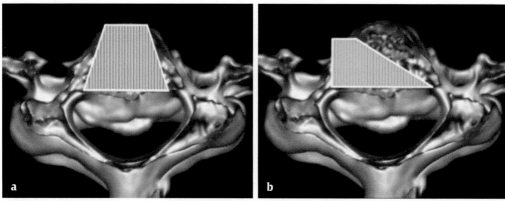

Fig. 12.2 Schematic view on a reconstructed vertebral body (VB) representing the amount of bone removed in a classical corpectomy **(a)** and in an oblique corpectomy (OC) **(b)**. Note that by drilling through an oblique orientation, a triangle shape of bone is removed but leaving > 50% of VB intact.

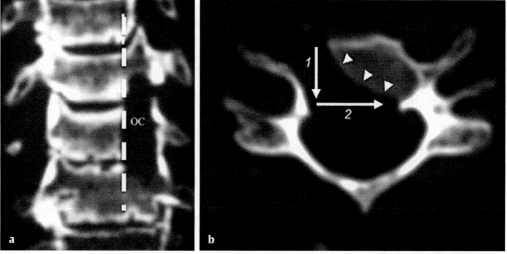

Fig. 12.3 Coronal **(a)** and axial **(b)** postoperative bone window CT scans showing the entry zone on the anterior wall of the vertebral body (VB) giving access to the oblique drilling. Note that most of the anterior longitudinal ligament and anterior vertebral wall, medial to the dashed white line, are preserved, contributing to postoperative stability. 1-2: sagittal and coronal measurements of the wedge hap-shaped corpectomy.

posterior cortical bone nor the posterior longitudinal ligament. Drilling must include all pathological segments with about 50% of vertebral bodies and intervertebral discs left untouched. Horizontal drilling should stop at the contralateral pedicle. Further drilling might be done with a diamond burr, and residual disc material or bone spurs can then be removed. The amount of bone drilling is tailored to the needs of the patients, as exemplified in **Fig. 12.4**.

Afterward, the posterior longitudinal ligament (PLL) may be opened and removed, enlarging thus the diameter of the spinal canal (**Fig. 12.5**). It is advised to perform this gesture from distal to proximal, because bulging of the dural sac may impair visualization and hinder proper decompression.

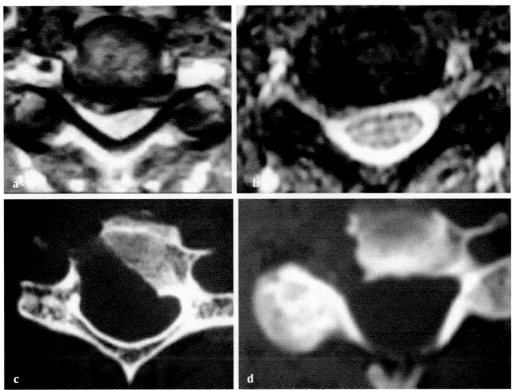

Fig. 12.4 Oblique corpectomy (OC): the extent of bone drilling and vertebral artery (VA) exposure depends on the clinical and imaging settings. (**a, b**): pre- and postoperative myelopathy case with the necessary bone removal to expose the anterior spinal cord. (**c, d**): pre-and postoperative radiculopathy case with the drilling limited to the exposure of the nerve root under control of vertebral artery (VA).

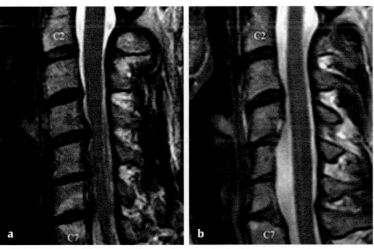

Fig. 12.5 Note the generous increase in the spine canal diameter after a two-level C5–6–7 oblique corpectomy (OC). Sagittal T2-weighted MRI pre- (**a**) and postoperative (**b**).

Even though this can sometimes be difficult because of calcification and adherence of the PLL to the overlying dura. Cervical nerve root decompression can be achieved only on the operating side, with foraminectomy releasing the nerve root from its exit laterally on the dural sac of the spinal cord to the medial aspect of the VA (**Fig. 12.6**).

Closure is done with an absorbable suture in the platysma and in the subcutaneous tissue, intradermal suture or staples to close the skin. A drain is sometimes left in place for 24 hours; early mobilization and ambulation are indicated, and no cervical collar is needed.

Clinical and Radiological Outcomes after Oblique Corpectomy

In their first paper, George et al (*n* = 101) reported a clinical improvement in the Japanese Orthopaedic Association (JOA) and Nurick grade (NG) scales, at a mean follow-up of 37 months (range 2–66 months), in 82 and 67% of patients, respectively, and worsening in 8% in both scales (level IV of evidence).[5]

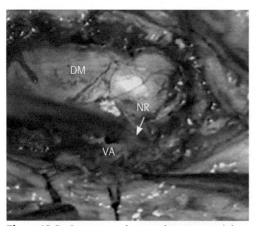

Fig. 12.6 Intraoperative microscope view showing the ventral dura mater (DM), spinal cord and the nerve root (NR) decompressed. Note the relationship between the vertebral artery (VA) and the nerve root. The anterolateral approach is the only anterior approach that can effectively expose the full length of the nerve root.

Chibarro et al confirmed these results later in the largest series published so far, enrolling 477 patients with similar inclusion criteria and 111 months of mean follow-up (range 9–202 months). They found an overall excellent recovery rate, but noticed that patients presenting radiculopathy had better results than myelopathic patients (88% vs. 95%, respectively) (level IV of evidence).[14] A significant improvement in neck disability index (NDI) score was seen at 6 weeks after surgery. The best clinical outcomes were reported by Kiris et al which showed a JOA score improvement in 92.5% of patients at 6 months of follow-up, worsening in 2.5%, and no changes in 5%. The mean preoperative JOA score of 12.8 ± 3.1 significantly changed to 14.9 ± 2.6 postoperatively (level IV of evidence).[15] Globally, OC offers a clinical improvement of 86% of myelopathic symptoms and long-term stability of 98 to 100%.[16,17]

These overall excellent clinical outcomes derive from the fact that OC is a very effective technique in producing a wide canal decompression, as reported by Koç et al. They found (*n* = 26) a postoperative increase in the mean Pavlov ratio (the ratio between the spinal canal and the vertebral body [VB] diameter) by 76.2% from 0.72 to 1.26 and a sagittal cervical canal diameter improvement with an average of 67% (level IV of evidence).[18] Sarkar at al presented the radiological and clinical results of OC in 56 myelopathic patients, showing that surgical decompression reverses the extensive cord edema with diffuse changes on MRI, and leaving behind small residual focal, necrotic and cavitatory lesions (level IV of evidence).[19] A regression of the increased signal intensity (ISI) by > 50% at 18 months of follow-up predicts better functional outcomes.

Besides the control of VA, the other major difficulty of the surgery during bone drilling is intraoperative navigation. There is a compromise between not removing too much bone, which may cause instability, nor leaving bone, which might anteriorly compress the spinal cord. The precise knowledge of the right amount of bone to be removed comes from experience; however, the learning curve could also be abbreviated by the use of navigation tools. Moses et al used intraoperative ultrasound (IU) to identify the VA, which they could do in all cases, but most importantly to identify residual bone compression. They found a good accuracy of IU measurement of the width of the oblique corpectomy compared with postoperative CT and MRI measurements. No significant difference in incidence of residual bony compression in cases operated with and without IU was found (level III of evidence).[20] Lee et al performed a study randomizing patients with OPLL (*n* = 22) by using image-guided navigation. They used a standard anterior approach, instead of an anterolateral, for OC, and used C-arm-based intraoperative navigation in half of their cases, leading to a more complete OC (level IV of evidence).[21] They were able to preserve the entire anterior portion of the upper and/or lower end of decompression through undermining drilling on sagittal oblique plane.

Biomechanics and Biokinematics of Oblique Corpectomy

Biomechanical testing showed less instability and altered kinematics compared to corpectomy with fusion. Cagli et al were the first to study the biomechanics and kinematic parameters of multilevel OC on a human cadaveric model (C3–T1). Compared to intact cervical spine, OC induced a greater range of motion (mean of 15°) in all motion directions (15% flexion, 18% extension, 11% lateral bending, 18% axial rotation), whereas the standard corpectomy without plate fixation originated a three times higher increase in motion.[22]

Turel et al in a study enrolling 28 patients with cervical myelopathy found that global and segmental range of motion decreased significantly by 11.2° and 10.9°, respectively, at mean follow-up of 45 months (level IV evidence).[23] The reduction in the range of motion (ROM) was associated with extensive osteophyte progression and ossification of the anterior longitudinal ligament in two-thirds of cases more pronounced at index level. Similar results were reported by Chacko et al, who described a significant decrease in flexion and extension by a mean of 2.5° and 7°, respectively, representing a loss of 33%. The loss of motion is inversely related to the number of operated segments (single-level 40%, two-level 33%, and for three-level 26%).[24] Regarding the impact in the postoperative sagittal balance, it seems that OC produces a kyphotic effect without clinical worsening, not correlated with the number of operated levels. Chacko et al found that 30% of patients with preoperative lordosis developed a straight spine and 5% became kyphotic. None of the patients developed spinal instability (level IV evidence).[24] George et al reported cervical spine instability in three cases.[5]

If no more bone than the necessary is removed to decompress, instability is not to be expected, as oblique drilling preserves most of the stabilizing bone and ligaments, at least 50% on anterior elements, without disrupting the posterior elements. Several biomechanical studies and case series demonstrated that OC results in no instability of the operated segments.[7,22,25] However, stability and weight-bearing capacity depends not only upon the amount of resected bone but also on bone density. Before applying oblique corpectomy on a larger scale in patients with high risk of pseudarthrosis (elders, diabetic, long-standing smokers) due to osteoporotic bone, a 3D finite element analysis (FEA) should be done in the future to test the stability after an oblique cervical corpectomy.

Complications

OC evades the complications related to bone site harvesting as well as those related with cervical spine reconstruction with cylinder or plate and screws.[26] The specific complications related to OC are Horner syndrome (HS), VA injury, and postoperative instability.[27]

Among these, the most frequent is by far HS, with an incidence of 3 to 57% of transient HS[5,24] and 0.4 to 8% permanent.[7,16,17,27] In the largest cohort of patients (n = 465), the cumulative rate of transient HS was 15.7% and permanent 3.4%.[7] A good knowledge of the anatomy of the CST is very important to reduce the morbidity. CST has a craniocaudal and lateromedial course over the LC muscle, a small percentage can even run posterior to carotid sheath.[28] A technical tip by making a longitudinal incision in the longus colli sheath and retracting with a suture, the CST medially may help to reduce the incidence of this complication when compared to dissection.[24]

So far, only one case of VA injury during dissection of the longus colli was reported.[24] A careful review of preoperative MRI, looking for the VA course and its anatomical variations, is advisable. Intraoperative use of the laser Doppler or ultrasonography may also be of great help to identify the artery.[20] It is also recommended to start the division of longus colli over the top of the transverse foramen once an intraforaminal course of the VA is confirmed. The skeletonization of the VA should be stated with a subperiosteal dissection inside the transverse foramen to avoid vascular injury.

Otherwise, OC is a safe technique with a low-rate incidence of additional complications such as axial pain (8%), kyphosis causing pain (4%), persistent brachialgia (4%), cerebrospinal fluid (CSF) fistula (4%), contralateral foraminal stenosis (4%), hematoma (2.5%), nerve root injury, and perforation of the lymphatic duct in one case.[5,15,16,24] Patients with OPLL had significantly higher rate of postoperative complications, including CSF leak and radicular deficit at last follow-up.[7] C5 radiculopathy is reported to be 7,3% for anterior corpectomy and fusion, while Chacko et al reported 3,7% (5/153) patients developed a C5 radiculopathy in the immediate postoperative period, four of which improved to normal in 6 months.[24,29]

Conclusion

Despite being a challenging technique, OC is a safe and reliable procedure and an alternative to conventional approaches for spondylotic cervical myelopathy with predominant anterior compression. With a good knowledge of the surgical anatomy and of the technique itself, the associated risk of VA injury and HS can be mitigated to a very low incidence. Multilevel OC is also a versatile technique that can be applied to various pathologies of the cervical spine, including intradural tumors.

Long-term neurological outcomes achieved are similar to long-term stability on flexion/extension compared to conventional anterior cervical corpectomy and fusion (ACCF) surgery. Under microscopic view and using a high-speed drill through an oblique inclination, a wedged hap-shaped part of the vertebral body (< 50%) is removed to adequately decompress the spinal cord. As the anterior longitudinal ligament and more than half of VB remain intact, reconstruction with implants, plates and screws are not needed. Thus, the main advantage of this technique is the adequate ventral decompression of the spinal cord and of the ipsilateral nerve root without the need of fusion and fixation. Accordingly, this procedure is a good alternative in patients with osteoporotic bone in whom implants are prone to fail.

OC, especially in less wealthy countries, may significantly reduce the costs of surgery for spondylotic cervical myelopathy, as no implants are used and serial radiographs scheduled to monitor for pseudarthrosis are not needed.

Take-home Points

- The indications for OC are the presence of a predominantly anterior compression of the spinal cord, which could be associated with unilateral radiculopathy, presence of hard collapsed discs, a straight or kyphotic spine curvature, a high risk for pseudarthrosis, and the absence of instability.

- OC is performed once an anterolateral approach of the cervical spine is completed. At this point, the lateral border of the classical anterior approach is no more than the medial border of the anterolateral approach.

- A key maneuver to effectively control the VA is the subperiosteal dissection of the VA inside the transversarium foramen.

- It is mandatory, in every case, to identify the location and course of the VA on the preoperative cervical MRI or CT, especially its entry point in the transverse foramen, in order to avoid major vascular complications.

- Under microscopic view and using a high-speed drill through an oblique inclination, a wedged hap-shaped part of the vertebral body (< 50%) is removed to adequately decompress the spinal cord. Horizontal drilling should stop at the contralateral pedicle.

- The PLL may be opened and removed, thereby enlarging the diameter of the spinal canal. This gesture should be performed from distal to proximal.

- OC offers a clinical improvement of 86% of myelopathic symptoms and long-term stability of 98 to 100%.

- Biomechanical testing showed less instability and altered kinematics for oblique corpectomy compared to corpectomy with fusion.

- OC produces a kyphotic effect without clinical worsening, not correlated with the number of operated levels.

- Postoperative instability is not to be expected, as oblique drilling preserves most of the stabilizing bone and ligaments, at least 50% on anterior elements, without disrupting the posterior elements.

- OC evades the complications related to bone site harvesting as well as those related with cervical spine reconstruction with cylinder or plate and screws. The specific complications related to oblique corpectomy are Horner syndrome (HS) and VA injury.

- The cumulative rate of transient HS was 15.7% and permanent 3.4%.

Acknowledgments

I, Oscar L. Alves, would like to express my sincere gratitude toward Prof. Bernard George, one of the most important scholars ever in neurosurgery, who taught me the oblique corpectomy technique, and made several other contributions in this field. Prof. George has always been very supportive and I must thank him for giving us permission to use some of the pictures and illustrations from his personal archive.

I would also like to thank Ms. Sonia Macedo for editing and reviewing the manuscript for language.

References

1. Tetreault L, Goldstein CL, Arnold P, et al. Degenerative Cervical myelopathy: a spectrum of related disorders affecting the aging spine. Neurosurgery 2015;77(Suppl 4): S51–S67

2. Luo J, Cao K, Huang S, et al. Comparison of anterior approach versus posterior approach for the treatment of multilevel cervical spondylotic myelopathy. Eur Spine J 2015;24(8):1621–1630

3. Wang S, Xiang Y, Wang X, et al. Anterior corpectomy comparing to posterior decompression surgery for the treatment of multilevel ossification of posterior longitudinal

ligament: A meta-analysis. Int J Surg 2017; 40:91–96

4. George B, Zerah M, Lot G, Hurth M. Oblique transcorporeal approach to anteriorly located lesions in the cervical spinal canal. Acta Neurochir (Wien) 1993;121(3-4):187–190

5. George B, Gauthier N, Lot G. Multisegmental cervical spondylotic myelopathy and radiculopathy treated by multilevel oblique corpectomies without fusion. Neurosurgery 1999;44(1):81–90

6. Bruneau M, Cornelius JF, George B. Multilevel oblique corpectomies: surgical indications and technique. Neurosurgery 2007; 61(3, Suppl):106–112, discussion 112

7. Chacko AG, Joseph M, Turel MK, Prabhu K, Daniel RT, Jacob KS. Multilevel oblique corpectomy for cervical spondylotic myelopathy preserves segmental motion. Eur Spine J 2012;21(7):1360–1367

8. Kunert P, Prokopienko M, Nowak A, Czernicki T, Marchel A. Oblique corpectomy for treatment of cervical spine epidural abscesses: Report on four cases. Neurol Neurochir Pol 2016;50(6):491–496

9. Radek M, Grochal M, Tomasik B, Radek A. The antero-lateral approach with corpectomy in the management of the ventral meningioma of the spinal canal. Neurol Neurochir Pol 2016;50(3):226–230

10. Delfini R, Marruzzo D, Tarantino R, Marotta N, Landi A. Multilevel oblique corpectomies as an effective surgical option to treat cervical chordoma in a young girl. World J Clin Cases 2014;2(3):57–61

11. Fontaine D, Lot G, George B. Intramedullary cavernous angioma. Resection by oblique corpectomy. Surg Neurol 1999;51(4): 435–441, discussion 441–442

12. Lot G, George B. Cervical neuromas with extradural components: surgical management in a series of 57 patients. Neurosurgery 1997;41(4):813–820, discussion 820–822

13. Salvatore C, Orphee M, Damien B, Alisha R, Pavel P, Bernard G. Oblique corpectomy to manage cervical myeloradiculopathy. Neurol Res Int 2011;2011:734232

14. Salvatore C, Orphee M, Damien B, Alisha R, Pavel P, Bernard G. Oblique corpectomy to manage cervical myeloradiculopathy. Neurol Res Int 2011;2011:734232

15. Kiris T, Kilinçer C. Cervical spondylotic myelopathy treated by oblique corpectomy:

a prospective study. Neurosurgery 2008; 62(3):674–682, discussion 674–682

16. Chibbaro S, Mirone G, Makiese O, George B. Multilevel oblique corpectomy without fusion in managing cervical myelopathy: long-term outcome and stability evaluation in 268 patients. J Neurosurg Spine 2009; 10(5):458–465

17. Rocchi G, Caroli E, Salvati M, Delfini R. Multilevel oblique corpectomy without fusion: our experience in 48 patients. Spine 2005;30(17):1963–1969

18. Koç RK, Menkü A, Akdemir H, Tucer B, Kurtsoy A, Oktem IS. Cervical spondylotic myelopathy and radiculopathy treated by oblique corpectomies without fusion. Neurosurg Rev 2004;27(4):252–258

19. Sarkar S, Turel MK, Jacob KS, Chacko AG. The evolution of T2-weighted intramedullary signal changes following ventral decompressive surgery for cervical spondylotic myelopathy: Clinical article. J Neurosurg Spine 2014;21(4):538–546

20. Moses V, Daniel RT, Chacko AG. The value of intraoperative ultrasound in oblique corpectomy for cervical spondylotic myelopathy and ossified posterior longitudinal ligament. Br J Neurosurg 2010;24(5):518–525

21. Lee H-Y, Lee S-H, Son HK, et al. Comparison of multilevel oblique corpectomy with and without image guided navigation for multisegmental cervical spondylotic myelopathy. Comput Aided Surg 2011;16(1):32–37

22. Cagli S, Chamberlain RH, Sonntag VKH, Crawford NR. The biomechanical effects of cervical multilevel oblique corpectomy. Spine 2004;29(13):1420–1427

23. Turel MK, Sarkar S, Prabhu K, Daniel RT, Jacob KS, Chacko AG. Reduction in range of cervical motion on serial long-term follow-up in patients undergoing oblique corpectomy for cervical spondylotic myelopathy. Eur Spine J 2013;22(7):1509–1516

24. Chacko AG, Turel MK, Sarkar S, Prabhu K, Daniel RT. Clinical and radiological outcomes in 153 patients undergoing oblique corpectomy for cervical spondylotic myelopathy. Br J Neurosurg 2014;28(1):49–55

25. Karalar T, Unal F, Güzey FK, Kiris T, Bozdag E, Sünbüloglu E. Biomechanical analysis of cervical multilevel oblique corpectomy: an in vitro study in sheep. Acta Neurochir (Wien) 2004;146(8):813–818

26. Vaccaro AR, Falatyn SP, Scuderi GJ, et al. Early failure of long segment anterior cervical plate fixation. J Spinal Disord 1998;11(5):410–415

27. Tykocki T, Poniatowski ŁA, Czyz M, Wynne-Jones G. Oblique corpectomy in the cervical spine. Spinal Cord 2018;56(5):426–435

28. Balak N, Baran O, Denli Yalvac ES, Esen Aydin A, Tanriover N. Surgical technique for the protection of the cervical sympathetic trunk in anterolateral oblique corpectomy: a new cadaveric demonstration. J Clin Neurosci 2019;63:267–271

29. Shou F, Li Z, Wang H, Yan C, Liu Q, Xiao C. Prevalence of C5 nerve root palsy after cervical decompressive surgery: a meta-analysis. Eur Spine J 2015;24(12):2724–2734

13 Anterior Controllable Antedisplacement and Fusion Surgery for Multisegmented OPLL

Zhenlei Liu, Zan Chen, and Fengzeng Jian

Introduction

Ossification of the posterior longitudinal ligament (OPLL) of cervical spine refers to the pathological process that involves ectopic bone formation of ligaments, causing stenosis of spinal canal and compression of spinal cord. The etiology of OPLL remains undefined, and surgical intervention is the main treatment modality for this disease.[1,2]

A variety of surgical approaches have been reported including anterior, posterior, and combined anterior and posterior approaches, each with multiple techniques and different advantages and disadvantages. For patients with canal occupancy of 60% or more, cervical kyphosis, and (-) K line, anterior approach is suggested with advantages such as direct decompression, better alignment, and superior clinical outcomes. However, dural tear is a common complication (up to 20%), even for the "floating" technique. Primary repair of dura is highly technique-demanding and actually impossible under common clinical settings.[2]

In this context, anterior controllable antedisplacement and fusion (ACAF) is one of the most recent techniques reported in the literature to not only achieve anterior direct decompression, but also avoid dural tear. Sun et al[3] reported the preliminary clinical results of this technique. A series of 15 patients with multilevel OPLL and myelopathy underwent ACAF and were followed for a mean follow-up duration of 9 months. The study demonstrated excellent postoperative outcomes with decompression of spinal cord, recovery of neurological deficits, and bony fusion achieved 6 months postoperatively. Almost

at the same time, Lee et al[4] reported a similar technique, which they named vertebral body sliding osteotomy (VBSO), with 14 patients afflicted with cervical myelopathy caused by OPLL, demonstrating excellent outcomes. By virtue of the efforts of Prof. Jian-gang Shi's team, the technique has become increasingly ready for common clinical application.

Anatomy

Sun et al[5] studied the morphometry of uncinate process (UP) in 20 OPLL patients and concluded that UP can serve as the landmark for lateral osteotomy in the ACAF procedure. The average base distance of the UP ranges from 14.6 mm at C3 to 22.7 mm at C7. The maximal width of OPLL is 13.2 mm on average. Thus, the width of the vertebrae-OPLL complex with UP as lateral osteotomy margin is adequate for decompression.

The transverse foramen (TF) to UP distance ranges from 4.6 to 7.2 mm,[5] and the distance of lateral wall of osteotomy slot to TF is larger than 2 mm at all levels.[6] Thus, it is safe in terms of avoiding injury of vertebral artery when using the UP as the landmark of longitudinal osteotomy.

Surgical Procedure

The key steps of ACAF are reported as follows[7–12]:

- After general anesthesia and intubation, the patient was placed in a supine position.
- A right-sided Smith–Robinson approach with a transverse or longitudinal incision was performed to expose

the cervical vertebrae, and intraoperative fluoroscopy was used to confirm surgical levels.

- Multiple discectomies were implemented **(Fig. 13.1a)**. The posterior longitudinal ligament at the cephalic and caudal end should be incised to expose the dura, while the ossified ligament at the middle disc levels were only partially removed for implantation of cages.
- The anterior portion of the vertebral bodies with OPLL was quantitatively removed. according to the thickness of ossification **(Fig. 13.1b)**.

- Proper cage filled with autologous bone fragments was implanted at each disc level **(Fig. 13.1c)**.
- On the left side of each vertebra, medial to the UP, high-speed burr and Kerrison rongeur were used to create a 2-mm-wide osteotomy slot. Intraoperative palpation of the integrity of lateral wall of slot was advocated during the whole process **(Fig. 13.1d)**.
- An appropriately curved cervical plate is fixed to the cephalic and caudal vertebrae. On the middle vertebrae, screws were inserted halfway for temporary fixation **(Figs. 13.1e and 13.1f)**.

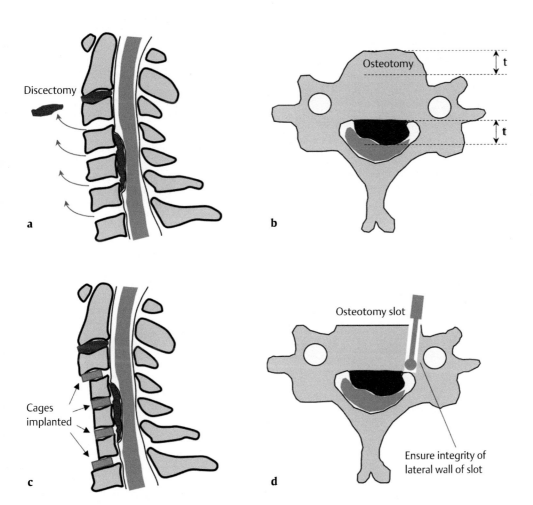

Fig. 13.1 **(a–d)** Key steps of ACAF. t, thickness of OPLL. (Adapted from Yang et al. Journal of Clinical Neuroscience, 2018)[12] (*Continued*)

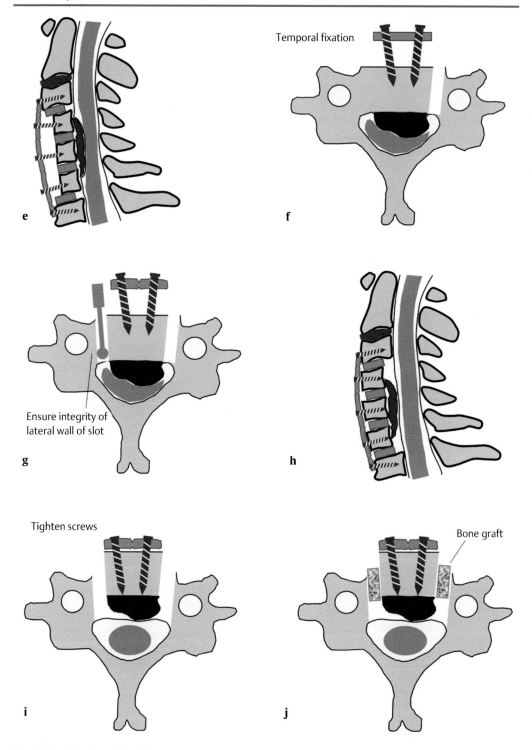

Fig. 13.1   (*Continued*) **(e–j)** Key steps of ACAF. t, thickness of OPLL. (Adapted from Yang et al. Journal of clinical neuroscience, 2018)

- On the right side of the vertebrae, as had been performed on the left side, an osteotomy slot was created. Now the vertebrae-OPLL complex were completely isolated **(Fig. 13.1g)**.
- The loose screws on the middle vertebrae were tightened to achieve a gradual antedisplacement of the vertebrae-OPLL complex, resulting in expansion of spinal canal and decompression of spinal cord **(Figs. 13.1h and 13.1i)**.
- Bone graft was implanted into the slot to ensure fusion **(Fig. 13.1j)**.

Safety and Efficacy

Sun et al[13] retrospectively studied 43 patients who underwent ACAF for OPLL. Mean time of surgery and blood loss is 168 minutes and 334 ml, respectively. All patients had satisfactory decompression with a mean change of occupying rate by 45%. Japanese Orthopaedic Association (JOA) score/recovery rate averaged 72%. A total of 5 complications occurred, including 2 cerebrospinal fluid (CSF) leakage (4.6%), 1 C5 nerve palsy (2.3%), and 2 slippages of screws (4.6%).

Anterior Controllable Antedisplacement and Fusion (ACAF) vs. Anterior Cervical Corpectomy and Fusion (ACCF)

In a retrospective comparison study on severe OPLL patients with occupying rate of 50%, Yang et al[14] reported better JOA score at 6 months follow-up in ACAF group (34 patients) than that in ACCF group (36 patients). Decompression width (17.9 ± 1.0 vs. 15.1 ± 0.8 mm; $p < 0.01$), spinal canal area (150.4 ± 31.6 vs. 127.0 ± 270.2; $p < 0.01$), and anteroposterior spinal cord diameter (5.4 ± 0.6 vs. 5.0 ± 1.1 mm; $p < 0.05$) were significantly greater in the ACAF group. Five patients (13.9%) developed CSF leakage and 1 patient (2.8%) had spinal cord injury in the ACCF group, whereas only 2 patients (5.9%)

in the ACAF group had CSF leakage and none had spinal cord injury. Further, 2 patients presented with subsidence of the titanium mesh in ACCF group, and all ACAF patients had solid fusion, with no pseudarthrosis at 6-month follow-up. Later, the same author[15] reviewed 28 ACAF and 31 ACCF surgeries for OPLL with dura ossification (double-layer sign on axial CT images). Seven (22.6%) patients had CSF leakage in ACCF group, while only one (3.6%) in the ACAF group.

Lee et al[16] retrospectively compared 24 VBSO patients and 38 ACCF patients. The VBSO group showed a shorter mean operating time and less blood loss. Sixteen patients in the ACCF group experienced various complications, namely, neurologic deficit (2), CSF leakage (4), graft migration (3), and pseudarthrosis (7). In the VBSO group, only pseudarthrosis occurred only in 2 patients.

ACAF vs. Posterior Laminoplasty

Sun et al[17] reported a retrospective cohort of 80 OPLL patients and compared ACAF with single open-door laminoplasty. ACAF could achieve better clinical outcomes and relatively lower incidence of C5 palsy (1/42) compared with laminoplasty (4/38).

Chen et al[7] reported a prospective 1:1 randomized controlled study to compare ACAF with laminoplasty in the treatment of multilevel OPLL. C5 palsy (3/38 vs. 1/39) and axial pain (7/38 vs 2/39) occurred more commonly in laminoplasty group, whereas dysphagia (6/39 vs. 0/38) and hoarseness (4/39 vs. 1/38) appeared more commonly in ACAF group. At 1-year follow-up, the final JOA score and recovery rate were significantly higher in ACAF group when occupying ratio ≥ 60%, or K-line was negative.

ACAF vs. Posterior Laminectomy

Sun et al[8] retrospectively compared ACAF (38 patients) with posterior laminectomy (33 patients) for OPLL. At the final follow-up,

ACAF group achieved better cervical alignment and JOA improvement. As of complications, one dysphagia, one CSF leakage, and one C5 palsy occurred in ACAF group (7.8%), while there were one CSF leakage, one hematoma, and three C5 palsy in laminectomy group (15%).

ACAF as Revision Surgery

As a revision surgical technique after initial posterior surgery for OPLL, Yang et al[12] reported a cohort of 13 patients, in which the mean postoperative JOA score at last follow-up was significantly better than preoperation (14.8 ± 2.5 vs. 8.5 ± 2.7, $p < 0.01$), with a mean improvement rate of 75.3% ± 12.2%. No complications such as CSF leakage, spinal cord or nerve injury, subsidence and pseudoarthrosis occurred. Li et al[9] reviewed 10 patients with cervical OPLL who underwent ACAF revision surgery after initial posterior surgery with similar clinical outcome as Yang's report. One case of CSF leakage occurred.

ACAF for Degenerative Kyphosis and Stenosis

In a consecutive cohort of 49 patients with degenerative cervical kyphosis and stenosis, Yang et al[18] reported a mean JOA improvement rate of 79.8% (14.9 points vs. 9.0 points, $p < 0.01$). No surgery-related complications such as C5 palsy, hematoma, and spinal cord injury and infection occurred.

Case Presentation

Case 1 is a 58-year-old male patient with OPLL. He underwent posterior laminoplasty 8 years ago. Unfortunately, he experienced progressive neck pain, numbness, and weakness at all limbs after 4 years. On physical examination, he had decreased sensation below clavicle, increased tendon reflexes, and positive Hoffmann sign and Babinski sign. CT scan of cervical spine showed mixed type of OPLL from C4 through C7, with occupancy ratio of 53%, negative K-line, and double-layer

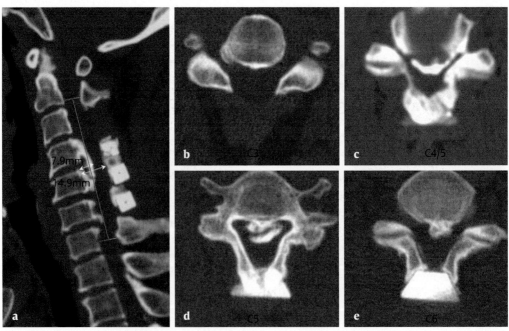

Fig. 13.2 Preoperative CT of a 58-year-old male OPLL patient. Sagittal view showed mixed type of OPLL from C4 through C7, with occupancy ratio of 53%, negative K-line (**a**). Axial view at C3 with laminectomy (**b**). The canal is most stenotic at C4/5 disc level (**c**). Double-layer sign at C5 level (**d**). OPLL at C6 after laminoplasty (**e**).

sign (**Fig. 13.2**). ACAF was planned and implemented uneventfully. The patient experienced immediate relief of all his symptoms after the surgery. Postoperative CT showed antedisplacement of C4-C6 vertebra-OPLL complex and apparent enlargement of spinal canal. Comparison of MRI before and after ACAF showed sufficient decompression of spinal cord (**Fig. 13.3**).

Case 2 is a 73-year-old male OPLL patient who endured numbness at bilateral upper extremities for 6 years. He reported a feeling of stepping on cotton while walking and gait disturbance for 11 months. Physical examination revealed increased tendon reflexes and positive Babinski sign bilaterally. Image workup concluded disc herniation at C3/4 and OPLL at C5 to C6 (**Fig. 13.4**). Hybrid surgery of ACAF and ACDF was conducted, and his symptoms were relieved.

Conclusion

ACAF is a safe and effective alternative for multilevel OPLL. ACAF exhibits more superior outcomes in the cases with large occupying ratio ($\geq 60\%$), negative K-line,[19] and cervical kyphosis. This technique may decrease complications such as dural tear and C5 nerve palsy. It can also serve as a revision surgical technique after initial posterior surgery for OPLL.

Take-home Points

- ACAF is a safe and effective alternative for multilevel OPLL.

- ACAF exhibits more superior outcomes in cases with large occupying ratio ($\geq 60\%$), negative K-line, and cervical kyphosis.

- ACAF may decrease complications such as dural tear and C5 nerve palsy.

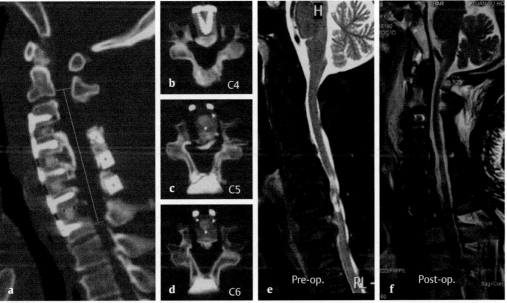

Fig. 13.3 Postoperative CT and MRI images of Case 2. Sagittal view after ACAF revealed enlargement of canal, and K-line changed to positive (**a**). Axial view of C4-C6 vertebrae showed the osteotomy slots bilaterally and antedisplacement of vertebra-OPLL complex (**b–d**). Preoperative MRI showed compression on spinal cord at C4–5 to C6–7 disc level. Hyperintense signal of spinal cord indicates chronic injury of spinal cord (**e**). Postoperative MRI exhibited excellent decompression of spinal cord (**f**).

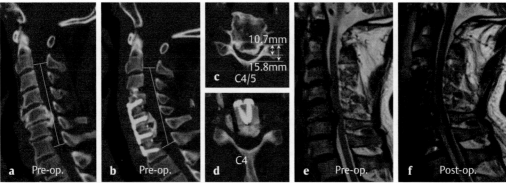

Fig. 13.4 Images of a 73-year-old male patient with OPLL and cervical disc herniation. Preoperative CT: sagittal view showed OPLL at C5 to C6 with a negative K-line; axial view at the most stenotic C4–5 disc level revealed wide ossification base and an occupancy ratio of 67.7% (**a, c**). After ACAF at C4 through C7 and ACDF at C3–4, postoperative CT exhibited enlargement of spinal canal and better cervical alignment (**b, d**). Preoperative MRI showed disc herniation at C3–4 and OPLL at C5 and C6 compressing spinal cord (**e**). Postoperative MRI indicated good decompression of spinal cord (**f**).

References

1. Wu J-C, Chen Y-C, Huang W-C. Ossification of the posterior longitudinal ligament in cervical spine: prevalence, management, and prognosis. Neurospine 2018;15(1):33–41

2. Boody BS, Lendner M, Vaccaro AR. Ossification of the posterior longitudinal ligament in the cervical spine: a review. Int Orthop 2019;43(4):797–805

3. Sun J, Shi J, Xu X, et al. Anterior controllable antidisplacement and fusion surgery for the treatment of multilevel severe ossification of the posterior longitudinal ligament with myelopathy: preliminary clinical results of a novel technique. Eur Spine J 2018;27(6): 1469–1478

4. Lee D-H, Cho JH, Lee CS, Hwang CJ, Choi SH, Hong CG. A novel anterior decompression technique (vertebral body sliding osteotomy) for ossification of posterior longitudinal ligament of the cervical spine. Spine J 2018; 18(6):1099–1105

5. Sun JC, Yang HS, Shi JG, et al. Morphometric analysis of the uncinate process as a landmark for anterior controllable antedisplacement and fusion surgery: a study of radiologic anatomy. World Neurosurg 2018;113:e101–e107

6. Kong Q-J, Sun X-F, Wang Y, et al. Risk assessment of vertebral artery injury in anterior controllable antedisplacement and fusion (ACAF) surgery: a cadaveric and radiologic study. Eur Spine J 2019;28(10):2417–2424

7. Chen Y, Sun J, Yuan X, et al. Comparison of anterior controllable antedisplacement and fusion with posterior laminoplasty in the treatment of multilevel cervical ossification of the posterior longitudinal ligament: a prospective, randomized, and control study with at least 1-year follow up. Spine 2020;45(16):1091–1101

8. Sun K, Wang S, Huan L, et al. Analysis of the spinal cord angle for severe cervical ossification of the posterior longitudinal ligament: comparison between anterior controllable antedisplacement and fusion (ACAF) and posterior laminectomy. Eur Spine J 2020;29(5):1001–1012

9. Li H-D, Zhang Q-H, Xing S-T, Min JK, Shi JG, Chen XS. A novel revision surgery for treatment of cervical ossification of the posterior longitudinal ligament after initial posterior surgery: preliminary clinical investigation of anterior controllable antidisplacement and fusion. J Orthop Surg Res 2018;13(1):215

10. Miao J, Sun J, Shi J, Chen Y, Chen D. A Novel Anterior Revision surgery for the treatment of cervical ossification of posterior longitudinal ligament: case report and review of the literature. World Neurosurg 2018;113:212–216

11. Yang H, Yang Y, Shi J, et al. Anterior Controllable Antedisplacement fusion as a choice for degenerative cervical kyphosis with stenosis: preliminary clinical and radiologic results. World Neurosurg 2018; 118:e562–e569

12. Yang H, Guo Y, Shi J, et al. Surgical results and complications of anterior controllable antedisplacement fusion as a revision surgery after initial posterior surgery for cervical myelopathy due to ossification of the posterior longitudinal ligament. J Clin Neurosci 2018;56:21–27

13. Sun J, Sun K, Wang Y, et al. Quantitative anterior enlargement of the spinal canal by anterior controllable antedisplacement and fusion for the treatment of cervical ossification of the posterior longitudinal ligament with myelopathy. World Neurosurg 2018;120:e1098–e1106

14. Yang H, Sun J, Shi J, Shi G, Guo Y, Yang Y. Anterior controllable antedisplacement fusion (ACAF) for severe cervical ossification of the posterior longitudinal ligament: comparison with anterior cervical corpectomy with fusion (ACCF). World Neurosurg 2018; 115:e428–e436

15. Yang H, Sun J, Shi J, et al. Anterior controllable antedisplacement fusion as a choice for 28 patients of cervical ossification of the posterior longitudinal ligament with dura ossification: the risk of cerebrospinal fluid leakage compared with anterior cervical corpectomy and fusion. Eur Spine J 2019; 28(2):370–379

16. Lee D-H, Riew KD, Choi SH, et al. Safety and efficacy of a novel anterior decompression technique for ossification of posterior longitudinal ligament of the cervical spine. J Am Acad Orthop Surg 2020;28(8):332–341

17. Sun K, Wang S, Sun J, et al. Surgical outcomes after anterior controllable antedisplacement and fusion compared with single open-door laminoplasty: preliminary analysis of postoperative changes of spinal cord displacements on T2-weighted magnetic resonance imaging. World Neurosurg 2019; 127:e288–e298

18. Yang H, Sun J, Shi J, et al. In situ decompression to spinal cord during anterior controllable antedisplacement fusion treating degenerative kyphosis with stenosis: surgical outcomes and analysis of C5 nerve palsy based on 49 patients. World Neurosurg 2018;115:e501–e508

19. Sun JC, Zhang B, Shi J, et al. Can K-Line predict the clinical outcome of anterior controllable antedisplacement and fusion surgery for cervical myelopathy caused by multisegmental ossification of the posterior longitudinal ligament? World Neurosurg 2018;116:e118–e127

14 The Role of Cervical Arthroplasty in the Surgical Treatment of Cervical Spondylotic Myelopathy

Óscar L. Alves and Rui Reinas

Introduction

Cervical spondylotic myelopathy (CSM) is the leading cause of adult spinal cord dysfunction worldwide, and surgical decompression remains the core treatment to arrest the progression of neurological deterioration. Short-term neurological improvement is directly related to the quality and extent of surgical decompression, which can be achieved by all classical surgical techniques.

When considering the anterior approach techniques to treat CSM, compressing the neural elements solely at the disc level, the options for reconstruction of the disc space are either interbody fusion or motion-preservation devices. Single- and multi-level anterior cervical discectomy and fusion (ACDF) have been considered the gold standard technique to treat cervical spondylosis. In the past two decades, the emerging technology of cervical arthroplasty has become a popular surgical option to treat cervical disc herniation or spondylosis, particularly for radiculopathy. When compared biomechanically to ACDF, cervical arthroplasty better mimics normal spine kinematics by preserving cervical motion segments, without compromising spinal cord and/or nerve roots decompression.[1] CSM being a multilevel disease affecting discs in different pathological stages, fusion may not be the universal answer. This opens the door to multilevel cervical arthroplasty and hybrid constructs as alternative techniques to preserve index level motion and putatively protect adjacent levels.[2] The interest of these techniques is evident in the face of growing incidence of

CSM among younger patients who will poorly tolerate multilevel fusion.[3]

Although many of the cervical arthroplasty clinical trials have included patients with medical refractory cervical radiculopathy, myelopathy, or both, caused by one- or two-level cervical disc herniation or spondylosis, none of these trials have specifically addressed patients with only myelopathy.[4–6] Not much evidence has been published to support cervical arthroplasty in the setting of CSM. For this reason, it remains largely intangible as to whether cervical arthroplasty is equally safe and effective as ACDF in management of patients with cervical myelopathy. On the other hand, the evolution of the biomechanical properties of the successive generations of cervical disc prosthesis offered the surgeon the possibility to expand the indications of arthroplasty in patients afflicted with cervical myelopathy. In this chapter, the authors review the major different aspects related to the use of cervical arthroplasty in myelopathic patients.

Clinical- and Imaging-Based Indications and Contraindications

Cervical arthroplasty is used in patients with radiculopathy or myelopathy due to compressive disc disease, and patients who have failed a course of optimized conservative treatment (rehabilitation and analgesic therapy). The Food and Drugs Administration (FDA) trials that enrolled adult patients excluded patients over 60 years old because they have a higher probability of presenting osteoporosis, facet joint arthrosis, or fusion, either favoring implant subsidence or limiting the range of motion (ROM) after cervical arthroplasty surgery.

The MRI is the gold standard for diagnosis and grading spinal canal and foraminal compression. Facet degeneration related to axial neck pain, advanced disc degenerative Modic changes (> grade 2), as well as a circumferential cord compression with a section around the cord (SAC) < 6 mm are contraindications for cervical arthroplasty. A study of patients with three-level myelopathy from congenital spinal stenosis found that hybrid two-level cervical arthroplasty with one-level ACDF had similar long-term outcomes as three-level ACDF, even though the postoperative cervical ROM improved.[7] Inclusion criteria for participation in this study were age (being less than 50 years) and cervical canal stenosis as defined by a Pavlov ratio ≤ 0.82.

The preoperative CT scans are useful for the detection of calcified disc, osteophytes, ossification of the posterior longitudinal ligament (OPLL), and facet arthropathy. Cervical arthroplasty has been shown to be effective in cervical myelopathy due to OPLL.[8] A study of patients with severe three-level cervical myelopathy from OPLL found that hybrid surgery with cervical arthroplasty combined with one-level anterior cervical corpectomy resulted in improvement in neck disability index (NDI), modified Japanese Orthopaedic

Association (mJOA) score, and preserved ROM across the cervical arthroplasty level at 12 months postoperatively.[9] However, OPLL, other than the localized type behind the disc, is a contraindication for cervical arthroplasty.

Both anteroposterior and lateral cervical radiographs information is of utmost importance to assess suitability of cervical arthroplasty. Preexisting cervical kyphotic deformity > 15°, ankylosis and spondylosis with disc height < 3 mm are considered contraindications for cervical arthroplasty.[10] On the dynamic lateral radiographs, one should value either the instability (> 3 mm translation/subluxation) or the restriction to motion due to facet joint arthrosis, both precluding cervical arthroplasty surgery. In multilevel disc disease, as for the single-level scenario, each level considered for operation needs to be carefully evaluated to rule out the contraindications for cervical arthroplasty in myelopathic patients, as summarized in **Box 14.1**.

Whenever translational instability is present, it should be underlined that nonconstrained implants are not recommended, since they are placed under a biomechanical stress beyond their capacity to maintain stability.[11] Regarding the significant loss of disc height (< 3 mm), considered to be a highway leading to ACDF, Patwardhan et al reported in six patients the feasibility of applying compressible disc prosthesis to slit

---

Box 14.1 Exclusion criteria for cervical arthroplasty in CSM

MRI: significant facet joint degeneration, Modic changes > 2, SAC < 6 mm
CT: large osteophytes, diffuse OPLL, ankylosis, facet arthropathy
Cervical radiographs: kyphotic deformity > 15°, spondylosis with disc height < 3 mm
Dynamic cervical radiographs: segmental motion restriction due to fused facets, instability (> 3 mm translation/subluxation)
Significant osteoporosis/osteopenia
Active infection at the operative site
Allergy to the implant components

Abbreviations: CSM, cervical spondylotic myelopathy; OPLL: ossification of posterior longitudinal ligament (other than type localized); SAC: section around the cord.

discs, with a significant increase in ROM and gain of disc height.[12]

A comprehensive knowledge of these factors reduces the rates of reoperation and complications in the long run and provides the patient with realistic expectations. As newer implants become available with a better biomechanical profile, clinical and radiological contraindications will be scrutinized and eventually revised.

Surgical Technique and Implant Options for Cervical Arthroplasty

In general, the surgical technique for cervical arthroplasty is far more demanding than ACDF, since the surgery aims to restore the physiological ROM while maintaining stability. However, the patient's positioning and the anterior approach, initial steps for cervical arthroplasty, are identical to a standard ACDF procedure. Caution should be taken to avoid overextension of the cervical spine, preventing intraoperative neural damage and the late occurrence of segmental kyphosis. As in myelopathic patients, more spondylotic slit discs are expected, a 4-mm burr drill should be used with care to reformat disc space, thus avoiding damaging the endplates; otherwise, the risk of implant subsidence would increase. A perfect, flat and smooth endplate preparation helps primary stability of parallel end plates cervical disc prosthesis (**Fig. 14.1**).

In multilevel cases, surgical decompression is always started from the inferior to the superior levels or at the most compressive level to release the spinal cord first. The insertion of cervical disc prosthesis always starts in the inferior levels, progressing upward with the aim of reconstructing the disc height, according to the healthy individuals disc height, since caudal discs tend to be higher than the more cephalad ones.[13]

For cervical arthroplasty surgery, resection of the posterior longitudinal ligament is recommended for a liberal decompression of the dura. Unlike ACDF, which partially relies on indirect decompression by distraction of the disc space with a tall bone graft or cage, cervical arthroplasty depends largely on direct decompression. Consequently, a resection of the bilateral uncovertebral joints, beyond the preexisting foraminal compression, is essential to ensure adequate decompression of neural foramen, in order to avoid recurrent radicular symptoms, resulting from nerve impingement during extreme motion after cervical arthroplasty.[14]

To achieve the best biokinematic outcome (ROM and center of rotation [COR] location) of cervical arthroplasty surgery, the prosthesis should be inserted properly, including centering, positioning, and alignment. Thus, a permanent notion of the midline throughout the surgery is important. Although there is no literature demonstrating the superiority of one implant over the other, it is advised to avoid using implants with keel, fin, or screws in myelopathic patients who are prone to osteopenia in order to avoid vertebral body fracture, subsidence, or loss of anterior body height in the long-term. Cervical

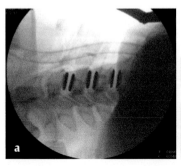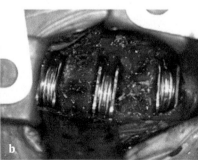

Fig. 14.1 Intraoperative views of a three-level cervical arthroplasty in a cervical myelopathy case. (**a**) lateral cervical radiograph view; (**b**) microscope view.

disc prosthesis with the proper height, commonly 6 mm high or less in most patients, and the largest footprint possible should be chosen to avoid complications such as subsidence, migration, heterotopic calcification, or absence of segmental motion by splaying the facet joints.[15]

Clinical Evidence in Favor of Cervical Arthroplasty in Cervical Spondylotic Myelopathy

Cervical Arthroplasty versus ACDF in Single-Level Surgery

In the literature, there is significant evidence, both with high-level quality and long-term follow-up, that speaks in favor of cervical arthroplasty in the treatment of single-level disc disease causing radiculopathy or myelopathy.[16–18] These prospective, randomized controlled trials include both myelopathic and nonmyelopathic patients, but without stratifying the results by each group. During flexion and extension, an averaged ROM preservation of 7 to 10 degrees per index level was consistently demonstrated unanimously across different devices in the long-term follow-up. Not surprisingly, cervical arthroplasty results in significant improvements in NDI, visual analogue scale (VAS)-arm pain, and VAS-neck pain in both myelopathy and nonmyelopathy populations. However, significant improvements are seen faster in nonmyelopathy populations.[19]

Cervical Arthroplasty versus ACDF in Multilevel Surgery

ACDF, considered the gold standard treatment option for multilevel degenerative disc disease, is associated with important caveats such as higher rates of pseudarthrosis and hardware failures, which are incremental with the number of operated levels, up to 26% and 44% of cases, respectively.[20,21] Moreover, the stiffness and rigidity created by multilevel fusion negatively impacts on neck mobility and on patient's quality of life, affecting clinical outcomes and the probability of reoperation at adjacent level.[22]

In recent years, data supporting the use of cervical arthroplasty for multilevel disc disease has increased. In their review of literature that included three prospective randomized studies and several retrospective studies (n = 1554, of which 947 were multilevel), Joaquim et al added evidence in favor of cervical arthroplasty for multilevel disc disease.[23]

Cervical Arthroplasty versus ACDF in Myelopathic Patients

No randomized trial to evaluate the efficacy of cervical arthroplasty over ACDF exclusively on myelopathic patients has been done so far. However, such randomized trials would not probably need a large number of patients to power it, as the minimal clinically important differences (MCID) between cervical arthroplasty and ACDF in the management of CSM would likely be more evident in multiple levels of disease in which case more segmental mobility is maintained by cervical arthroplasty. For one-level fusion, a loss of 7 to 10 degrees of ROM is often imperceptible. As CSM often affects several disc levels, the advantage of motion preservation in cervical arthroplasty surgery becomes more evident when compared to two- or three-level fusion (**Fig. 14.2**).

Regarding cervical arthroplasty for multilevel degenerative disc disease causing myelopathy, the results of the few prospective nonrandomized studies and randomized control trials unanimously demonstrated the improvement of neurological function after cervical arthroplasty.[7,24–28] Improvements in gait and neurologic function and rates of reoperation were also similar between cervical arthroplasty and ACDF at both 2- and 7-year follow-up. A retrospective study examined outcomes for cervical arthroplasty versus ACDF in patients with myelopathy and

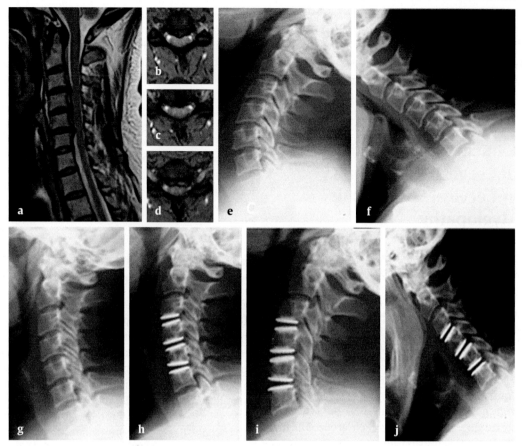

Fig. 14.2 Cervical arthroplasty in a three-level cervical spondylotic myelopathy (CSM) case. A 45-year-old, female, presenting with neck pain (visual analogue scale [VAS] score 7) and bilateral pain (VAS 8) and radiculopathy, with a modified Japanese Orthopaedic Association (mJoA) score = 14. The patient became asymptomatic and fully recovered with fine motor skills. Sagittal T2-weighted MRI showing spinal cord compression at disc level from C3–6 (**a**); Axial T2-weighted MRI confirming spinal cord and nerve roots compression (**b–d**); Lateral dynamic cervical radiographs exhibiting a fairly normal range of motion (ROM) and ruling out major instability (**e–g**); 3 years postoperative lateral dynamic cervical radiographs showing proper mobility of the disc prosthesis, absence of heterotopic calcification, and improvement of sagittal balance parameters on neutral view (**h–j**).

found surgery time to be longer for cervical arthroplasty but with lower rates of serious adverse events.[29] In 72 myelopathic patients treated with cervical arthroplasty, Fay et al reported at 3 years follow-up, a significant improvement on the average NDI and mJOA scores.[2] Only 4.2% (3/72) of the patients showed no movement across the prostheses despite heterotopic ossification being observed in 47.2% of patients.

Patients undergoing cervical arthroplasty seem to have superior outcomes on the mJOA, Nurick, and NDI/Oswestry disability index (ODI) scales according to some long-term retrospective cohort studies, but pooled analysis has not provided a clear superiority of cervical arthroplasty over ACDF or vice versa.[30,31] A meta-analysis (based on eight studies with a minimum 4-year follow-up) demonstrated a significantly higher index or adjacent level reoperation rate with ACDF (16.8%) when compared to cervical arthroplasty (7.4%).[32] However, prospective studies with long-term follow-up are required, including studies of hybrid constructs combining fusion and arthroplasty.

Hybrid constructs (combining in the same construct cervical arthroplasty and ACDF) have also been studied recently and may constitute a valid option for patients with different stages of spondylosis progression (**Fig. 14.3**). Cervical arthroplasty may be used in levels that are less spondylotic or expected to have a higher ROM (C5–6 as opposed to C6–7), whereas fusion can be applied in the more spondylotic, less mobile or high slippage levels. Hybrid constructs are described in literature as having a favorable biomechanical

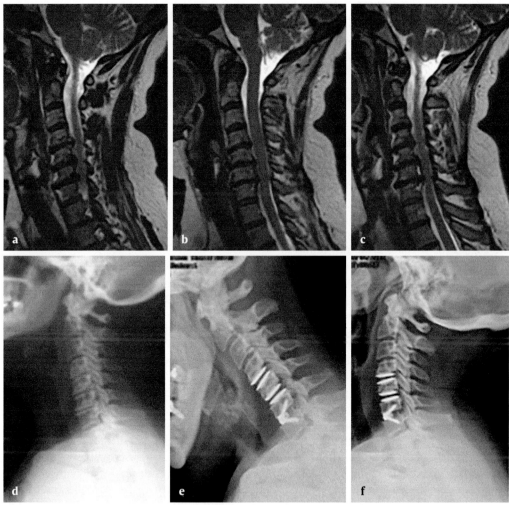

Fig. 14.3 Hybrid construct for three-level cervical spondylotic myelopathy (CSM), including cervical arthroplasty at C4–5 and C5–6, and ACDF at C6–7. A 55-year-old, female presenting with neck pain (visual analogue scale [VAS] score 6), multiradicular arm pain (VAS 8), and myelopathic signs (modified Japanese Orthopaedic Association (mJoA) score = 13). Cervical T2-weighted MRI sagittal views showing compression from C4 to C7 **(a–c)**; Preoperative neutral lateral cervical radiograph denoting an increased sagittal vertical alignment (SVA) **(d)**; 5 years postoperative dynamic, flexion and extension, lateral cervical radiographs showing a good sagittal balance and proper function of the cervical disc prosthesis **(e, f)**.

profile, since they preserve ROM at the index and adjacent natural level with minimal changes in center of rotation.[33,34] Not surprisingly, there is mounting evidence regarding better clinical outcomes with hybrid construct. In their meta-analysis comparing multilevel ACDF, cervical arthroplasty, and hybrid constructs in 442 patients, Hollyer et al found improvement in both global and segmental ROM and a shorter return to work compared to ACDF, while NDI and VAS were similar to those of multilevel cervical arthroplasty.[35] On the other hand, Hung et al found hybrid construct superior compared to two-level cervical arthroplasty in restoring cervical lordosis and sagittal vertical alignment (SVA).[34]

Cervical Arthroplasty in Patients with Milder Forms of Myelopathy

Patients with mild-to-moderate myelopathy are more likely to achieve a postoperative mJOA ≥ 16 or ≥ 12 after surgery for CSM if their preoperative baseline mJOA scores are higher, or if their symptom duration is shorter.[35,36] Furthermore, patients with mild CSM are usually younger in age with a substantial disease burden when assessed using quality of life scales such as the short form-36 (SF-36) v2 or SF-6D, as demonstrated by Badhiwala et al.[37] Surgery produced a dramatic improvement in these measures at 2-year follow-up, sometimes up to four times the MCID (SF-6D). Cervical arthroplasty may represent a window of opportunity to treat earlier patients with milder forms of myelopathy, achieving an MCID on the mJOA scale. Typically, these are patients with greater life expectancy, not affected by osteoporosis, and minimal facet joint degeneration.

Cost-effectiveness of Cervical Arthroplasty Surgery

One economic and decision analysis found that for radiculopathy patients, cervical arthroplasty resulted in lower long-term costs compared with ACDF.[38] Despite higher initial costs, as prosthesis tends to be more expensive than fusion cages, evidence for multilevel cervical arthroplasty may follow a similar trend. In the 2019 outcomes review by the Health Quality Ontario, two-level arthroplasty was found to be superior to fusion regarding not only clinical outcomes (greater satisfaction at 2 years of follow-up) but also lower costs over a span of 5 years.[39]

Biokinematic ROM and COR—Effect of Cervical Arthroplasty

Besides static compressive factors (osteophytes, congenital stenotic canal and OPLL) of the spinal cord, segmental instability also contributes to the pathophysiology of CSM.[40] However, there is no compelling evidence as to whether fusion is always mandatory after the decompression for cervical myelopathy, especially taking into consideration the prospect of hypermobility over the extremities of the fusion construct that may aggravate myelopathy in the long-term. On the other hand, cervical arthroplasty devices tend to mimic the quantity and the quality of motion at the index level, with a lasting effect in the majority of surgical levels for 5 to 10 years. The strategy of motion preservation yielded similar improvements of cervical myelopathy to motion elimination (ACDF) in patients with central canal stenosis, while the theoretical benefit of reducing adjacent segment disease (ASD), by limiting hypermobility, required further validation.[7] Besides ROM, quality of motion is critical for the outcome of cervical arthroplasty surgery. Liu et al found that a posterior location of the COR was associated with worse SF-36 and Nurick scores.[41] Consequently, an altered COR may affect negatively segmental and global ROM as shown by Lee et al.[42] Artificial discs with a mobile core having an additional degree of freedom, the anterior-posterior translation, will significantly provide more movement between the two vertebras. In addition to the mobile core, a cervical arthroplasty device with a compressible property will allow a more "physiological" COR that will effectively lower the mechanical load over adjacent discs, features that may be significant in mye-lopathic patients.[43]

Effect of Cervical Arthroplasty on Cervical Sagittal Balance

Cervical spine kyphosis plays a crucial role in the development and progression of CSM, as it leads to an anterior shift in the spinal cord, making it susceptible to anterior compres-sion and stretching, with the potential for ischemic phenomena.[44] A kyphotic deform-ity has a significant negative impact on the quality of life scores, and on the inability to maintain horizontal gaze and pain scores.[45] By projecting more anteriorly the axial load vector of the head, kyphosis produces through the loss of anterior vertebral height, with more and more kyphosis in the long term. Moreover, an SVA > 4 cm is associated with worsening of myelopathy scores.[46]

Uchida et al showed the benefit of align-ment correction in maximizing the potential for clinical improvement in patients with preoperative cervical kyphosis ≥ 10°, con-firming the importance of sagittal deform-ity correction.[47] Cervical arthroplasty may restore lordosis in selected CSM patients as shown by Park et al. They described in their series of 464 patients (n = 272 cervical arthro-plasty patients vs. n = 181 ACDF patients) an increase in segmental and global lordo-sis along with a marginal anteroinferior dis-placement of COR.[48] As shown in **Fig. 14.4**, from authors' own experience, based on a cohort of multilevel patients (n = 32, includ-ing three-level and four-level patients), an increase in segmental and global lordosis and a reduction of SVA compared to preoperative status while preserving ROM was demon-strated.[13] There is also evidence that it may be effective in segmental kyphosis caused by disc degeneration as reported by Kim et al.[49] Authors' own data showed compelling evi-dence of segmental kyphosis correction in 23 patients from a mean preoperative index

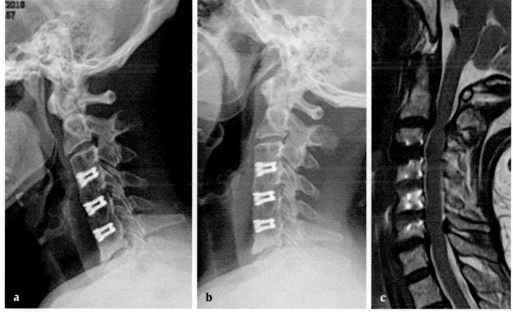

Fig. 14.4 Adjacent segment disease at the extremity levels (C2–3 and C6–7) of a three-level cervical fusion 5-years later.

level kyphosis of – 3.9° ± 3.52 to a lordosis of 3.4° ± 5.31 (in press).

When counseling patients for cervical arthroplasty surgery, it is worth knowing that the effect on sagittal alignment may not be immediate. As reported by Ahn et al, it may take weeks or months until the implant interface is fully integrated to the endplate and the structures of the functional segmental unit (FSU) adapt to the gain in mobility offered by the cervical arthroplasty, leading to a correction toward the physiological alignment of the patient.[50]

Relationship between Cervical Arthroplasty and Adjacent Segment Disease

Adjacent segment disease (ASD) is an elusive concept resulting either from the natural progression of cervical spondylosis or from the stiffness created by fusion at the index level, in an uncertain relative contribution of both factors (**Fig. 14.4**). The reports of ASD, and related reoperation rates, in the literature are biased according to patients' perceptions of the outcome and from the surgeons' expectations about the technique being used. The incidence of ASD is different if we consider radiological or clinical definitions. However, it seems clear that the majority of radiological ASD has no clinical translation. With these concepts in mind, it is very difficult to evaluate the real and meaningful incidence of ASD in cervical Arthroplasty when compared to ACDF.

As reported by Kong et al in a meta-analysis, including a total of 83 studies, the prevalence of radiographic ASD, symptomatic ASD, and reoperation ASD after cervical surgery was 28.3%, 13.3% and 5.8%, respectively, in a general analysis.[51] It was found that 2.8%, 1.4%, and 0.2% additions per year of follow-up in the incidence of radiographic ASD, symptomatic ASD, and reoperation ASD, respectively. Limitation of this study is the pooling of data from patients with different characteristics, devices, and surgical techniques.

Another meta-analysis included 11 studies with 2632 patients; comparing cervical arthroplasty against ACDF, the overall rate of ASD in cervical arthroplasty group was lower than ACDF group ($p < 0.00001$). Both the incidence of adjacent segment degeneration (ASDeg) and the reoperation rate were statistically lower in the cervical arthroplasty group than in the ACDF group ($p < 0.00001$ and $p = 0.01$, respectively). Subgroup analysis was performed according to the follow-up time, showing that the rate of ASDeg was lower in patients who underwent cervical arthroplasty no matter the follow-up time, and cervical arthroplasty tended to increase the superiority across time.[52]

In a smaller study of cervical arthroplasty patients, no significant differences were identified in 7-year clinical outcomes or adjacent level surgery for patients with or without myelopathy.[29] Due to the preservation of quality and the range of motion at the index level along with sagittal rebalancing, it would be expected a lower incidence of ASD in patients who underwent cervical arthroplasty than in those who underwent ACDF, especially in myelopathic patients. Thus, it may seem licit to select cervical arthroplasty purely in terms of mitigation of ASD in cervical myelopathy.

An interesting topic in evolving CSM context is the surgical management of ASD next to a prior fusion (**Fig. 14.5**). According to Lu et al, cervical arthroplasty confers similar surgical and postoperative outcomes in the treatment of ASD as ACDF. Both procedures lead to improvement in all performance outcomes.[53]

Long-term Tolerability and Safety of Multilevel Cervical Arthroplasty

As cervical arthroplasty patients tend to be younger than patients submitted to ACDF, with an increased life expectancy, doubts about safety and durability of cervical arthroplasty implants are pertinent. Additionally,

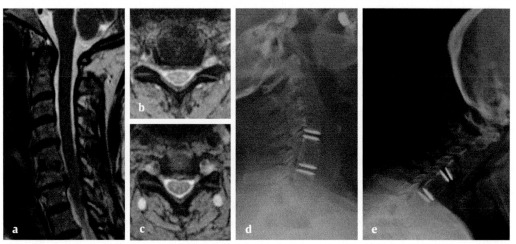

Fig. 14.5 A 50-year-old female admitted in 2010 to a C5–6 fusion, with neck pain (visual analogue scale [VAS] score 8) and L-arm pain (VAS 9) due to adjacent segment disease at C4–5 and C6–7 levels. Sagittal and axial T2-weighted cervical MRI showing compression at C4–5 and C6–7 levels **(a–c)**; 3 years postoperative dynamic, flexion and extension, lateral cervical radiographs showing two-level cervical arthroplasty next to an intermediate level previous fusion **(d, e)**.

this subgroup of patients may have a more demanding lifestyle, imposing increased stress loads, sometimes in extremes of the ROM, on their cervical disc prosthesis. Chen et al in a systematic review and a network meta-analysis, including 12 randomized control trials with follow-up from ranging 2 to 7 years, found that cervical arthroplasty implants, despite their differences in design and materials, are more durable than ACDF implants.[54] Cervical arthroplasty devices' durability is enhanced by a precise size selection, a proper surgical technique, as well as biomechanical profile that is closer to a normal cervical disc and that seems to be better achieved by semiconstrained structural devices.

Materials used in the manufacturing of these implants account for the durability with a plethora of polymers and alloys being used (cobalt-chromium, titanium, stainless steel, polyurethane, polyethylene).[15] Metal-on-metal interfaces display less wear and debris production than metal-on-polymer, but are susceptible to corrosion.[15,55] Osteolysis, mainly of upper endplate, has been described, without association with implant failure or overt infection.[56] Most studies published on

this issue have not disclosed significant negative clinical consequences, with revision surgeries being rare.[57]

Complications of Cervical Arthroplasty in Cervical Myelopathy

Medical and Postoperative Complications

Both ACDF and cervical arthroplasty have comparable postoperative complications and outcomes of patient with cervical radiculopathy or myelopathy.[58] As reported by Samuel et al, based on a large national cohort, medical complications were similarly low in both myelopathy and nonmyelopathy groups after cervical arthroplasty. There was no significant difference in discharge disposition to outside facility (1.2% vs. 1.7%, $p = 0.76$), serious medical complications (0.2% vs. 0.2%, p = 0.96), venous thromboembolism (0.1% vs. 0.2%, $p = 0.50$), surgical site infection (0.4% vs. 0.2%, $p = 0.66$), or blood transfusion (0.5% vs. 0.0%, $p = 0.15$).[19]

In one large cohort of ACDF patients, the presence of myelopathy was associated with increased rates of serious complications and death.[59] Contrary to what has been shown with ACDF patients in this study, myelopathy is not associated with increased perioperative morbidity and complications after cervical arthroplasty.[19] In their own local cohort, there were no intraoperative complications in any patients, including incidental durotomy, hematoma, neurological deficit, or surgical site infection.[19] In the national cohort (with 411 myelopathy patients out of 3023), Samuel et al reported no differences in complications between myelopathy and nonmyelopathy patients ($p > 0.05$), despite longer operative times and length of stay for the former ($p < 0.05$).[19]

Heterotopic Ossification (HO)

The ectopic bone formation around the cervical disc prosthesis may jeopardize the function of the device, attenuating the biokinematic advantage. The real impact of HO on the clinical outcome after cervical arthroplasty remains a debatable question. Actually, depending on the grade, HO formation is not always impeditive of a "useful" ROM. The incidence of HO varies in the literature largely, because it depends on the method of detection. Kong et al estimated progression of HO toward higher rates in their meta-analysis to be 0.63% per month.[60] Despite evidence that HO reduces ROM, its clinical significance is still under debate.[61,62]

Although the clinical outcomes are similar, it was reported that the incidence of HO formation after cervical arthroplasty was higher either in patients with soft disc herniation compared to spondylotic or calcified discs or in patients with multilevel disc herniation compared to single-level disease.[63,64] The device anchoring mechanism (more HO is associated with keel than with spikes), extent of noncovered endplate, as well as kyphotic positioning are other possible risk factors associated with HO.[15,65] Less violation of the endplate may be associated with lower rates HO.[66] Surgical technique may also be a determinant in the development of HO. Profuse irrigation to remove bone dust when implanting a cervical arthroplasty, waxing the exposed surface of cancellous bone, as well as giving nonsteroidal anti-inflammatory drugs (NSAIDs) postoperatively during 3 weeks will decrease the incidence of HO.[67] As authors reported in their review of multilevel cervical arthroplasty, the systematic removal of posterior ligament, which may act as a scaffold for ectopic bone formation, and the extensive removal of anterior and posterior osteophytes, are of utmost importance in reducing the rates of HO to 9.9% with at least 2 years follow-up.[14] Huppert et al found HO to be less prevalent in multilevel than single-level cervical arthroplasty over 24 months (175 patients single-level versus 56 patients two-level), while Zhao et al found no significant differences between both groups.[68,69]

Anterior Bone Loss of Vertebral Body

Anterior bone loss (ABL) after cervical arthroplasty may be a relevant complication in the context of CSM, as the disease courses with loss of vertebral body height. Kieser et al in a retrospective study with nonkeeled cervical arthroplasty ($n = 146$) and with a minimum follow-up of 5 years found that ABL is common (57.1%).[70] It occurs at an early stage (within 3 months) and typically follows a nonprogressive natural history with stable radiographic features after the first year. Most ABL cases are mild, but severe ABL occurs in approximately 3% of cervical arthroplasty patients. The greater the number of levels operated, the higher the risk of developing ABL. The development of ABL has no long-term effect on the mechanical functioning of the disc or necessity for revision surgery, although it may increase the rate of fusion.[70]

Conclusion

As long as myelopathy is caused by pathology situated exclusively behind the disc level and there is no rigidity or major instability, it should be amenable to treatment by arthroplasty. Once the compressive pathology, soft disc, or hard spurs is removed, the myelopathy should resolve. When multilevel disease is present, fusion is not mandatory after decompression for cervical myelopathy, especially in younger patients.

There is no question that relatively less evidence has been published to support the use of cervical arthroplasty in the setting of CSM compared to fusion. Further literature with robust evidence needs to be gathered on the efficacy of combining neural decompression with motion preservation and appropriate and enduring sagittal alignment. The current available technology, a generous decompression of the neural elements, accurate sizing of the device, and appropriately centered implant placement are the cornerstones of successful cervical arthroplasty surgery, especially in myelopathic patients.

The prospect of a widespread use of cervical arthroplasty in the treatment strategy of CSM may represent a significant paradigm shift that would allow patients to be treated at earlier stages of the disease with an expected improvement on the outcome. Nevertheless, the key to successful and widespread cervical arthroplasty surgery in myelopathic patients depends on strict patient selection and further developing of custom-made implants, better materials and devices design.

Take-home Points

- Contraindications for cervical arthroplasty are:
  - Axial neck pain related to facet degeneration.
  - Advanced disc degeneration; Modic changes > grade 2.
  - Circumferential cord compression with a section around the cord (SAC < 6 mm).
  - OPLL, other than the localized type, behind the disc.
  - Preexisting cervical kyphotic deformity > 15°
  - Ankylosis and spondylosis with disc height < 3 mm.
  - Instability (> 3 mm translation/subluxation).
  - Restriction to motion due to facet joint arthrosis.
- Unlike ACDF, which partially relies on indirect decompression by distraction of the disc space with a tall bone graft or cage, cervical arthroplasty depends largely on direct decompression. Consequently, a resection of the bilateral uncovertebral joints, beyond the preexisting foraminal compression, is essential to ensure adequate decompression of neural foramen, in order to avoid recurrent radicular symptoms resulting from nerve impingement during extreme motion after cervical arthroplasty.
- Cervical disc prosthesis should be inserted properly, including centering, positioning and alignment in order to achieve the best biokinematic outcome (ROM and COR location) of cervical arthroplasty surgery.
- Cervical disc prosthesis with the proper height, commonly 6 mm high or less in most patients, and the largest footprint possible should be chosen to avoid complications such as subsidence, migration, heterotopic calcification, or absence of segmental motion by splaying the facet joints.
- Cervical arthroplasty results in significant improvements in NDI, VAS-arm pain, and VAS-neck pain in both myelopathy and nonmyelopathy populations in single-level disc disease.
- As CSM often affects several disc levels, the advantage of motion preservation in cervical arthroplasty surgery becomes more evident when compared to two- or three-level fusion.

- Hybrid constructs (combining cervical arthroplasty and ACDF in the same construct) constitute a valid option for patients with different stages of spondylosis progression. Cervical arthroplasty may be used in levels that are less spondylotic or expected to have a higher ROM (C5–6 as opposed to C6–7), whereas fusion can be applied in the more spondylotic, less mobile or high slippage levels.

- Cervical arthroplasty represents a window of opportunity to treat earlier patients with milder forms of myelopathy, achieving a MCID on the mJOA scale.

- Two-level arthroplasty is superior to fusion regarding not only clinical outcomes (greater satisfaction at 2 years of follow-up), but also lower costs over the span of 5 years.

- In addition to the mobile core, a cervical arthroplasty device with a compressible property will allow a more "physiological" COR, which will effectively lower the mechanical load over adjacent disc features that may be significant in myelopathic patients.

- An increase in segmental and global lordosis and a reduction of SVA compared to preoperative status, while preserving ROM, were demonstrated with cervical arthroplasty

- The rate of ASDeg is lower in patients who underwent cervical arthroplasty no matter the follow-up time, and cervical arthroplasty tended to increase the superiority across time.

- Cervical arthroplasty implants, despite their differences in design and materials, are more durable than ACDF implants. Cervical arthroplasty devices durability is enhanced by a precise size selection, a proper surgical technique, as well as biomechanical profile that is closer to a normal cervical disc and that seems to be better achieved by semiconstrained structural devices.

- Myelopathy is not associated with increased perioperative morbidity and complications after cervical arthroplasty.

- The incidence of heterotopic ossification (HO) varies largely, because it depends on the method of detection. Despite evidence that HO reduces ROM, its clinical significance is still under debate.

- The incidence of HO formation after cervical arthroplasty was higher either in patients with soft disc herniation compared to spondylotic or calcified discs or in patients with multilevel disc herniation compared to single-level disease. Surgical technique may be also determinant in the development of HO. The device anchoring mechanism (more HO is associated with keel than with spikes), the extent of noncovered endplate, endplate violation, as well as kyphotic positioning are other possible risk factors associated to HO.

References

1. Chang CC, Huang WC, Wu JC, Mummaneni PV. The option of motion preservation in cervical spondylosis: cervical disc arthroplasty update. Neurospine 2018;15(4):296–305

2. Fay LY, Huang WC, Wu JC, et al. Arthroplasty for cervical spondylotic myelopathy: similar results to patients with only radiculopathy at 3 years' follow-up. J Neurosurg Spine 2014; 21(3):400–410

3. Amenta PS, Ghobrial GM, Krespan K, Nguyen P, Ali M, Harrop JS. Cervical spondylotic myelopathy in the young adult: a review of the literature and clinical diagnostic criteria in an uncommon demographic. Clin Neurol Neurosurg 2014;120:68–72

4. Coric D, Guyer RD, Nunley PD, et al. Prospective, randomized multicenter study of cervical arthroplasty versus anterior cervical discectomy and fusion: 5-year results with a metal-on-metal artificial disc. J Neurosurg Spine 2018;28(3):252–261

5. Hisey MS, Zigler JE, Jackson R, et al. Prospective, randomized comparison of one-level Mobi-C cervical total disc replacement vs. anterior cervical discectomy and fusion: results at 5-year follow-up. Int J Spine Surg 2016;10:10

6. Gornet MF, Burkus JK, Shaffrey ME, Nian H, Harrell FE Jr. Cervical disc arthroplasty with prestige LP disc versus anterior cervical discectomy and fusion: seven-year outcomes. Int J Spine Surg 2016;10:24

7. Chang PY, Chang HK, Wu JC, et al. Is cervical disc arthroplasty good for congenital cervical stenosis? J Neurosurg Spine 2017; 26(5):577–585

8. Wu JC, Chen YC, Huang WC. Ossification of the posterior longitudinal ligament in cervical spine: prevalence, management, and prognosis. Neurospine 2018;15(1):33–41

9. Chang HC, Tu TH, Chang HK, et al. Hybrid corpectomy and disc arthroplasty for cervical spondylotic myelopathy caused by ossification of posterior longitudinal ligament and disc herniation. World Neurosurg 2016;95:22–30

10. Koreckij TD, Gandhi SD, Park DK. Cervical disc arthroplasty. J Am Acad Orthop Surg 2019;27(3):e96–e104

11. Sears WR, McCombe PF, Sasso RC. Kinematics of cervical and lumbar total disc replacement. Semin Spine Surg 2006;18:117–129

12. Patwardhan AG, Carandang G, Voronov LI, et al. Are collapsed cervical discs amenable to total disc arthroplasty?: analysis of prospective clinical data with 2-year follow up. Spine 2016;41(24):1866–1875

13. Reinas R, Kitumba D, Pereira L, Baptista AM, Alves OL. Multilevel cervical arthroplasty-clinical and radiological outcomes. J Spine Surg 2020;6(1):233–242

14. Tu TH, Chang CC, Wu JC, Fay LY, Huang WC, Cheng H. Resection of uncovertebral joints and posterior longitudinal ligament for cervical disc arthroplasty. Neurosurg Focus 2017;42(VideoSuppl1):V2

15. Taksali S, Grauer JN, Vaccaro AR. Material considerations for intervertebral disc replacement implants. Spine J 2004; 4(6, Suppl)231S–238S

16. Vaccaro A, Beutler W, Peppelman W, et al. Long-term clinical experience with selectively constrained SECURE-C cervical artificial disc for 1-level cervical disc disease: results from seven-year follow-up of a prospective, randomized, controlled investigational device exemption clinical trial. Int J Spine Surg 2018;12(3):377–387

17. Burkus JK, Traynelis VC, Haid RW Jr, Mummaneni PV. Clinical and radiographic analysis of an artificial cervical disc: 7-year follow-up from the Prestige prospective randomized controlled clinical trial: clinical article. J Neurosurg Spine 2014;21(4):516–528

18. Turel MK, Kerolus MG, Adogwa O, Traynelis VC. Cervical arthroplasty: what does the labeling say? Neurosurg Focus 2017;42(2):E2

19. Samuel AM, Moore HG, Vaishnav AS, et al. Effect of myelopathy on early clinical improvement after cervical disc replacement: a study of a local patient cohort and a large national cohort. Neurospine 2019;16(3):563–573

20. Buttermann GR. Anterior cervical discectomy and fusion outcomes over 10 years: a prospective study. Spine 2018;43(3):207–214

21. Laratta JL, Reddy HP, Bratcher KR, McGraw KE, Carreon LY, Owens RK II. Outcomes and revision rates following multilevel anterior cervical discectomy and fusion. J Spine Surg 2018;4(3):496–500

22. Wang QL, Tu ZM, Hu P, et al. Long-term results comparing cervical disc arthroplasty to anterior cervical discectomy and fusion: a systematic review and meta-analysis of randomized controlled trials. Orthop Surg 2020;12(1):16–30

23. Joaquim AF, Riew KD. Multilevel cervical arthroplasty: current evidence. A systematic review. Neurosurg Focus 2017;42(2):E4

24. Chen YC, Kuo CH, Cheng CM, Wu JC. Recent advances in the management of cervical spondylotic myelopathy: bibliometric analysis and surgical perspectives. J Neurosurg Spine 2019;31(3):299–309

25. Chang HK, Huang WC, Wu JC, et al. Should cervical disc arthroplasty be done on patients with increased intramedullary signal intensity on magnetic resonance imaging? World Neurosurg 2016;89:489–496

26. Riew KD, Buchowski JM, Sasso R, Zdeblick T, Metcalf NH, Anderson PA. Cervical disc arthroplasty compared with arthrodesis for the treatment of myelopathy. J Bone Joint Surg Am 2008;90(11):2354–2364

27. Sekhon LH. Cervical arthroplasty in the management of spondylotic myelopathy. J Spinal Disord Tech 2003;16(4):307–313

28. Chang HK, Chang CC, Tu TH, et al. Can segmental mobility be increased by cervical arthroplasty? Neurosurg Focus 2017;42(2):E3

29. Gornet MF, McConnell JR, Riew KD, et al. Treatment of cervical myelopathy: long-term outcomes of arthroplasty for myelopathy versus radiculopathy, and arthroplasty

versus arthrodesis for myelopathy. Clin Spine Surg 2018;31(10):420–427

30. Traynelis VC, Arnold PM, Fourney DR, Bransford RJ, Fischer DJ, Skelly AC. Alternative procedures for the treatment of cervical spondylotic myelopathy: arthroplasty, oblique corpectomy, skip laminectomy: evaluation of comparative effectiveness and safety. Spine 2013; 38(22, Suppl 1):S210–S231

31. Zheng B, Hao D, Guo H, He B. ACDF vs TDR for patients with cervical spondylosis - an 8 year follow up study. BMC Surg 2017;17(1):113

32. Wu TK, Liu H, Wang BY, Meng Y. Minimum four-year subsequent surgery rates of cervical disc replacement versus fusion: A meta-analysis of prospective randomized clinical trials. Orthop Traumatol Surg Res 2017;103(1):45–51

33. Laratta JL, Shillingford JN, Saifi C, Riew KD. Cervical disc arthroplasty: a comprehensive review of single-level, multilevel, and hybrid procedures. Global Spine J 2018;8(1):78–83

34. Hung CW, Wu MF, Yu GF, Ko CC, Kao CH. Comparison of sagittal parameters for anterior cervical discectomy and fusion, hybrid surgery, and total disc replacement for three levels of cervical spondylosis. Clin Neurol Neurosurg 2018;168:140–146

35. Hollyer MA, Gill EC, Ayis S, Demetriades AK. The safety and efficacy of hybrid surgery for multilevel cervical degenerative disc disease versus anterior cervical discectomy and fusion or cervical disc arthroplasty: a systematic review and meta-analysis. Acta Neurochir (Wien) 2020;162(2):289–303

36. Tetreault L, Wilson JR, Kotter MR, et al. Predicting the minimum clinically important difference in patients undergoing surgery for the treatment of degenerative cervical myelopathy. Neurosurg Focus 2016;40(6):E14

37. Badhiwala JH, Witiw CD, Nassiri F, et al. Efficacy and safety of surgery for mild degenerative cervical myelopathy: results of the AOSpine North America and international prospective multicenter studies. Neurosurgery 2019;84(4):890–897

38. Ghori A, Konopka JF, Makanji H, Cha TD, Bono CM. Long term societal costs of anterior discectomy and fusion (ACDF) versus cervical disc arthroplasty (CDA) for treatment of

cervical radiculopathy. Int J Spine Surg 2016;10:1

39. Health Quality Ontario. Cervical artificial disc replacement versus fusion for cervical degenerative disc disease: a health technology assessment. Ont Health Technol Assess Ser 2019;19(3):1–223. eCollection 2019

40. Matsunaga S, Sakou T, Taketomi E, Yamaguchi M, Okano T. The natural course of myelopathy caused by ossification of the posterior longitudinal ligament in the cervical spine. Clin Orthop Relat Res 1994; (305):168–177

41. Liu S, Lafage R, Smith JS, et al. Impact of dynamic alignment, motion, and center of rotation on myelopathy grade and regional disability in cervical spondylotic myelopathy. J Neurosurg Spine 2015;23(6):690–700

42. Lee JH, Lee JH. The feasibility of optimal surgical result prediction according to the center of rotation shift after multilevel cervical total disc replacement. Asian Spine J 2020;14(4):445–452

43. Patwardhan AG, Tzermiadianos MN, Tsitsopoulos PP, et al. Primary and coupled motions after cervical total disc replacement using a compressible six-degree-of-freedom prosthesis. Eur Spine J 2012;21(Suppl 5):S618–S629

44. Chavanne A, Pettigrew DB, Holtz JR, Dollin N, Kuntz C IV. Spinal cord intramedullary pressure in cervical kyphotic deformity: a cadaveric study. Spine 2011; 36(20):1619–1626

45. Tan LA, Riew KD, Traynelis VC. Cervical spine deformity-part 1: biomechanics, radiographic parameters, and classification. Neurosurgery 2017;81(2):197–203

46. Smith JS, Lafage V, Ryan DJ, et al. Association of myelopathy scores with cervical sagittal balance and normalized spinal cord volume: analysis of 56 preoperative cases from the AOSpine North America Myelopathy study. Spine 2013; 38(22, Suppl 1):S161–S170

47. Uchida K, Nakajima H, Sato R, et al. Cervical spondylotic myelopathy associated with kyphosis or sagittal sigmoid alignment: outcome after anterior or posterior decompression. J Neurosurg Spine 2009; 11(5):521–528

48. Park DK, Lin EL, Phillips FM. Index and adjacent level kinematics after cervical disc

replacement and anterior fusion: in vivo quantitative radiographic analysis. Spine 2011;36(9):721–730

49. Kim SW, Shin JH, Arbatin JJ, Park MS, Chung YK, McAfee PC. Effects of a cervical disc prosthesis on maintaining sagittal alignment of the functional spinal unit and overall sagittal balance of the cervical spine. Eur Spine J 2008;17(1):20–29

50. Ahn PG, Kim KN, Moon SW, Kim KS. Changes in cervical range of motion and sagittal alignment in early and late phases after total disc replacement: radiographic follow-up exceeding 2 years. J Neurosurg Spine 2009;11(6):688–695

51. Kong L, Cao J, Wang L, Shen Y. Prevalence of adjacent segment disease following cervical spine surgery: A PRISMA-compliant systematic review and meta-analysis. Medicine (Baltimore) 2016;95(27):e4171

52. Xu S, Liang Y, Zhu Z, Qian Y, Liu H. Adjacent segment degeneration or disease after cervical total disc replacement: a meta-analysis of randomized controlled trials. J Orthop Surg Res 2018;13(1):244

53. Lu VM, Mobbs RJ, Phan K. Clinical outcomes of treating cervical adjacent segment disease by anterior cervical discectomy and fusion versus total disc replacement: a systematic review and meta-analysis. Global Spine J 2019;9(5):559–567

54. Chen C, Zhang X, Ma X. Durability of cervical disc arthroplasties and its influence factors: A systematic review and a network meta-analysis. Medicine (Baltimore) 2017;96(6):e5947

55. Michel R, Hofmann J, Löer F, Zilkens J. Trace element burdening of human tissues due to the corrosion of hip-joint prostheses made of cobalt-chromium alloys. Arch Orthop Trauma Surg 1984;103(2):85–95

56. Harati A, Oni P, Oles L, Reuter T, Hamdan M. Vertebral body osteolysis 6 years after cervical disc arthroplasty. J Neurol Surg A Cent Eur Neurosurg 2020;81(2):188–192

57. Cavanaugh DA, Nunley PD, Kerr EJ III, Werner DJ, Jawahar A. Delayed hyper-reactivity to metal ions after cervical disc arthroplasty: a case report and literature review. Spine 2009;34(7):E262–E265

58. Hu Y, Lv G, Ren S, Johansen D. Mid- to long-term outcomes of cervical disc arthroplasty versus anterior cervical discectomy and fusion for treatment of symptomatic cervical disc disease: a systematic review and meta-analysis of eight prospective randomized controlled trials. PLoS One 2016;11(2):e0149312

59. Lukasiewicz AM, Basques BA, Bohl DD, Webb ML, Samuel AM, Grauer JN. Myelopathy is associated with increased all-cause morbidity and mortality following anterior cervical discectomy and fusion: a study of 5256 patients in American College of Surgeons National Surgical Quality Improvement Program (ACS-NSQIP). Spine 2015;40(7):443–449

60. Kong L, Ma Q, Meng F, Cao J, Yu K, Shen Y. The prevalence of heterotopic ossification among patients after cervical artificial disc replacement: A systematic review and meta-analysis. Medicine (Baltimore) 2017;96(24):e7163

61. Yang X, Bartels RHMA, Donk R, et al. Does Heterotopic Ossification in Cervical Arthroplasty Affect Clinical Outcome? World Neurosurg 2019;131:e408–e414

62. Barbagallo GM, Corbino LA, Olindo G, Albanese V. Heterotopic ossification in cervical disc arthroplasty: Is it clinically relevant? Evid Based Spine Care J 2010;1(1):15–20

63. Wu JC, Huang WC, Tu TH, et al. Differences between soft-disc herniation and spondylosis in cervical arthroplasty: CT-documented heterotopic ossification with minimum 2 years of follow-up. J Neurosurg Spine 2012;16(2):163–171

64. Wu JC, Huang WC, Tsai HW, et al. Differences between 1- and 2-level cervical arthroplasty: more heterotopic ossification in 2-level disc replacement: Clinical article. J Neurosurg Spine 2012;16(6):594–600

65. Yang MMH, Ryu WHA, Casha S, DuPlessis S, Jacobs WB, Hurlbert RJ. Heterotopic ossification and radiographic adjacent-segment disease after cervical disc arthroplasty. J Neurosurg Spine 2019 (e-pub ahead of print). doi:10.3171/2019.5.SPINE19257

66. Mehren C, Wuertz-Kozak K, Sauer D, Hitzl W, Pehlivanoglu T, Heider F. Implant design and the anchoring mechanism influence the incidence of heterotopic ossification in cervical total disc replacement at 2-year follow-up. Spine 2019;44(21):1471–1480

67. Tu TH, Wu JC, Huang WC, Wu CL, Ko CC, Cheng H. The effects of carpentry on heterotopic ossification and mobility in cervical arthroplasty: determination by computed tomography with a minimum 2-year follow-up: clinical article. J Neurosurg Spine 2012;16(6):601–609

68. Huppert J, Beaurain J, Steib JP, et al. Comparison between single- and multi-level patients: clinical and radiological outcomes 2 years after cervical disc replacement. Eur Spine J 2011;20(9):1417–1426

69. Zhao H, Cheng L, Hou Y, et al. Multi-level cervical disc arthroplasty (CDA) versus single-level CDA for the treatment of cervical disc diseases: a meta-analysis. Eur Spine J 2015;24(1):101–112

70. Kieser DC, Cawley DT, Fujishiro T, et al. Risk factors for anterior bone loss in cervical disc arthroplasty. J Neurosurg Spine 2018; 29(2):123–129

15

Cervical Laminoplasty

Se-Hoon Kim and Maurizio Fornari

Introduction

Degenerative cervical myelopathy (DCM) causes compression of the spinal cord, posing significant problems and resulting in daily dysfunction. DCM includes cervical spondylotic myelopathy (CSM), ossification of the posterior longitudinal ligament (OPLL), ossification of ligamentum flavum (OLF), and degenerative disk disease (DDD) (**Fig. 15.1**).[1-4]

Cervical laminoplasty aims to enlarge the spinal canal, provide spinal stability, and preserve the spine's protective function.

Mobility preservation of the spine is also the goal of this procedure for multiple-level involvement.

Selection of the Surgical Approach in Degenerative Cervical Myelopathy

Operative treatment is chosen if the symptoms of CSM or OPLL are disturbing the patient significantly. Surgery is a common treatment choice for patients with severe

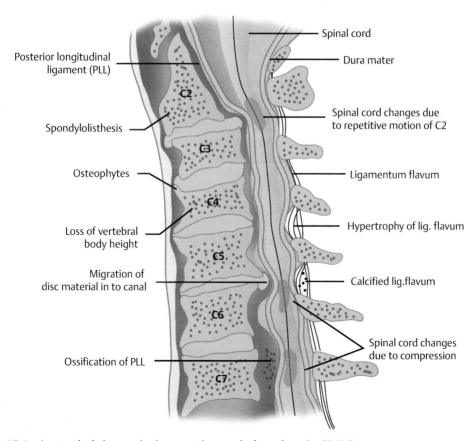

Fig. 15.1 Anatomical changes in degenerative cervical myelopathy (DCM).[4]

myelopathy symptoms, mainly if an imbalance in walking and hand function loss develops. Surgical management of CSM patients aims to decompress the spinal cord, provide sagittal alignment, and stabilize the spine.[4] There are mainly two treatment options: anterior and posterior approaches. For this decision, one should consider several factors: (1) sagittal curvature, (2) location of the compression, (3) the number of levels affected, and (4) the patient's comorbidities.[4,5] Some other factors affecting the surgeon's choice of approach include the extent of ventral compression (modified K-line +/−)[6,7] and the presence of radiculopathy, including pain, numbness, or weakness.[4]

Background

The primary approach to the cervical spinal canal was the anterior approach developed by Smith and Robinson[8] and Cloward.[9] A broad and extensive laminectomy was necessary for an adequate dorsal shift of the spinal cord and if the stability of the spine was provided. The so-called laminectomy membrane, which is a thick epidural scar formation due to laminectomy hematoma, could occasionally cause a worse outcome.[10]

Due to the poor results of conventional laminectomy for CSM, Japanese spine surgeons introduced laminoplasty procedures in the 1970s.[11,12] To avoid distortion of the spinal cord by the resected laminae edges, Kirita and Miyazaki developed simultaneous decompression laminectomy.[13,14] Oyama et al improved a laminoplasty technique by Z-plasty of the thinned laminae and preservation of the dorsal wall of the spinal canal, which is called Z-shaped laminoplasty.[10,15]

Hirabayashi et al introduced a new laminoplasty technique in 1977, which was called expansive open-door laminoplasty.[10–12] The advantages of the procedure included simultaneous decompression of multilevel spinal cord, earlier mobilization of the patients, better neck support, prevention of kyphotic deformity, and restriction of mobility of the cervical spine, which are useful to prevent

late neurologic deterioration and progression of OPLL.[10–12]

The laminoplasty technique introduced by Hirabayashi has had various modifications since then to improve the safety and efficacy of posterior decompression and stability of the cervical spine.[10,16]

Cervical Laminoplasty for CSM and OPLL

The anterior, posterior, and combined approaches have some advantages and disadvantages. The optimal approach for handling multilevel CSM is still under discussion. The anterior approach has some advantages: easy removing of disk herniation, osteophytes, and OPLL; it can relieve postoperative pain. The anterior approach is also preferred for CSM with kyphosis. However, many studies have stated that the posterior approach should be considered for multilevel CSM.[4,17] Anterior decompression with graft placement and fusion is preferred in CSM cases with a kyphotic and straightened cervical spine along with compression at fewer than three levels. Such an intervention should be done to relieve pressure in the nerve and spinal cord. The anterior approach effectively reduces the clinical symptoms of cervical radiculopathy and anterior midline and/or paramedian compressive pathology. On the other hand, posterior decompression should be chosen in case of cervical lordosis, with more than three levels of compression and posterior ligamentous hypertrophy and ossification.[4,18]

Advantages and Disadvantages of Laminoplasty

The spinal canal expands more at its central part in bilateral hinge laminoplasty. However, the expansion of the canal is maximum at its opening side in unilateral hinge laminoplasty. In unilateral open-door laminoplasty, a significant increase of the cervical spinal canal has been demonstrated using CT scan.[19] A dorsal migration of the spinal cord has also been confirmed with CT myelography after both laminoplasty types.[20,21] In the unilateral hinge type laminoplasty, a nerve root decompression can be done by a careful partial facetectomy.[10]

Major disadvantages of a laminectomy are the development of kyphosis and a thick epidural scar, which causes late neurologic worsening. However, after laminoplasty, the spared laminae shield the spinal cord from the pressure of hematoma during the early postoperative periods and prevent scar tissue in the late period.[10]

The theoretical advantages of laminoplasty include the fact that the spinal cord can be indirectly decompressed, and the spondylotic protrusions impinging on the neural tissue are left intact. During anterior decompression, removing hard tissues of osteophytes and cartilages encroaching on the already compromised neural tissue is the riskiest portion of the surgery.[10] A second advantage is that laminoplasty facilitates obtaining hemostasis around the affected spinal cord. Hemostasis during anterior surgery for CSM or OPLL should be done more carefully and meticulously. Such procedures may threaten the spinal cord that is already distressed.[10] A third advantage is that laminoplasty allows some other nerve root decompression procedures or reinforcement of spinal stability. Partial facetectomy to decompress the roots on the opening side may also be done. To provide stability, bone grafting in either side and one segment or multiple segments may also be applied.[10]

There are mainly two disadvantages of laminoplasty; first, the cervical spine range of motion (ROM) is reduced, particularly in extension, lateral bending, and rotation.[10,19,22] This restriction is more prominent when laminotomy or hinges are located at the facet in either expansive open-door laminoplasty or spinous process-splitting laminoplasty. The second disadvantage is the discomfort of the neck or axial neck pain after laminoplasty. Neck pain is one of the most discouraging complications.[10,23]

Indications and Contraindications of Laminoplasty

General indications for laminoplasty are continuous or mixed type of OPLL, multilevel (> 2 vertebrae) CSM, or congenital spinal canal stenosis (AP canal diameter < 13 mm) with posterior compression and syringomyelia.[4,24] The best candidates for laminoplasty are patients with multisegmental OPLL and a developmentally narrow spinal canal which do not exhibit significant kyphosis of the cervical spine. Laminoplasty also helps reach the spinal cord in tumors, vascular problems, and functional surgery, in which procedures such as laminectomy are difficult.[4,10,25]

For one- or two-level CSM without developmental spinal canal stenosis, anterior discectomy and arthrodesis would be the treatment of choice rather than laminoplasty. A kyphotic cervical spine is a contraindication for laminoplasty. Laminoplasty cannot correct a fixed kyphotic deformity to a lordotic curve.[10]

Techniques of Laminoplasty and the Modifications of the Procedures

None of the laminoplasty types has been proven to have statistical superiority to any of the other procedures with regard to the neurologic and radiological outcomes.

The patient is placed in the prone position on an operating table to decrease the abdominal pressure. A three-point Mayfield pin fixation of the head is strongly recommended to secure the head. The cervical spine must be kept in a neutral position or slight extension.

Through a dorsal midline skin incision, the nuchal ligament is divided at the midline. In most CSM cases, the extent of decompression should be from C3 to C6, in order to provide a complete dorsal migration of the spinal cord. Surgeons may differ regarding placement and the laminotomy method for the opening side and the gutter for the hinge.

Unilateral Hinge Laminoplasty

Expansive Open-Door Laminoplasty by Hirabayashi

Hirabayashi performed the first case of open-door laminoplasty in a patient with OPLL in 1977 and named the technique "expansive laminoplasty". In 1982, he described the first series of patients treated using expansive laminoplasty with encouraging results.[12,26]

The spinous processes are exposed taking care so as not to damage the supraspinous and interspinous ligaments.[27] A gutter is then created at the junction of the lamina and articular processes with a burr. The laminotomy is then performed along the gutter with a thin-bladed Kerrison rongeur on the opening side. Another gutter is created on the hinge side. This gutter should better be more lateral than the gutter on the opening side.

The laminae's opening is secured by sutures placed on the facet joint capsule on the hinge side and the corresponding laminae.[10,26,27]

The author performs a safe preparation of the gutter on the hinge side using a 2-mm sized high-speed drill burr, and laminotomy on the opening side using a novel ultrasonic osteotome or ultrasonic bone curette device (**Fig. 15.2**). A gentle elevation of the laminae is performed using a Raney applier (**Fig. 15.3**).[19]

Modifications to Expansive Open-Door Laminoplasty

In 1973, Hattori et al developed an expansive laminoplasty involving Z-plasty of the laminae.[15] This technique provided a reconstruction of the complete cervical spinal canal except for the spinous processes. However, this technique did not become popular since it required highly meticulous skill and was time-consuming.

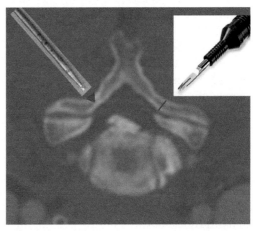

Fig. 15.2 Safe preparation of gutters for laminoplasty. Preparation of gutter on the hinge side is made using a 2-mm diameter high-speed drill and laminotomy on the opening side, using a novel ultrasonic osteotome or ultrasonic bone-cutter device.[19]

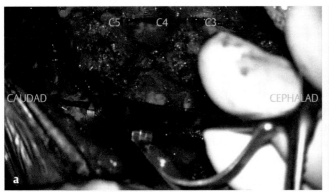
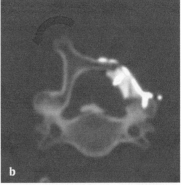

Fig. 15.3 Gentle elevation of lamina using Raney applier. After making laminotomy on the opening side using a novel ultrasonic osteotome, a Raney applier is inserted into the lamina opening, with gentle pressure on each spinous process toward hinge side to separate bony edges (**a**). A properly selected hydroxyapatite spacer and a malleable titanium miniplate complex are secured on the opening side using miniscrews (**b**).[19]

If the elevated laminae are not fixed firmly, the enlargement of the spinal canal may be reduced, and the resultant "spring-back closure of lamina" occurs. Since 1977, when the original expansive laminoplasty was devised, the open-door technique itself has also undergone a variety of modifications by many surgeons throughout the world, including the use of bone grafts, spacers, titanium mini plates, and other instrument systems, to address problems of spring-back closure of lamina or an established kyphotic deformity.[19,22,28,29–35]

Itoh and Tsuji described "en-bloc laminoplasty," in which the spinous processes are cut at their bases and preserved for bone grafting through a conventional posterior midline approach.[28] The laminae are lifted en-bloc, usually from C3 to C7. The grafts prepared from the resected spinous processes are placed between the edges of laminae at C4 and C6 and the articular processes. The grafts support the elevated lamina. The laminae and bone grafts are then secured in position with steel wires.[28]

Bilateral Hinge Laminoplasty

Spinous Process-Splitting Laminoplasty by Kurokawa

A standard posterior approach is made along the nuchal ligament to the line of the spinous processes. The spinous processes are cut in the midline with a high-speed burr to split them sagittally. Bilateral gutters for the hinges are crafted again with a high-speed burr at the transitional area between the facet joint and lamina; spinal canal enlargement is achieved by opening the split laminae bilaterally with a spreader and placing corticocancellous iliac crest autografts, which are held in place with sutures or wire.[10,36] Foraminotomy is often very difficult to perform in the bilateral hinge laminoplasty, compared to unilateral hinge laminoplasty. With unilateral open laminoplasty, foraminotomy or facetectomy can be performed on the side.[10]

A hydroxyapatite spacer can also be substituted for an autogenous bone graft.[37] Tomita modified the spinous process splitting procedure using a thread-wire saw in expansive midline "T-saw laminoplasty," with the advantages of reducing mean surgery time and mean blood loss compared to the original method.[38]

Modifications and Supplementary Procedures to Laminoplasty

The nuchal muscles and ligaments play an important role in the stabilization of the cervical spine. After laminoplasty, the nuchal muscles are reattached to their origins by suturing the bony fragments to the spinous process' tip. Ono reported that C3–C6 laminoplasty, in which the C7 spinous process is preserved, reduces invasion of the nuchal muscles.[39]

To preserve the spinous process–ligament–muscle complex, the laminae on one side are exposed, and the nuchal, supraspinous, and interspinous ligaments are kept intact; the spinous processes are then cut at their bases, and the laminae on the opposite side are exposed by retracting the nuchal muscles laterally with the resected spinous process.[40]

Several procedures of less invasive laminoplasty have been developed to decrease axial pain and maintain cervical ROM. Takeuchi modified conventional C3–C7 laminoplasty to C4–C7 laminoplasty with C3 laminectomy, and found that the modified laminoplasty, preserving the semispinalis cervicis inserted into C2, reduced the postoperative axial symptoms compared to conventional C3–C7 laminoplasty, reattaching the muscle to C2.[41] Hosono et al prospectively reduced the range of laminoplasty from C3–C7 to C3–C6, preserving muscles attached to the C2 and C7 spinous processes. They found that preservation of the C7 process was beneficial to reduce the axial pain and C3–C6 laminoplasty maintained satisfactory long-term neurologic improvement and recommended that C3–C6 laminoplasty is a promising alternative to conventional C3–C7 laminoplasty for treatment of multisegmental compression myelopathy.[42,43]

Kim developed a new method, myoarchitectonic spinolaminoplasty, which preserves all of the nuchal muscles and reconstitutes all musculoskeletal couplings to the posterior elements of the vertebrae. He found that myoarchitectonic spinolaminoplasty effectively preserved the volume and functions of the nuchal musculature and helped to minimize postoperative musculoskeletal complaints, with significantly reduced incidence of neck pain and shoulder strain.[16]

Outcomes of Laminoplasty

Clinical Outcome

Very few studies have been conducted concerning differences in surgical outcome based on the particular procedure used. The recovery rate after various laminoplasties is reported to range from 50 to 70%. So far, no approach has been proven to be statistically superior to the others, suggesting that the outcome is likely to be identical, provided that the procedure is done correctly.

Herkowitz compared the outcomes of anterior cervical fusion, laminectomy, and laminoplasty for multiple cervical spondylotic radiculopathy. He concluded that although anterior cervical fusion provided the best results, laminoplasty provided an effective alternative to anterior fusion.[10,44]

Radiological Outcome

None of the laminoplasty types can guarantee lifelong spinal stability, except when it is supplemented with spinal fusion. Although laminoplasty relatively preserves the posterior elements compared to laminectomy, postoperative ROM decrease after laminoplasty has been frequently described in the literature.[19,45] The type of laminoplasty, the extent of exposure, the location of laminotomy, the use of bone grafting, and the postoperative rehabilitation program, including the period of neck immobilization, may influence the degree of ROM loss.[10] There are several reported reasons for the decrease of ROM after laminoplasty. Seichi et al said that only 22% of preoperative ROM was maintained after laminoplasty.[36] They mentioned that the facet joints' unexpected fusion caused the loss of ROM after laminoplasty. The high-fusion rate in their series may have occurred because they used the iliac crest as struts for the laminoplasty.[36] Meyer noted that plated laminoplasty led to a loss of ROM in extension.[46] In the author's study of modified open-door laminoplasty using hydroxyapatite laminar spacers and titanium miniplates, the percentage of ROM preservation was 73.32%. Authors assumed that this decrease of ROM might have occurred partly as a result of impingement of the opened lamina, leading to mild restriction of extension.[19]

The authors fixated the lifted lamina with a spacer at the lamina-facet junction using miniscrews.

When it is fixed with a miniplate, it provides immediate and rigid stabilization of the posterior elements of the cervical spine. It helps to maintain continuous expansion of lamina, even in hinge-side fracture during laminar elevation. The authors note that it is a technically safe technique, as it provides a stable construct, avoiding reclosure and dislodgement (**Figs. 15.4** and **15.5**).[19]

Complications of Cervical Laminoplasty

Yonenobu et al reported that patients who underwent laminoplasty demonstrated a significantly lower complication rate than those who underwent corpectomy (7 vs. 29%).[4,24] Reported complications resulting from cervical laminoplasty include injury to the spinal

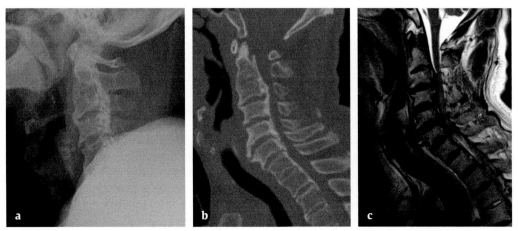

Fig. 15.4 A 70-year-old man with severe ossification of the posterior longitudinal ligament (OPLL) slipped on ice and exhibited cervical myelopathy and tetraparesis. Preoperative lateral radiograph (**a**) and sagittal CT scan (**b**) delineating extensive OPLL. Preoperative T2-weighted sagittal MR image (**c**).

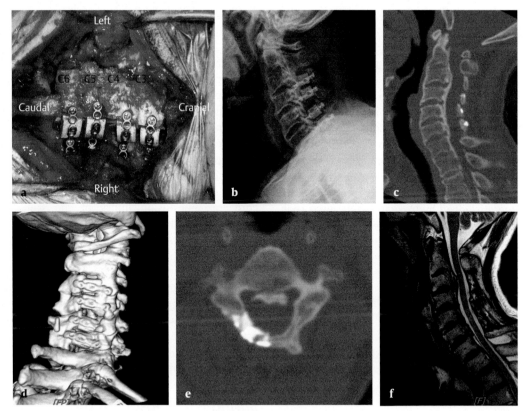

Fig. 15.5 An illustrative case of a successful four-level open-door laminoplasty (C3–6) using hydroxyapatite (HA) spacers and titanium miniplates. Intraoperative photo (**a**), 1-year postoperative lateral radiograph (**b**), sagittal CT scan (**c**), 3D CT scan (**d**), axial CT scan (C4 level) (**e**), and T2-weighted sagittal MR image (**f**).

cord and nerve roots, nerve root palsy (typically C5 palsy), spring-back closure of the elevated lamina, and complications related to laminar spacers.[4]

Spinal Cord Injury

Although iatrogenic spinal cord damage is most commonly attributed to direct mechanical trauma, such as inadvertent cord manipulation, blunt forces directly onto the spinal cord, and introducing of an instrument under the lamina, vascular or ischemic factors, such as intraoperative hypotension and over distraction, may also contribute to neurologic compromise.[47] It is also notable that the hyperextension of the neck required for intubation could cause compression of the spinal cord, resulting in a central cord injury in a patient with a severely stenotic cervical spinal canal.[48–50]

Spinal cord injury can be caused by fracture of a hinge or loss of spinal canal enlargement after laminoplasty, resulting from the insufficient fixation of the lifted laminae and the lamina's consequent migration into the spinal canal. Immediate and rigid stabilization of the reconstructed laminae has also been proposed in a laminoplasty using titanium miniplates.[19,32] Several cases of delayed dural damage and spinal cord compression from dislodged hydroxyapatite laminar spacers due to absorption of the tip of the spinous process have been reported following double-door laminoplasty.[51,52]

Nerve Root Palsy

Postoperative motor root deficits, typically involving the C5 root (C5 palsy), can highly vary from 5.5 to 15% and are significantly more frequent after posterior procedures compared to anterior ones.[47,53] The incidence of C5 palsy from dorsal approaches has been reported to range from 0 to 30%, with an average of 4.6%.[54–58] In a recent meta-analysis on the incidence of C5 palsy for patients after cervical surgery, the incidence after

laminoplasty was 4.4% and the one after laminectomy and fusion was 12.2%.[59]

The postoperative C5 palsy has been defined as postoperative upper extremity paresis, mainly the deltoid muscle and biceps brachii muscle, without accompanying deterioration of the underlying myelopathy symptoms. Several investigations revealed that upper extremity palsy after laminoplasty developed in other cervical nerve roots (C6, C7, or C8) in isolation or in combination, associated with high-signal intensity areas in the spinal cord on T2-weighted MR imaging.[10,60,61]

The postoperative C5 palsy onset is most often within the first week, but the delayed presentation has been reported from 2 to 6 weeks postoperatively.[54,56–58]

Although not all cases fully recover, with conservative treatment and time, most nerve root palsies resolve spontaneously within 3 to 6 months postoperatively, sometimes within 2 years.[47,57,62]

Sakaura et al have suggested five possible pathways that may contribute to postoperative C5 palsy. These include intraoperative accidental injury to the nerve root, traction or tethering of the nerve root from an excessive dorsal shift of spinal cord after decompression, ischemia to the nerve root and spinal cord from the decreased blood supply, segmental dysfunction of the spinal cord, or reperfusion injury of the spinal cord.[54,58] According to Pan et al, foraminotomy and intraoperative neuromonitoring are the two main methods used to prevent C5 palsy.[4,63]

Since the exact etiology of the segmental motor palsy may be controversial and multifactorial, and no preventive tools have been established, the potential risk of nerve root palsy after laminoplasty should be informed to patients preoperatively.

Spring-Back Closure of the Elevated Lamina

Spring-back closure of the elevated lamina has a reported rate of 40% after laminoplasty.[4,64] However, this complication has only been reported with suture fixation and has yet to be observed in modern screw or plate fixation.[4,65]

Durotomy and Cerebrospinal Fluid (CSF) Leakage

The incidental dural tears can occur while an electrocautery device is used during a posterior exposure, while a Kerrison rongeur is used during a posterior foraminotomy, and while the lamina is elevated during a laminoplasty.[66]

The prevalence of cervical dural tears has been reported to range from 0.5 to 3%.[66–68]

The durotomy's potential etiologies include monopolar cautery slipping between the lamina and injury with the high-speed drill or Kerrison rongeur. Most durotomies are small, and the CSF leak is usually easily controlled with gel foam tamponade and tight closure of the fascia. Compared with the use of the high-speed drill, applying an ultrasonic osteotome or ultrasonic bone curette in patients undergoing cervical laminoplasty could reduce the incidence of inadvertent durotomy.[69]

Fracture of a Hinge

Fracture of a hinge and loss of spinal canal enlargement from the insufficient fixation of the elevated lamina can cause nerve root palsy or spinal cord compression when a lamina migrates into the spinal canal. To prevent the fracture of a hinge in laminoplasty, the lamina's inner cortex on the hinge side should be thinned step-by-step. At the same time, its mobility is assessed until the surgeon is very familiar with the procedure.[10]

In the case of hinge-side fracture, a salvage procedure of rigid fixation of the reconstructed laminae using titanium miniplates has been proposed in the literature.[19,32]

Hematoma

Neurologic deterioration from hematoma after cervical laminoplasty has decreased because reconstructed laminae still possesses a protective function that diminishes blood pooling and soft-tissue swelling after surgery.[10]

Ophthalmologic Complications

Important risk factors for developing postoperative visual loss include positioning and complexity of the surgery. Prone positioning without Mayfield pins was associated with higher incidences than anterior surgical approaches. The incidence of postoperative visual loss was three times higher with spinal fusion procedures than with simple decompression.[70,71] To prevent ophthalmologic complications, preoperatively, the surgeon should review and optimize a patient's medical comorbid conditions, particularly diabetes mellitus and glaucoma. Intraoperatively, the surgeon must place the patient's head in rest or clamp that minimizes direct pressure on the orbits, such as a Mayfield head-holder, in prone positioning.

Conclusion

Cervical laminoplasty for DCM, including CSM and OPLL, is a useful technique for improving patients' neurological function through spinal decompression.

After introducing the epoch-making laminoplasty by Hirabayashi, various modifications and supplementary procedures have been proposed to further improve the safety and efficacy of posterior decompression and the cervical spine's stability.

The advantages and disadvantages of each laminoplasty should be carefully considered along with proper indications and contraindications of the laminoplasty for a successful outcome.

Take-home Points

- Cervical laminoplasty must aim to expand the spinal canal, provide stability to the spine, and preserve the spine's protective function.

- After introducing the epoch-making expansive open-door laminoplasty by Hirabayashi in 1977, various modifications and supplementary procedures have been developed to further improve the safety and efficacy of posterior decompression and the stability of the cervical spine.

- General indications for laminoplasty are a continuous or mixed type of OPLL, multilevel (> 2 vertebrae) CSM, or congenital spinal canal stenosis (AP canal diameter < 13 mm) with posterior compression and syringomyelia.

- Possible cervical laminoplasty complications are injury to the spinal cord and nerve roots, nerve root palsy (typically C5 palsy), spring-back closure of the elevated lamina, durotomy and CSF leakage, fracture of the hinge, ophthalmologic complications, and so on.

References

1. Lad SP, Patil CG, Berta S, Santarelli JG, Ho C, Boakye M. National trends in spinal fusion for cervical spondylotic myelopathy. Surg Neurol 2009;71(1):66–69, discussion 69

2. Klineberg E. Cervical spondylotic myelopathy: a review of the evidence. Orthop Clin North Am 2010;41(2):193–202

3. Nouri A, Tetreault L, Singh A, Karadimas SK, Fehlings MG. Degenerative cervical myelopathy: epidemiology, genetics, and pathogenesis. Spine 2015;40(12):E675–E693

4. Bajamal AH, Kim SH, Arifianto MR, et al; World Federation of Neurosurgical Societies (WFNS) Spine Committee. Posterior surgical techniques for cervical spondylotic myelopathy: WFNS spine committee recommendations. Neurospine 2019;16(3):421–434

5. Bridges KJ, Simpson LN, Bullis CL, Rekito A, Sayama CM, Than KD. Combined laminoplasty and posterior fusion for cervical spondylotic myelopathy treatment: a literature review. Asian Spine J 2018;12(3):446–458

6. Fujiyoshi T, Yamazaki M, Kawabe J, et al. A new concept for making decisions regarding the surgical approach for cervical ossification of the posterior longitudinal ligament: the K-line. Spine 2008;33(26):E990–E993

7. Taniyama T, Hirai T, Yoshii T, et al. Modified K-line in magnetic resonance imaging predicts clinical outcome in patients with nonlordotic alignment after laminoplasty for cervical spondylotic myelopathy. Spine 2014;39(21):E1261–E1268

8. Smith GW, Robinson RA. The treatment of certain cervical-spine disorders by anterior removal of the intervertebral disc and interbody fusion. J Bone Joint Surg Am 1958;40-A(3):607–624

9. Cloward RB. The anterior approach for removal of ruptured cervical disks. J Neurosurg 1958;15(6):602–617

10. Wada E, Yonenobu K. Treatment of cervical myelopathy: laminoplasty. In: Benzel EC, ed. The Cervical Spine. 5th ed. Philadelphia, PA: Lippincott Williams & Wilkins; 2012: 980–994

11. Hirabayashi K, Miyakawa J, Satomi K, Maruyama T, Wakano K. Operative results and postoperative progression of ossification among patients with ossification of cervical posterior longitudinal ligament. Spine 1981; 6(4):354–364

12. Hirabayashi K, Watanabe K, Wakano K, Suzuki N, Satomi K, Ishii Y. Expansive open-door laminoplasty for cervical spinal stenotic myelopathy. Spine 1983;8(7):693–699

13. Kirita Y. Posterior decompression for cervical spondylosis and ossification of the posterior longitudinal ligament. [in Japanese] Shujutu. 1976;30:287

14. Miyazaki K, Kirita Y. Extensive simultaneous multisegment laminectomy for myelopathy due to the ossification of the posterior longitudinal ligament in the cervical region. Spine 1986;11(6):531–542

15. Oyama M, Hattori S, Moriwaki N. A new method of posterior decompression. [in Japanese] Chubuseisaisi. 1973;16:792

16. Kim P, Murata H, Kurokawa R, Takaishi Y, Asakuno K, Kawamoto T. Myoarchitectonic spinolaminoplasty: efficacy in reconstituting the cervical musculature and preserving

biomechanical function. J Neurosurg Spine 2007;7(3):293–304

17. Rhee JM, Basra S. Posterior surgery for cervical myelopathy: laminectomy, laminectomy with fusion, and laminoplasty. Asian Spine J 2008;2(2):114–126

18. Liu JK, Das K. Posterior fusion of the subaxial cervical spine: indications and techniques. Neurosurg Focus 2001;10(4):E7

19. Jin SW, Kim SH, Kim BJ, et al. Modified open-door laminoplasty using hydroxyapatite spacers and miniplates. Korean J Spine 2014;11(3):188–194

20. Aita I, Hayashi K, Wadano Y, Yabuki T. Posterior movement and enlargement of the spinal cord after cervical laminoplasty. J Bone Joint Surg Br 1998;80(1):33–37

21. Sodeyama T, Goto S, Mochizuki M, Takahashi J, Moriya H. Effect of decompression enlargement laminoplasty for posterior shifting of the spinal cord. Spine 1999;24(15): 1527–1531, discussion 1531–1532

22. Shin JW, Jin SW, Kim SH, et al. Predictors of outcome in patients with cervical spondylotic myelopathy undergoing unilateral open-door laminoplasty. Korean J Spine 2015;12(4):261–266

23. Hosono N, Yonenobu K, Ono K. Neck and shoulder pain after laminoplasty. A noticeable complication. Spine 1996;21(17):1969–1973

24. Yonenobu K, Hosono N, Iwasaki M, Asano M, Ono K. Laminoplasty versus subtotal corpectomy. A comparative study of results in multisegmental cervical spondylotic myelopathy. Spine 1992;17(11):1281–1284

25. Ghasemi AA, Behfar B. Outcome of laminoplasty in cervical spinal cord injury with stable spine. Asian J Neurosurg 2016; 11(3):282–286

26. Hirabayashi K, Watanabe K. A review of my invention of expansive laminoplasty. Neurospine 2019;16(3):379–382

27. Hirabayashi K. Expansive open door laminoplasty. In: Shark HH, et al. eds. The Cervical Spine. An Atlas of Surgical Procedures. Philadelphia, PA: JB Lippincott; 1994:233–250

28. Itoh T, Tsuji H. Technical improvements and results of laminoplasty for compressive myelopathy in the cervical spine. Spine 1985;10(8):729–736

29. Satomi K, Takahashi M, Ogawa J. Significances of using laminar spacer on postoperative cervical alignment in cervical expansive

laminoplasty. [in Japanese]. East Jpn J Clin Orthop. 1994;6:1–4

30. Tani S, Suetsua F, Mizuno J, et al. New titanium spacer for cervical laminoplasty: initial clinical experience. Technical note. Neurol Med Chir (Tokyo) 2010;50(12):1132–1136

31. Matsuoka H, Ohara Y, Kimura T, Kikuchi N, Nakajima Y, Mizuno J. Clinical outcome and radiological findings after cervical open door laminoplasty with titanium basket. J Clin Neurosci 2020;73:140–143

32. Frank E, Keenen TL. A technique for cervical laminoplasty using mini plates. Br J Neurosurg 1994;8(2):197–199

33. O'Brien MF, Peterson D, Casey AT, Crockard HA. A novel technique for laminoplasty augmentation of spinal canal area using titanium miniplate stabilization. A computerized morphometric analysis. Spine 1996;21(4):474–483, discussion 484

34. Wang JM, Roh KJ, Kim DJ, Kim DW. A new method of stabilising the elevated laminae in open-door laminoplasty using an anchor system. J Bone Joint Surg Br 1998;80(6):1005–1008

35. Kobayashi Y, Matsumaru S, Kuramoto T, et al. Plate fixation of expansive open-door laminoplasty decreases the incidence of postoperative C5 palsy. Clin Spine Surg 2019;32(4):E177–E182

36. Seichi A, Takeshita K, Ohishi I, et al. Long-term results of double-door laminoplasty for cervical stenotic myelopathy. Spine 2001; 26(5):479–487

37. Nakano K, Harata S, Suetsuna F, Araki T, Itoh J. Spinous process-splitting laminoplasty using hydroxyapatite spinous process spacer. Spine 1992; 17(3, Suppl):S41–S43

38. Tomita K, Kawahara N, Toribatake Y, Heller JG. Expansive midline T-saw laminoplasty (modified spinous process-splitting) for the management of cervical myelopathy. Spine 1998;23(1):32–37

39. Ono A, Tonosaki Y, Yokoyama T, et al. Surgical anatomy of the nuchal muscles in the posterior cervicothoracic junction: significance of the preservation of the C7 spinous process in cervical laminoplasty. Spine 2008;33(11):E349–E354

40. Liu J, Ebraheim NA, Sanford CG Jr, et al. Preservation of the spinous process-ligament-muscle complex to prevent kyphotic deformity following laminoplasty. Spine J 2007;7(2):159–164

41. Takeuchi K, Yokoyama T, Aburakawa S, et al. Axial symptoms after cervical laminoplasty with C3 laminectomy compared with conventional C3-C7 laminoplasty: a modified laminoplasty preserving the semispinalis cervicis inserted into axis. Spine 2005; 30(22):2544–2549

42. Hosono N, Sakaura H, Mukai Y, Fujii R, Yoshikawa H. C3-6 laminoplasty takes over C3-7 laminoplasty with significantly lower incidence of axial neck pain. Eur Spine J 2006;15(9):1375–1379

43. Sakaura H, Hosono N, Mukai Y, Iwasaki M, Yoshikawa H. C3-6 laminoplasty for cervical spondylotic myelopathy maintains satisfactory long-term surgical outcomes. Global Spine J 2014;4(3):169–174

44. Herkowitz HN. A comparison of anterior cervical fusion, cervical laminectomy, and cervical laminoplasty for the surgical management of multiple level spondylotic radiculopathy. Spine 1988;13(7):774–780

45. Ratliff JK, Cooper PR. Cervical laminoplasty: a critical review. J Neurosurg 2003; 98(3, Suppl):230–238

46. Meyer SA, Wu JC, Mummaneni PV. Laminoplasty outcomes: is there a difference between patients with degenerative stenosis and those with ossification of the posterior longitudinal ligament? Neurosurg Focus 2011;30(3):E9

47. Epstein NE. Cervical myelopathy: laminectomy. In: Benzel EC, ed. The Cervical Spine. 5th ed. Philadelphia, PA: Lippincott Williams & Wilkins; 2012:970–979

48. Rhee KJ, Green W, Holcroft JW, Mangili JA. Oral intubation in the multiply injured patient: the risk of exacerbating spinal cord damage. Ann Emerg Med 1990;19(5): 511–514

49. Muckart DJ, Bhagwanjee S, van der Merwe R. Spinal cord injury as a result of endotracheal intubation in patients with undiagnosed cervical spine fractures. Anesthesiology 1997;87(2):418–420

50. Saldua NS, Harrop JS. Iatrogenic spinal cord injuries. In: Benzel EC, ed. The Cervical Spine. 5th ed. Philadelphia, PA: Lippincott Williams & Wilkins; 2012:1321–1325

51. Ono A, Yokoyama T, Numasawa T, Wada K, Toh S. Dural damage due to a loosened hydroxyapatite intraspinous spacer after spinous process-splitting laminoplasty. Report of two cases. J Neurosurg Spine 2007; 7(2):230–235

52. Kanemura A, Doita M, Iguchi T, Kasahara K, Kurosaka M, Sumi M. Delayed dural laceration by hydroxyapatite spacer causing tetraparesis following double-door laminoplasty. J Neurosurg Spine 2008;8(2):121–128

53. Zdeblick TA, Zou D, Warden KE, McCabe R, Kunz D, Vanderby R. Cervical stability after foraminotomy. A biomechanical in vitro analysis. J Bone Joint Surg Am 1992; 74(1):22–27

54. Sakaura H, Hosono N, Mukai Y, Ishii T, Yoshikawa H. C5 palsy after decompression surgery for cervical myelopathy: review of the literature. Spine 2003;28(21):2447–2451

55. Greiner-Perth R, Elsaghir H, Böhm H, El-Meshtawy M. The incidence of C5-C6 radiculopathy as a complication of extensive cervical decompression: own results and review of literature. Neurosurg Rev 2005; 28(2):137–142

56. Takemitsu M, Cheung KM, Wong YW, Cheung WY, Luk KD. C5 nerve root palsy after cervical laminoplasty and posterior fusion with instrumentation. J Spinal Disord Tech 2008;21(4):267–272

57. Imagama S, Matsuyama Y, Yukawa Y, et al; Nagoya Spine Group. C5 palsy after cervical laminoplasty: a multicentre study. J Bone Joint Surg Br 2010;92(3):393–400

58. Dafford KA, Hart RA. Postsurgical C5 nerve root palsy. In: Benzel EC, ed. The Cervical Spine. 5th ed. Philadelphia, PA: Lippincott Williams & Wilkins; 2012:1316–1320

59. Wang T, Wang H, Liu S, Ding WY. Incidence of C5 nerve root palsy after cervical surgery: a meta-analysis for last decade. Medicine (Baltimore) 2017;96(45):e8560

60. Seichi A, Takeshita K, Kawaguchi H, Nakajima S, Akune T, Nakamura K. Postoperative expansion of intramedullary high-intensity areas on T2-weighted magnetic resonance imaging after cervical laminoplasty. Spine 2004;29(13):1478–1482, discussion 1482

61. Sakaura H, Hosono N, Mukai Y, Fujii R, Iwasaki M, Yoshikawa H. Segmental motor paralysis after cervical laminoplasty: a prospective study. Spine 2006;31(23):2684–2688

62. Sakaura H, Hosono N, Mukai Y, Ishii T, Iwasaki M, Yoshikawa H. Long-term outcome of laminoplasty for cervical myelopathy due

to disc herniation: a comparative study of laminoplasty and anterior spinal fusion. Spine 2005;30(7):756–759

63. Pan FM, Wang SJ, Ma B, Wu DS. C5 nerve root palsy after posterior cervical spine surgery. J Orthop Surg (Hong Kong) 2017; 25(1):2309499016684502

64. Mochida J, Nomura T, Chiba M, Nishimura K, Toh E. Modified expansive open-door laminoplasty in cervical myelopathy. J Spinal Disord 1999;12(5):386–391

65. Currier BL. Neurological complications of cervical spine surgery: C5 palsy and intra-operative monitoring. Spine 2012;37(5): E328–E334

66. Hannallah D, Lee J, Khan M, Donaldson WF, Kang JD. Cerebrospinal fluid leaks following cervical spine surgery. J Bone Joint Surg Am 2008;90(5):1101–1105

67. Graham JJ. Complications of cervical spine surgery. A five-year report on a survey of the membership of the Cervical Spine Research Society by the Morbidity and Mortality Committee. Spine 1989;14(10):1046–1050

68. Cammisa FP Jr, Girardi FP, Sangani PK, Parvataneni HK, Cadag S, Sandhu HS. Incidental durotomy in spine surgery. Spine 2000;25(20):2663–2667

69. Parker SL, Kretzer RM, Recinos PF, et al. Ultrasonic BoneScalpel for osteoplastic laminoplasty in the resection of intradural spinal pathology: case series and technical note. Neurosurgery 2013; 73(1, Suppl Operative):ons61–ons66

70. Shen Y, Drum M, Roth S. The prevalence of perioperative visual loss in the United States: a 10-year study from 1996 to 2005 of spinal, orthopedic, cardiac, and general surgery. Anesth Analg 2009;109(5):1534–1545

71. Slavin J, Lewis EM, Sansur CA. Complication avoidance in spine surgery. In: Winn HR, ed. Youmans and Winn Neurological Surgery. 7th ed. Philadelphia, PA: Elsevier; 2017:2344–2347

16 Cervical Laminectomy and Fusion

Krishna Sharma, Ibet Marie Y. Sih, and Karlo M. Pedro

Introduction

Cervical myelopathy due to spondylotic cervical canal stenosis, called degenerative cervical myelopathy (DCM), remains a major public health problem worldwide, mainly affecting the aged population. DCM is a major source of disability in this age group, especially for more than 50 years old, and is the leading cause of acquired spinal cord dysfunction.[1-4] There is an increased prevalence of severe symptomatic cervical stenosis, probably due to increasing aged population in the society. People are living longer because of better medical facilities, awareness, desire for good health, healthy lifestyles, as well as availability of better nutrition. The incidence of spondylotic cervical stenosis needing surgical decompression likewise has increased.[2,4] Spine surgeons must make expeditious efforts to diagnose this condition early and offer appropriate surgery in indicated individuals to prevent further progression of neurologic deficits, relieve pain, and prevent the development of deformity.

Background

The most common cause of cervical stenosis is degenerative changes. Cervical canal is normally more than 17 mm, although it varies at different levels, in different sexes and in different ages. In the spinal canal, 8 to 13 mm is normally occupied by the spinal cord in the anterior-posterior dimension, and soft tissues take up another 2 to 3 mm.[5]

There is relative stenosis if the anterior-posterior diameter is less than 13 mm and absolute stenosis when it is less than 10 mm.[6] Cervical canal stenosis may be present congenitally or may be acquired. In the presence of congenital stenosis, the myelopathic features appear at an earlier age and even after minor trauma. The acquired causes can include multilevel spondylosis with disc prolapse, ossification of the posterior longitudinal ligament (OPLL), inward shingling of the laminae, hypertrophied facet joints, and enfolding of hypertrophied or ossified yellow ligament (OYL). Most of the symptomatic cases of spondylotic cervical canal stenosis have congenital stenosis with superimposed acquired causes.[7] Cervical cord compression may be focal or circumferential by the above-mentioned pathologies. The compression may be static, being present at all times or dynamic wherein compression is present only either in flexion, extension, or rotation, compromising the canal dimensions.[8] Flexion movement increases axial tension and narrows the AP diameter of the cord, whereas extension of the cervical spine shortens and thickens the cord dimensions. The spondylotic myelopathy could be due to mechanical compression and/or due to vascular compromise, resulting in ischemia and gliosis.[7]

X-ray of the spondylotic cervical spine can show the presence of cervical spinal canal stenosis, causes of canal stenosis like osteophytes and OPLL, as well as different forms and extent of cervical sagittal alignment disturbances. There may be straightening of the cervical lordosis in 47%, lordotic cervical spine of less than 100 degrees in 29%, and kyphosis in 24% of cervical spine X-rays.[9] Lordosis of the cervical spine is a very important parameter that should be assessed to decide on the type of surgical approach to be chosen.

CT scan is the best investigative modality to document bony pathology, ossification/calcific changes measurement, OPLL, and OYL in addition to laminar shingling. It gives the most accurate AP diameter of the cervical spinal canal. Addition of CT-myelogram,

2D- and 3D-CT studies demonstrate the status of the cord and the cause of cord compromise in multiple planes in addition to the details of neural foraminal pathology better.

MRI can show cervical cord edema, gliosis, and atrophy due to compression. Atrophy is evident by the spinal fluid all around the cord, widened anterior fissure, and curved bean-shaped shrunken cord appearance.[10,11]

The effect of spondylotic cervical canal stenosis can be assessed by different scales and grades. The most popular evaluation methods are Nurick grading system, Ranawat scoring system, Japanese Orthopedic Association (JOA) scoring system, and modified Japanese Orthopedic Association (mJOA) scoring system.[12–16]

Conservative Management

The indications of conservative management are mild myelopathy (mJOA score > 12), elderly patients of more than 70 years of age, and medically unfit individuals with increased comorbid factors like cardiac disease, peripheral vascular disease, obstructive pulmonary disease, diabetes, stroke, hypertension, and alcoholism. Conservative treatment in appropriate indication can maintain or even improve functional status in patients.[17] A relative indication is severely atrophied cord or myelomalacia, where the possibility of improvement after decompressive surgery is minimal. Severe "painless" myelopathic deficits like significant quadriparesis and "useless hands" with marked loss of function in either one or both hands, where the result of surgery is very poor in terms of reversibility of the deficits, should be managed conservatively. Patients on anticoagulation or on antiplatelet agents are advised to stop these medicines at least for a week before the surgery, or till the coagulation parameters are stabilized. Those with a recent history of reversible ischemic neurologic deficit or stroke, unstable atrial fibrillation, and active myocardial or peripheral vascular arterial or venous disease should also refrain from surgery.[11,18–21]

Conservative treatment modalities include cervical collars, short-term steroids, long-term non-steroid anti-inflammatory drugs (NSAIDs), physiotherapy, biofeedback techniques, and epidural steroid injections.

Surgery

Individuals with spondylotic cervical canal stenosis having moderate-to-severe cervical myelopathy (mJOA score < 12), rapidly progressive neurological deficit, and long duration of symptoms can benefit from surgical decompression. These patients have been shown to significantly improve functional status and improved pain.[17,22,23]

Clinical features of moderate-to-severe cervical myelopathy are: difficulty in walking, loss of balance, bladder and bowel involvement, and progressive long tract signs. As much as 15% of these have "double crush syndrome," presenting with clinical features of both myeloradiculopathy and carpal tunnel syndrome (CTS), which need to be thoroughly assessed before planning for surgery. About 10 to 15% of these patients also have significant coexisting lumbar lateral recess stenosis and may also need lumbar spine surgery for the expected improvement in symptoms.[24]

The type of surgery for DCM with canal stenosis is classified into anterior, posterior, or combined anterior and posterior approaches. All the three methods have been shown to be efficacious in the treatment of cervical spondylotic myelopathy (CSM), and each has its merits, indications and relative contraindications.[25–27] There is a lack of consensus on the optimal surgical approach for the management of spondylotic cervical canal stenosis. The choice of surgical approach depends on the location of compressive pathology, spinal alignment, number of levels of compression, clinical variables like age, surgeon's preference and experience, and also patient preference in selective cases. The factors contributing to which approach is to be chosen are depicted in **Table 16.1**.

The pros and cons of anterior cervical decompression have already been

Table 16.1 Factors that would promote anterior versus posterior surgery in cervical spinal stenosis

Factors	Variables	Decision
Sagittal Alignment	Kyphosis	Fixed: anterior
		Flexible: anterior or posterior with fusion
	Neutral or lordotic	Posterior (laminoplasty)
Involved Levels	3 or more levels	Posterior (laminoplasty)
	up to 2 levels	Anterior
Age	Elderly	Posterior
	Young	Anterior
Preoperative Pain	Moderate to high	Anterior or posterior with fusion
	None to low	Posterior (laminoplasty) or anterior
Instability	Yes	Anterior or posterior with fusion
	No	Posterior (laminoplasty) or anterior

discussed.[28] In this section, posterior laminectomy and fusion techniques will be reviewed. Several factors must be considered when laminectomy is chosen as the treatment modality for DCM. These factors include the following: K-line, sagittal vertical axis (SVA), location of compression, and the number of segments involved.

K-line

The concept of K-line is to assess the extent of cervical lordosis. It was introduced by Fujiyoshi in 2008 as a single measure of cervical alignment and effect of OPLL size.[29] Assessment of K-line is important to decide the type of surgical approach. It is taken with X-ray lateral view or CT scan. K-line is the line joining the midpoint of cervical canal at C2 and C7 levels. If the K-line is touched or crossed by the dorsal surface of vertebral body of a kyphotic spine, thickened OPLL, or large osteophytes, K-line is said to be negative. With K-line negative, laminectomy is not beneficial as the spinal cord cannot shift further posteriorly after laminectomy and remains plastered against the ventral spinal canal, making the process of decompression ineffective. Thus, successful decompression in these cases with negative K-line cannot

be accomplished by merely removing the dorsal spinal elements. Patients with positive K-line on the other hand have their compressive pathology ventral to this line, and laminectomy releases the ventral pressure on the cord by allowing the spinal cord to shift posteriorly. This is illustrated in **Fig. 16.1**.

Sagittal Vertical Axis (SVA)

The C2–C7 SVA also plays a decisive role in choosing the approach (**Fig. 16.2**). This parameter shows the cervical regional alignment, and it is defined as the horizontal distance between the C2 vertical line (extending downwards from the center of the C2 vertebral body) and the posterior superior endplate of C7. The SVA value was shown by Smith and colleagues to be well correlated with the severity of myelopathy in a North American cohort of DCM patients.[30] A value > 40 mm has shown to be statistically correlated with poor functional outcomes after cervical laminectomy.[31]

The surgical options for posterior approaches in spondylotic cervical stenosis are as follows:[32,33]

- Laminoplasty.
- Laminectomy.
- Laminectomy and fusion.

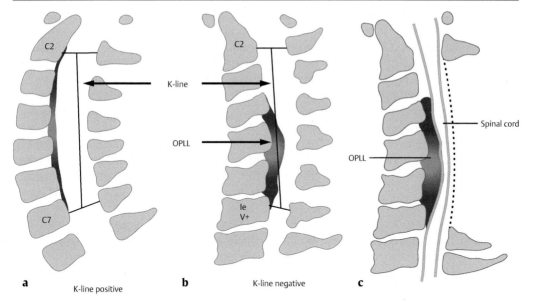

Fig. 16.1 **(a)** K-line (+) does not touch the dorsal surface of vertebral body or OPLL. **(b)** K-line (–) is seen when ossification of the posterior longitudinal ligament (OPLL) crosses K-line. **(c)** Persistent cord compression after laminectomy in K-line (–)

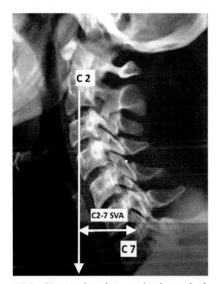

Fig. 16.2 X-ray showing sagittal vertical axis (SVA).

Laminoplasty will be discussed in chapter 15. Posterior approaches were the earliest techniques employed in the cervical spine, and laminectomy is considered to be the oldest form in this category. Cervical laminectomy and fusion is now the most commonly performed (70%) posterior procedure, followed by laminoplasty (23%), and laminectomy alone (7%).[34,35]

Cervical laminectomy is a decompressive procedure for symptomatic and progressive cervical canal stenosis. The first successful laminectomy was performed in 1828 by an American surgeon, Alban G. Smith, in a patient who became paraplegic after falling from a horse.[36] The patient was documented to have an improvement in motor function after his surgery, which entailed removal of fractured spinous process and lamina.

Laminectomy immediately releases a compressive force from posterior side and increases the space available for the spinal cord, which falls back posteriorly, getting relieved from the ventral mechanical compression, both in static and dynamic states.[37] For this, cervical lordosis should be adequately sufficient, that is, more than 10 degrees, and the thickness of ventrally situated osteophytes or OPLL be less than 7 mm, in order to allow the cord to shift sufficiently away from ventrally situated compressive pathologies.[10,38–41] Both these parameters can be assessed by K-line and SVA. Laminectomy also improves cord perfusion as axial tension is released. It is a safe, very effective, and direct method for decompression in suitable patients and is particularly useful in the geriatric age group where there are many associated comorbidities.[42,43] Large case series have been published on cervical laminectomy from the 1960s and thereafter. It still is a very viable option for surgical management of CSM due to cervical canal stenosis.

Indications for laminectomy can be summarized as cervical cord compression by disc prolapse at more than three levels, significantly compromising the cervical canal, thick (> 7mm) OPLL, K-line positive, and SVA less than 40 mm with moderate-to-severe myelopathy.[43] Laminectomy is also indicated for posterior compressive pathologies like OYL or laminar shilling.

Operative Procedure

Cervical laminectomy is performed under general anesthesia. During intubation of severely myelopathic patients, extreme extension is avoided. It remains crucial to have a well-documented neurological examination of the patient, especially of the motor function, prior to putting the patient to sleep. A good routine is to allow the patient to perform full range of neck movements as tolerated to have an estimate of the extent of safe neck manipulation during intubation and positioning. Awake fiberoptic intubation with adequate local analgesia is recommended in severely myelopathic patients or those with difficult airway. Arterial line monitoring is highly recommended to avoid and quickly correct hypotension. Myelopathic patients have a compromised anterior blood circulation due to ongoing OPLL compression on the cord. Hence, efforts must be exerted to avoid additional cord injury secondary to hypotension, and blood pressure (BP) should be maintained at normal or about 20% above the normal level. Vasopressors must likewise always be made ready in case it is needed.

Good communication between the surgeon and anesthesiologist is critical, especially at certain stages of surgery where a drop in BP might be expected (e.g., prone positioning and reverse Trendelenburg positioning).

Proper patient positioning is essential to avoid intraoperative and postoperative complications. The patient must be placed on a Mayfield head holder or tongs to adequately maintain the head and neck in desired position and avoid pressure on the face and eyes. It is essential to keep the Mayfield head clamp freely rotatable over the patient's nose once the patient is positioned prone. The single pin of the head clamp is placed above the pinna, superior to the temporal line just above the insertion of the temporalis muscle. The two rocker pins are placed coaxially on the opposite side of the calvarium, avoiding thin bone plates or the temporalis muscle, to prevent slippage.

The patient is then logrolled prone onto a radiolucent spine table with well-padded bolsters. During this maneuver, it is important that the surgeon is in complete control of the head with the Mayfield head clamp in place. The Mayfield is then connected to the bed and locked in place. The bed is placed in reverse Trendelenburg position to help facilitate venous outflow from the head and neck and subsequently avoid excessive bleeding from the epidural venous plexus. The abdomen must be freely hanging in between bolsters to avoid increase in venous pressure. The elbows and wrist are likewise well padded and the arms are tucked to the sides. Knees are padded with foam donuts and two to three pillows are used underneath the legs and feet to avoid excessive stretch on the sciatic nerve. Mechanical compression devices are then placed over bilateral legs. The final position of the patient prepared for laminectomy can be seen in **Fig. 16.3**.

Cervical laminectomy is almost always done in prone position. Sitting position has been described with its advantage of reducing intraoperative bleeding, particularly in obese patients with short thick necks. The intraoperative ventilation is also easier for

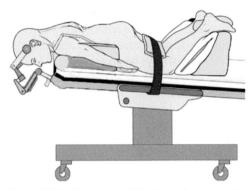

Fig. 16.3 Prone positioning for cervical laminectomy. The patient is placed on Mayfield head clamp with adequate provision for padding of pressure points as well as retraction of shoulders downward to maximize exposure of the subaxial spine.

those with pulmonary disease, and there is greater accessibility for cardiac massage should cardiac arrest occur.[44,45] However, sitting position is very rarely used because of potential risks of air embolism, hypotension, stroke, cervical cord ischemia, particularly in older individuals with significant cardiovascular pathology.[46]

The neck position during surgery is dependent on the goal of surgery. In patients undergoing occiput-C2 decompression, the chin must be slightly flexed to allow visualization of the occipito–cervical junction and avoid overlap of the inferior lamina, which will make laminectomy technically demanding. If fusion is planned, on the other hand, it is imperative to keep the neck neutral or slightly extended to create the desired cervical lordosis and maintain horizontal gaze. A comparison between prepositioning and postpositioning signals of somatosensory-evoked potential (SSEP) or motor-evoked potential (MEP) can help in detecting any neurophysiologic changes secondary to improper neck alignment after prone positioning. To increase visualization of the lower cervical level, the shoulders are held down using 4-inch cloth tape unrolled over the patient's back and fastened toward the end of the operating table. After ensuring that all

lines and tubes are patent, a radiograph is taken to confirm proper level of surgery.

Prophylactic administration of 1 gm of intravenous (IV) methylprednisolone has been suggested before laminectomy in cases of severely compressed spinal cord but there is no Class I evidence to support this practice.[47]

Spinal cord monitoring during cervical spine surgery is usually in the form of SSEP or MEP. This is often reserved for the severely myelopathic patients with extremely tight stenosis to monitor for any neurologic deficits prior to and during surgery. It may also be used to avoid brachial plexopathies that may incur during positioning. It must be started preoperatively to obtain the baseline data about muscle and nerve status, and the monitoring is continued throughout the procedure. SSEP monitoring is used to monitor the median, ulnar, and posterior tibial nerve function throughout the operation.[48] Any change in amplitude by > 50% or 10% prolongation of latency is considered significant. If this occurs, resuscitative efforts must be immediately instituted, which includes cessation of manipulation, release of any traction, screw/rod repositioning, warm irrigation, induction of hypertension, increase in oxygenation, infusion of methylprednisolone, and/or decrease in inhalational or intravenous anesthetic. MEPs, on the other hand, is considered more important mode of monitoring for cervical degenerative myelopathy, as it is able to reflect anterior cord function directly compared to SSEP. During laminectomy, when a very compressed cord is acutely decompressed, the MEP and SEP signals may transiently drop out. It is important to wait for MEP/SEP baselines to return to normal before proceeding with further dissection.

Routine use of multimodality intraoperative monitoring (MIOM) in cervical surgery remains controversial. A recent systematic review on this topic provided evidence that both SSEP and MEP have high sensitivity and specificity in detecting neurologic injury when either of these modalities is used in surgery. There is no evidence, however, that their combined use leads to a higher and early detection rate.[49] The most recent guideline drafted for MIOM supports the use of MEP and SSEP recording during spinal surgery for diagnostic purposes with level I evidence.[50] Despite this recommendation, however, there is still no strict criteria as to what subset of patients benefit from monitoring.

Local anesthesia should be administered to the skin along the incision and paracervical musculature with 0.5% bupivacaine HCL and 1:200,000 epinephrine. A midline incision from C2 to T1 levels is made. To avoid excessive bleeding, it is important to maintain a midline trajectory and dissect over the avascular median raphe. The fascia is incised in midline over the spinous process of the desired cervical level, sparing the muscular attachment at C2 and T1 level. Wide subperiosteal stripping of paraspinal muscles is done (**Fig. 16.4**). It is important to note that C2–C6 spinous processes are bifid in various configurations. Hence, their careful dissection and exposure is needed to proceed further deep into the paraspinal muscles. When releasing the ligaments inserted on the spinous processes, it is important to proceed in craniocaudal direction and not in the opposite direction to avoid plunging into the spinal canal, which is unprotected in the midline. Dissection is carried laterally up to the lateral margin of the lateral masses. Cerebellar retractors are helpful in maintaining adequate exposure at

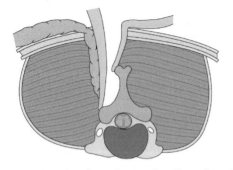

Fig. 16.4 Subperiosteal muscle dissection is accomplished using electrocautery, following the lamina of the desired level and extended up to the lateral end of the facet joint.

this point. Intermittent release of retractors is also recommended to avoid denervation of erector spinae muscles. At any level, the facet capsule must always be preserved.

Laminectomy is performed two levels above and below the site of maximal cord compression. Laminectomy is commenced by removing the outer half of the spinous process. Bilateral troughs are then created using high-speed drills with 4-mm diamond burr tips. The goal is to slightly decorticate the bone until a thin layer of inner bone is left and can be removed using 2 or 1 mm Kerrison rongeur. It must be noted that the morphology of the lamina is oval in cross-section with bicortical bone layer in midportion and single thick cortex toward the end. The cephalad portion is also ventral to the overlying lamina, hence more drilling work is necessary at this portion (**Fig. 16.5**).

Once bilateral troughs are created, the lamina can be circumferentially freed. The remaining island of bone is removed using Kerrison rongeurs, carefully taking into consideration that dense adhesion may form on its underside with the adjacent dura and ligamentum flavum. This dense adhesion can be carefully separated using Penfield No.1 and pituitary rongeur. Laminectomy is complete when the dorsal thecal sac is visible in the operative field and its lateral borders are freely palpable with a nerve hook.

Foraminotomy and Facet Resection

Patients with radiculopathy may benefit from additional foraminotomy after successful laminectomy. A neural foramen is identified by following the course of a nerve root by a probe. The medial third to half of the facet joint is removed using high-speed drill or Kerrison punch. This maneuver effectively unroofs the foramen and decompresses the exiting nerve root. It is important to avoid taking more than 50% of the facet as this has been shown to increase instability in cervical spine.[51,52] A 45-degree-angled nerve

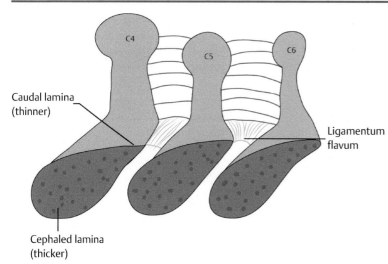

Caudal lamina
(thinner)

Ligamentum
flavum

Cephaled lamina
(thicker)

Fig. 16.5 Sagittal representation of the lamina. Note that the cephalad portion of the lamina is thicker than caudal end also covered partially by the superior lamina. The ligamentum flavum is absent underneath the most cephalad portion of the lamina.

hook is used to palpate for the neural foramen and assess adequacy of decompression. Any bleeding from epidural venous plexus is controlled using Gelfoam and cotton patties. Bipolar cautery on low setting can be used if the source of bleeding can be identified.

Prophylactic laminectomy may be done in cases of significant spinal canal stenosis with soft neurological signs. It may also be done for asymptomatic severe congenital stenosis where there is a high chance of trauma producing severe cervical cord injury. In these cases, dynamic forces (e.g., shear, distraction, and stretch injury) can cause severe deficits.[8]

Standalone cervical laminectomy is not highly favored because of the associated potential complications like instability, kyphosis, and neurological deficits.[53–57]

Complications of Foraminotomy and Facet Resection

1. **Instability:** Postlaminectomy instability of the cervical spine occurs in 14 to 47%, especially after a wide laminectomy or when more than 50% facetectomy is performed.[52,58,59] Nowinski and colleagues have documented instability with facetectomies of even as little as 25%.[60] A preexisting instability due to extensive degeneration or loss of posterior band may be aggravated

further after laminectomy. Removal of lamina therefore increases instability of the spine, especially when ≥ 3 levels are removed.[61] Instability can be better diagnosed by dynamic imaging and characterized by more than 3.5 mm of subluxation, more than 20 degrees of angulation, and more than 1 to 2 mm of motion demonstrated between the tips of adjacent spinous processes.[32,34,52]

2. **Kyphotic deformity:** The incidence and causes of postlaminectomy kyphosis in adults and children vary. In adults, the estimated incidence ranges from 6 to 47%.[62] It is thought to result from the loss of posterior tension band and weakening of posterior cervical musculature after laminectomy (**Fig. 16.6**).[63] In children, the rate of postlaminectomy kyphosis is higher, almost approaching close to 100%. This is secondary to combination of wedging of the vertebral body and secondary subluxation from the loss of interspinous ligament during laminectomy as well as the inherent mobility of ligaments in children, which potentially weakens the posterior facet joint.[64] Risk factors identified in the development of postoperative kyphosis after laminectomy include: straight or kyphotic spine, wide laminectomies,

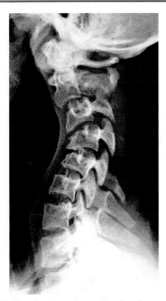

Fig. 16.6 Postlaminectomy kyphosis.

young patient with neck hypermobility, as well as laminectomies including C2 and the cervicothoracic junction. The cervical spine is known to transmit 36% of the compressive force through the vertebral body, whereas 64% is transmitted by the posterior elements.[65,66] Removing the posterior tension band during laminectomy would therefore lead to increasing compressive loads over the disc and vertebral body, resulting in progressive kyphotic deformity. In addition, the subperiosteal stripping of muscle, especially if performed at C2 and C7, can lead to postoperative loss of lordosis and can also contribute to new or persistent axial neck pain.[67] The kyphosis is higher if the preoperative cervical alignment is straight than with normal lordosis. However, no study has clearly demonstrated a relationship between postlaminectomy kyphosis and deterioration in quality of life.[53,55–57]

3. **Neurological deficit**: Appearance of new neurological deficits after cervical laminectomy or aggravation of preexisting neurological deficit occurs in 5.5%. This could be due to direct trauma to the cervical cord, blood vessels or roots during laminectomy, rapid posterior cord migration of cervical cord, especially affecting C5 roots, or due to aggravation of deformity and instability.[68] Delayed deterioration has been observed in an average of 7.35 years postoperatively, which is significantly higher (10% to 23%) in older individuals with high comorbid status. It is more common in those with severe original myelopathy and history of recent trauma. Delayed deterioration due to continued progression of OPLL after laminectomy may also be seen in as high as 70% of patients.[54,69]

4. **Postlaminectomy membrane**: The concept of "postlaminectomy membrane" was introduced by LaRocca and MacNab based on observation in dogs.[70] This adherent membrane, which covered the epidural space extending into the canal bilaterally, was postulated to arise from the fibrous tissue elements of the paraspinal muscle in contact with the dura. The significance of this membrane has been controversial, as this was rarely encountered in postoperative imaging and even during reoperation.[71] Recently, however, a report on a case of recurrent myelopathy due to postlaminectomy membrane was reported, which was discovered after dynamic imaging and has paved the way for renewed interest in this topic.[72] Several authors have postulated this to be due to scarring from epidural hematoma or some foreign body reaction in the peridural space.[73] Due to this report, some authors have advocated not to use any form of barrier between muscle and dura to aid in reducing the constrictive effect of this scarring on the dura postoperatively.[71]

Due to these limitations and complications, instead of standalone laminectomy, cervical laminectomy followed by fusion procedure has become the standard procedure in the treatment of cervical spondylotic stenosis with moderate-to-severe myelopathy.[71,74] When laminectomy is performed at the cervicothoracic junction, the incidence of instability and deformity is higher and thus it warrants simultaneous fusion procedure. With an increase in the incidence of aged population with significant CSM and a greater desire for a better quality of life, posterior cervical fusion is more frequently performed nowadays. In addition, with greater number of trained manpower, safer anesthesia, better surgical instrumentation and technique, and better perioperative care, cervical laminectomy and fusion has become the preferred and standard procedure.[4]

Cervical laminectomy with fusion, decompresses the cord, provides a rigid stabilization of the spine, and corrects deformity without significant increase in morbidity and mortality.[3,4,75] By providing a very rigid fixation, laminectomy and fusion limits movement between the vertebral bodies and prevent further progression of degenerative cervical myelopathy.

Cervical laminectomy and fusion are indicated in CSM requiring multilevel (more than three levels) laminectomies, instability, especially if facetectomy of more than 50% is done, and cervical malalignment with instability and subluxation.[9] It is suitable for elderly patients who have osteoporotic bone and need more rigid fixation. Even in cases of severe kyphosis with K-line negative and if the cervical kyphosis is not fixed, laminectomy with fusion can still be performed, as fusion and fixation recorrects the cervical lordosis in addition to decompression of the cervical cord.[76–78]

The procedure of laminectomy has already been described above. Different fusion techniques have been described, mainly fusion between vertebral bodies (e.g., interbody or anterior fusion), between laminae (posterior fusion), between the transverse processes (posterolateral fusion), or combination of any of these. Prior to the advent of screw fixation, fusion relied heavily on "in situ fusion" or the use of wiring techniques like facetal wiring technique.[32,79,80] In situ fusion utilized autologous bone graft along with prolonged postoperative external cervical immobilization. "In situ fusion" without fixation was associated with high rates of pseudoarthrosis, subluxation, graft displacement and instability. Thus, this technique was gradually replaced by the use of other constructs. Nowadays, fusion using polyaxial screw-rod constructs, mainly either with lateral mass or transpedicular screws, provides a very rigid fixation.[81–85] The details of these procedures will be described in subsequent chapters.

A summary of the factors that decide between laminectomy alone or laminectomy with fusion is summarized in **Table 16.2**.

Table 16.2 Recommendations for cervical laminectomy or laminectomy and fusion

Variables	Cervical laminectomy alone	Cervical laminectomy and fusion
Cervical lordosis	10° cervical lordosis	< 10° cervical lordosis or straight spine
Instability	None	Yes
Axial neck pain	None	Yes
Age	Elderly (> 70)	Younger (< 70)
Comorbidities	Cardiac disease, diabetes, coagulopathy, chronic obstructive pulmonary disease	Absence of comorbidities

A recent review on the outcomes following posterior cervical fusion and decompression has shown that for all surgical indications (myelopathy, OPLL, radiculopathy) the success rate of cervical laminectomy with fusion is much better, that is, 98.25%. Similarly, an overall pooled revision rate is 1.09% and complication rate is 9.02% (**Fig. 16.7**).[3,26,86,87]

Advantages of cervical laminectomy and fusion can be summarized as follows:

- It recreates the posterior column tension band, which is removed during laminectomy and thus maintains cervical stability and alignment in rotational, axial, and lateral bending. Hence, it corrects and prevents the occurrence of postlaminectomy kyphosis.[88]
- The fixation is very rigid and strong, especially with transpedicular fixation, which includes all the three columns of cervical spine. This limits and prevents repetitive microtrauma to a healing cord and delays neurological deterioration.
- The rigid fixation by screws and rods also prevents micromovements at the joints and fusion area and thus prevents development of pseudoarthrosis.
- Laminectomy and fusion lowers axial neck pain, compared to standalone laminectomy procedure.[89]

- The fixation recreates the posterior column, which bears 2/3 of the axial force transmitted from head onto the cervical spine and below.
- Due to its longer purchase in bone with better pullout strength, using these techniques, especially lateral mass or transpedicular fixation, cervical laminectomy and decompression can be performed even in osteoporotic spines.
- The revision rate (7.4% with a median follow-up of 70 months) and other complications are low.[90]

These advantages of fusion and fixation over standalone laminectomy, however, have not been accepted universally. The results of the LAMIFUSE trial showed that the outcomes after laminectomy alone did not significantly differ compared to laminectomy with instrumented fusion.[91] Similarly, other studies have shown equivalence of laminectomy with other techniques for DCM, except that "laminectomy alone" has a higher incidence of postoperative kyphosis.[56,62,92,93]

Fusion and fixation procedure after laminectomy has its own intrinsic complications like:

- Hardware problems.
  - Malposition, pull out, or avulsion of screws in 1.8%.

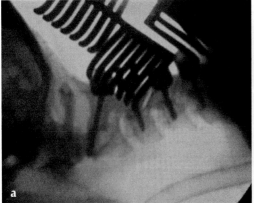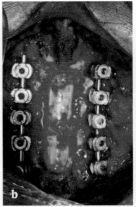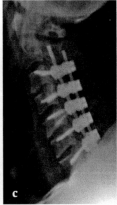

Fig. 16.7 Laminectomy and posterior fusion using transpedicular fixation for degenerative cervical canal stenosis. (**a**) Intraoperative X-ray with transpedicular screws in place, (**b**) intraoperative picture with transpedicular screws in place, (**c**) postoperative X-ray of transpedicular screw fixation.

– Implant failure like loosening (1.1%), breakage (4–7%), misplaced or displaced screws.
- Facet or lateral mass fracture and facet violation in 0.2%.
- Displacement of bone graft.
- Increase in wound infection (1.3%).[94,95]
- Nerve root injury (0.6%).
- Cervical cord injury (2.6%).
- Iatrogenic foraminal stenosis (2.6%) due to screw misplaced in the cervical spinal canal.
- Loss of reduction (2.6%).
- Adjacent segment disease (3.8%).
- Increased costs of the procedure.

Although the list of complications is long, their incidence is very low. Additionally, the use of image guidance has made this procedure even safer, reducing the complication rates further. Thus cervical laminectomy with fusion can be considered a safe procedure, improving functional outcome in most of the patients with CSM due to cervical canal stenosis.

Skip Laminectomies

This technique was introduced by Shiraishi in 2002 as a minimally invasive decompressive procedure for cervical myelopathy (**Fig. 16.8**).[96] The procedure entails laminectomy in focal segmental units of the spine where maximum compression is present along with minimal posterior muscle trauma.

Using this technique, a C3–C7 posterior cervical surgery, for example, is performed by removing only the C4 and C6 lamina, with the addition of partial laminectomy and flavum resection at adjacent levels, but all the posterior band elements at C3, C5 and C7 are preserved.[97] This has been indicated for patients with CSM and calcification of ligamentum flavum with no concomitant congenital narrowing of the spine. It is contraindicated, on the other hand, in patients with continuous OPLL. Two studies thus far have supported the superiority of skip laminectomy over laminoplasty for patients with CSM.[98,99] Another study has shown similar outcomes in terms of improvement in JOA score and neck visual analogue scale (VAS) score with skip laminectomy compared to laminoplasty.[100] In a recent prospective review with radiologic follow-up, Robins and colleague have shown that skip laminectomy showed no difference from conventional laminectomy in terms of patient outcomes, postoperative spinal alignment, and reoperation rates.[101]

Conclusion

Wide ranges and options are available to treat symptomatic degenerative cervical myelopathy with cervical canal stenosis. Cervical laminectomy with fusion when chosen for appropriate indications, avoiding its associated complications, can give a durable, safe, and effective solution to degenerative

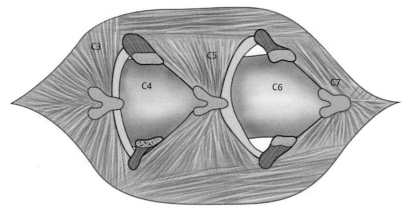

Fig. 16.8 C3–C7 decompression using skip laminectomy technique. The lamina of C4 and C6 are completely removed but the C3, C5 and C7 posterior arch as well as the muscular attachment over their respective spinous processes are preserved.

cervical canal stenosis. Cervical laminectomy allows adequate neural tissue decompression while posterior fusions ensure maintaining alignment and stability.

Take-home Points

- Patients with multilevel cervical myeloradiculopathy, and significant cord or root compression on MRI or CT scan studies, would benefit from multilevel cervical laminectomy.

- Adding fusion to multilevel laminectomy has become the standard of care, as it takes care of most of the limitations of standalone laminectomy.

- This is now considered the procedure of choice for the treatment of moderate-to-severe compressive myelopathy or radiculopathy.

- It has its own set of complications, mainly hardware-related.

- With increasing use of image guidance, the procedure has become safer. However, the cost and availability of these instrumentation and imaging systems are the limitations for their use.

References

1. Wilkinson M. Cervical spondylosis. Practitioner 1970;204(222):537–545
2. Liu JK, Das K. Posterior fusion of the subaxial cervical spine: indications and techniques. Neurosurg Focus 2001;10(4):E7
3. Salzmann SN, Derman PB, Lampe LP, et al. Cervical spinal fusion: 16-year trends in epidemiology, indications, and in-hospital outcomes by surgical approach. World Neurosurg 2018;113:e280–e295
4. Vonck CE, Tanenbaum JE, Smith GA, Benzel EC, Mroz TE, Steinmetz MP. Stein- metz MP. National trends in demographics and outcomes following cervical fusion for cervical spondylotic myelopathy. Global Spine J 2018;8(3):244–253
5. Breig A. The therapeutic possibilities of surgical bio-engineering in incomplete spinal cord lesions. Paraplegia 1972;9(4):173–182
6. Epstein JA, Epstein NE. The surgical management of cervical spinal stenosis, spondylosis, and myeloradiculopathy by means of the posterior approach. In: Clark CR, The Cervical Spine Research Society Editorial Committee, eds. The Cervical Spine. 2nd ed. Philadelphia: JB Lippincott; 1989:625–643
7. Ono K, Ota H, Tada K, Yamamoto T. Cervical myelopathy secondary to multiple spondylotic protrusions: a clinicopathologic study. Spine 1977;2:109–125
8. Henderson FC, Geddes JF, Vaccaro AR, Woodard E, Berry KJ, Benzel EC. Stretch-associated injury in cervical spondylotic myelopathy: new concept and review. Neurosurgery 2005;56(5):1101–1113, discussion 1101–1113
9. Chang V, Lu DC, Hoffman H, Buchanan C, Holly LT. Clinical results of cervical laminectomy and fusion for the treatment of cervical spondylotic myelopathy in 58 consecutive patients. Surg Neurol Int 2014;5(Suppl 3):S133–S137
10. Al-Mefty O, Harkey LH, Middleton TH, Smith RR, Fox JL. Myelopathic cervical spondylotic lesions demonstrated by magnetic resonance imaging. J Neurosurg 1988;68(2):217–222
11. Matsumoto M, Toyama Y, Ishikawa M, Chiba K, Suzuki N, Fujimura Y. Increased signal intensity of the spinal cord on magnetic resonance images in cervical compressive myelopathy. Does it predict the outcome of conservative treatment? Spine 2000;25(6):677–682
12. Nurick S. The pathogenesis of the spinal cord disorder associated with cervical spondylosis. Brain 1972;95(1):87–100
13. Ranawat CS, O'Leary P, Pellicci P, Tsairis P, Marchisello P, Dorr L. Cervical spine fusion in rheumatoid arthritis. J Bone Joint Surg Am 1979;61(7):1003–1010
14. Japanese Orthopaedic Association. Scoring system for cervical myelopathy. J Jpn Orthop Assoc. 1994;68:490–503
15. Benzel EC, Lancon J, Kesterson L, Hadden T. Cervical laminectomy and dentate ligament section for cervical spondylotic myelopathy. J Spinal Disord 1991;4(3):286–295
16. Tetreault L, Nouri A, Kopjar B, Côté P, Fehlings MG. The minimum clinically important difference of the modified Japanese

orthopaedic association scale in patients with degenerative cervical myelopathy. Spine 2015;40(21):1653–1659

17. Lawrence BD, Brodke DS. Posterior surgery for cervical myelopathy: indications, techniques, and outcomes. Orthop Clin North Am 2012;43(1):29–40, vii–viii

18. Saal JS, Saal JA, Yurth EF. Nonoperative management of herniated cervical intervertebral disc with radiculopathy. Spine 1996;21(16):1877–1883

19. Persson LC, Carlsson CA, Carlsson JY. Long-lasting cervical radicular pain managed with surgery, physiotherapy, or a cervical collar. A prospective, randomized study. Spine 1997;22(7):751–758

20. Nakamura K, Kurokawa T, Hoshino Y, Saita K, Takeshita K, Kawaguchi H. Conservative treatment for cervical spondylotic myelopathy: achievement and sustainability of a level of "no disability". J Spinal Disord 1998;11(2):175–179

21. Nelson BW, Carpenter DM, Dreisinger TE, Mitchell M, Kelly CE, Wegner JA. Can spinal surgery be prevented by aggressive strengthening exercises? A prospective study of cervical and lumbar patients. Arch Phys Med Rehabil 1999;80(1):20–25

22. Naderi S, Ozgen S, Pamir MN, Ozek MM, Erzen C. Cervical spondylotic myelopathy: surgical results and factors affecting prognosis. Neurosurgery 1998;43(1):43–49, discussion 49–50

23. Chiles BW III, Leonard MA, Choudhri HF, Cooper PR. Cervical spondylotic myelopathy: patterns of neurological deficit and recovery after anterior cervical decompression. Neurosurgery 1999;44(4):762–769, discussion 769–770

24. Epstein NE, Epstein JA, Carras R, Murthy VS, Hyman RA. Coexisting cervical and lumbar spinal stenosis: diagnosis and management. Neurosurgery 1984;15(4):489–496

25. Yalamanchili PK, Vives MJ, Chaudhary SB. Cervical spondylotic myelopathy: factors in choosing the surgical approach. Adv Orthop 2012;2012:783762

26. Fehlings MG, Wilson JR, Kopjar B, et al. Efficacy and safety of surgical decompression in patients with cervical spondylotic myelopathy: results of the AOSpine North America prospective multi-center study. J Bone Joint Surg Am 2013;95(18):1651–1658

27. Zhu B, Xu Y, Liu X, Liu Z, Dang G. Anterior approach versus posterior approach for the treatment of multilevel cervical spondylotic myelopathy: a systemic review and meta-analysis. Eur Spine J 2013;22(7):1583–1593

28. Bohlman H. Cervical Spondylosis with moderate to severe myelopathy: A report of 17 cases treated by Robinson anterior cervical discectomy and fusion. Spine 1977; 2:151–162

29. Fujiyoshi T, Yamazaki M, Kawabe J, et al. A new concept for making decisions regarding the surgical approach for cervical ossification of the posterior longitudinal ligament: the K-line. Spine 2008;33(26):E990–E993

30. Smith JS, Lafage V, Ryan DJ, et al. Association of myelopathy scores with cervical sagittal balance and normalized spinal cord volume: analysis of 56 preoperative cases from the AOSpine North America Myelopathy study. Spine 2013; 38(22, Suppl 1):S161–S170

31. Roguski M, Benzel EC, Curran JN, et al. Postoperative cervical sagittal imbalance negatively affects outcomes after surgery for cervical spondylotic myelopathy. Spine 2014;39(25):2070–2077

32. Bajamal AH, Kim SH, Arifianto MR, et al; World Federation of Neurosurgical Societies (WFNS) Spine Committee. Posterior surgical techniques for cervical spondylotic myelopathy: WFNS spine committee recommendations. Neurospine 2019;16(3):421–434

33. Rhee JM, Basra S. Posterior surgery for cervical myelopathy: laminectomy, laminectomy with fusion, and laminoplasty. Asian Spine J 2008;2(2):114–126

34. Manzano GR, Casella G, Wang MY, Vanni S, Levi AD. A prospective, randomized trial comparing expansile cervical laminoplasty and cervical laminectomy and fusion for multilevel cervical myelopathy. Neurosurgery 2012;70(2):264–277

35. Liu CY, Zygourakis CC, Yoon S, et al. Trends in utilization and cost of cervical spine surgery using the National Inpatient Sample Database, 2001 to 2013. Spine 2017;42(15): E906–E913

36. Patchell RA, Tibbs PA, Young AB, Clark DB, Alban G. Alban G. Smith and the beginnings of spinal surgery. Neurology 1987;37(10): 1683–1684

37. Levi L, Wolf A, Mirvis S, Rigamonti D, Fianfaca MS, Monasky M. The significance of dorsal

migration of the cord after extensive cervical laminectomy for patients with traumatic central cord syndrome. J Spinal Disord 1995; 8(4):289–295

38. Hamanishi C, Tanaka S. Bilateral multilevel laminectomy with or without posterolateral fusion for cervical spondylotic myelopathy: relationship to type of onset and time until operation. J Neurosurg 1996;85(3):447–451

39. Ishida Y, Ohmori K, Suzuki K, Inoue H. Analysis of dural configuration for evaluation of posterior decompression in cervical myelopathy. Neurosurgery 1999;44(1): 91–95, discussion 95–96

40. Yamazaki A, Homma T, Uchiyama S, Katsumi Y, Okumura H. Morphologic limitations of posterior decompression by midsagittal splitting method for myelopathy caused by ossification of the posterior longitudinal ligament in the cervical spine. Spine 1999; 24(1):32–34

41. Epstein N, Herkowitz HN, Rothman RH, Simeone FA, eds. Cervical myelopathy: posterior approach-laminectomy. Rothman-Simeone, The Spine. Philadelphia: Saunders Elsevier; 2006:864–76

42. Epstein NE. Laminectomy for cervical myelopathy. Spinal Cord 2003;41(6):317–327

43. Klineberg E. Cervical spondylotic myelopathy: a review of the evidence. Orthop Clin North Am 2010;41(2):193–202

44. Matjasko J, Petrozza P, Cohen M, Steinberg P. Anesthesia and surgery in the seated position: analysis of 554 cases. Neurosurgery 1985;17(5):695–702

45. Standefer M, Bay JW, Trusso R. The sitting position in neurosurgery: a retrospective analysis of 488 cases. Neurosurgery 1984; 14(6):649–658

46. Albin MS, Carroll RG, Maroon JC. Clinical considerations concerning detection of venous air embolism. Neurosurgery 1978; 3(3):380–384

47. Vidal PM, Ulndreaj A, Badner A, Hong J, Fehlings MG. Methylprednisolone treatment enhances early recovery following surgical decompression for degenerative cervical myelopathy without compromise to the systemic immune system. J Neuroinflammation 2018;15(1):222

48. Epstein NE, Danto J, Nardi D. Evaluation of intraoperative somatosensory-evoked potential monitoring during 100 cervical operations. Spine 1993;18(6):737–747

49. Di Martino A, Papalia R, Caldaria A, Torre G, Denaro L, Denaro V. Should evoked potential monitoring be used in degenerative cervical spine surgery? A systematic review. J Orthop Traumatol 2019;20(1):19

50. Hadley MN, Shank CD, Rozzelle CJ, Walters BC. Guidelines for the use of electrophysiological monitoring for surgery of the human spinal column and spinal cord. Neurosurgery 2017;81(5):713–732

51. Zdeblick TA, Zou D, Warden KE, McCabe R, Kunz D, Vanderby R. Cervical stability after foraminotomy. A biomechanical in vitro analysis. J Bone Joint Surg Am 1992; 74(1):22–27

52. Raynor RB, Pugh J, Shapiro I. Cervical facetectomy and its effect on spine strength. J Neurosurg 1985;63(2):278–282

53. Snow RB, Weiner H. Cervical laminectomy and foraminotomy as surgical treatment of cervical spondylosis: a follow-up study with analysis of failures. J Spinal Disord 1993;6(3):245–250, discussion 250–251

54. Kato Y, Iwasaki M, Fuji T, Yonenobu K, Ochi T. Long-term follow-up results of laminectomy for cervical myelopathy caused by ossification of the posterior longitudinal ligament. J Neurosurg 1998;89(2):217–223

55. Kaptain GJ, Simmons NE, Replogle RE, Pobereskin L. Incidence and outcome of kyphotic deformity following laminectomy for cervical spondylotic myelopathy. J Neurosurg 2000; **93**(2, Suppl)199–204

56. Anderson PA, Matz PG, Groff MW, et al; Joint Section on Disorders of the Spine and Peripheral Nerves of the American Association of Neurological Surgeons and Congress of Neurological Surgeons. Laminectomy and fusion for the treatment of cervical degenerative myelopathy. J Neurosurg Spine 2009;11(2):150–156

57. Ryken TC, Heary RF, Matz PG, et al; Joint Section on Disorders of the Spine and Peripheral Nerves of the American Association of Neurological Surgeons and Congress of Neurological Surgeons. Cervical laminectomy for the treatment of cervical degenerative myelopathy. J Neurosurg Spine 2009;11(2):142–149

58. Coe JD, Warden KE, Sutterlin CE III, McAfee PC. Biomechanical evaluation of cervical spinal stabilization methods in a human cadaveric model. Spine 1989;14(10):1122–1131

59. Grubb MR, Currier BL, Stone J, Warden KE, An KN. Biomechanical evaluation of posterior cervical stabilization after a wide laminectomy. Spine 1997;22(17):1948–1954

60. Nowinski GP, Visarius H, Nolte LP, Herkowitz HN. A biomechanical comparison of cervical laminaplasty and cervical laminectomy with progressive facetectomy. Spine 1993; 18(14):1995–2004

61. Sciubba DM, Chaichana KL, Woodworth GF, McGirt MJ, Gokaslan ZL, Jallo GI. Factors associated with cervical instability requiring fusion after cervical laminectomy for intradural tumor resection. J Neurosurg Spine 2008;8(5):413–419

62. McAllister BD, Rebholz BJ, Wang JC. Is posterior fusion necessary with laminectomy in the cervical spine? Surg Neurol Int 2012;3(Suppl 3):S225–S231

63. Saito T, Yamamuro T, Shikata J, Oka M, Tsutsumi S. Analysis and prevention of spinal column deformity following cervical laminectomy. I. Pathogenetic analysis of postlaminectomy deformities. Spine 1991; 16(5):494–502

64. Yasuoka S, Peterson HA, Laws ER Jr, MacCarty CS. Pathogenesis and prophylaxis of postlaminectomy deformity of the spine after multiple level laminectomy: difference between children and adults. Neurosurgery 1981;9(2):145–152

65. Albert TJ, Vacarro A. Postlaminectomy kyphosis. Spine 1998;23(24):2738–2745

66. Deutsch H, Haid RW, Rodts GE, Mummaneni PV. Postlaminectomy cervical deformity. Neurosurg Focus 2003;15(3):E5

67. Sakaura H, Hosono N, Mukai Y, Fujimori T, Iwasaki M, Yoshikawa H. Preservation of muscles attached to the C2 and C7 spinous processes rather than subaxial deep extensors reduces adverse effects after cervical laminoplasty. Spine 2010;35(16):E782–E786

68. Chang V, Lu DC, Hoffman H, Buchanan C, Holly LT. Clinical results of cervical laminectomy and fusion for the treatment of cervical spondylotic myelopathy in 58 consecutive patients. Surg Neurol Int 2014;5(Suppl 3):S133–S137

69. Kalb S, Martirosyan NL, Perez-Orribo L, Kalani MY, Theodore N. Analysis of demographics, risk factors, clinical presentation, and surgical treatment modalities for the ossified posterior longitudinal ligament. Neurosurg Focus 2011;30(3):E11

70. LaRocca H, Macnab I. The laminectomy membrane. Studies in its evolution, characteristics, effects and prophylaxis in dogs. J Bone Joint Surg Br 1974;56B(3):545–550

71. Herkowitz HN. Cervical laminaplasty: its role in the treatment of cervical radiculopathy. J Spinal Disord 1988;1(3):179–188

72. Kitahara T, Hanakita J, Takahashi T. Postlaminectomy membrane with dynamic spinal cord compression disclosed with computed tomographic myelography: a case report and literature review. Spinal Cord Ser Cases 2017;3:17056

73. Vender JR, Rekito AJ, Harrison SJ, McDonnell DE. The evolution of posterior cervical and occipitocervical fusion and instrumentation. Neurosurg Focus 2004;16(1):E9

74. Epstein JA, Epstein NE. The Cervical Spine. 2nd ed. Philadelphia: JB Lippincott; 1989

75. Abduljabbar FH, Teles AR, Bokhari R, Weber M, Santaguida C. Laminectomy with or without fusion to manage degenerative cervical myelopathy. Neurosurg Clin N Am 2018;29(1):91–105

76. Weiland DJ, McAfee PC. Posterior cervical fusion with triple-wire strut graft technique: one hundred consecutive patients. J Spinal Disord 1991;4(1):15–21

77. Lovely TJ, Carl A. Posterior cervical spine fusion with tension-band wiring. J Neurosurg 1995;83(4):631–635

78. Weis JC, Cunningham BW, Kanayama M, Parker L, McAfee PC. In vitro biomechanical comparison of multistrand cables with conventional cervical stabilization. Spine 1996;21(18):2108–2114

79. Epstein NE. Laminectomy with posterior wiring and fusion for cervical ossification of the posterior longitudinal ligament, spondylosis, ossification of the yellow ligament, stenosis, and instability: a study of 5 patients. J Spinal Disord 1999;12(6):461–466

80. González-Feria L. The effect of surgical immobilization after laminectomy in the treatment of advanced cases of cervical spondylotic myelopathy. Acta Neurochir (Wien) 1975;31(3-4):185–193

81. Graham AW, Swank ML, Kinard RE, Lowery GL, Dials BE. Posterior cervical arthrodesis and stabilization with a lateral mass plate. Clinical and computed tomographic evaluation of lateral mass screw placement and associated complications. Spine 1996;21(3):323–328, discussion 329

82. Kumar VG, Rea GL, Mervis LJ, McGregor JM. Cervical spondylotic myelopathy: functional and radiographic long-term outcome after laminectomy and posterior fusion. Neurosurgery 1999;44(4):771–777, discussion 777–778

83. Abumi K, Kaneda K. Pedicle screw fixation for nontraumatic lesions of the cervical spine. Spine 1997;22(16):1853–1863

84. Abumi K, Kaneda K, Shono Y, Fujiya M. One-stage posterior decompression and reconstruction of the cervical spine by using pedicle screw fixation systems. J Neurosurg 1999; 90(1, Suppl):19–26

85. Joaquim AF, Mudo ML, Tan LA, Riew KD. Posterior subaxial cervical spine screw fixation: A review of techniques. Global Spine J 2018;8(7):751–760

86. Youssef JA, Heiner AD, Montgomery JR, et al. Outcomes of posterior cervical fusion and decompression: a systematic review and meta-analysis. Spine J 2019;19(10): 1714–1729

87. Cole T, Veeravagu A, Zhang M, Azad TD, Desai A, Ratliff JK. Anterior versus posterior approach for multilevel degenerative cervical disease: a retrospective propensity score-matched study of the Market Scan database. Spine 2015;40(13):1033–1038

88. Tang JA, Scheer JK, Smith JS, et al; ISSG. The impact of standing regional cervical sagittal alignment on outcomes in posterior cervical fusion surgery. Neurosurgery 2015;76 (Suppl 1):S14–S21, discussion S21

89. Wang M, Luo XJ, Deng QX, Li JH, Wang N. Prevalence of axial symptoms after posterior cervical decompression: a meta-analysis. Eur Spine J 2016;25(7):2302–2310

90. Derman PB, Lampe LP, Hughes AP, et al. Demographic, clinical, and operative factors affecting long- term revision rates after cervical spine arthrodesis. J Bone Joint Surg Am 2016;98(18):1533–1540

91. Bartels RH, Groenewoud H, Peul WC, Arts MP. Lamifuse: results of a randomized controlled trial comparing laminectomy with and without fusion for cervical spondylotic myelopathy. J Neurosurg Sci 2017;61(2):134–139

92. Fehlings MG, Barry S, Kopjar B, et al. Anterior versus posterior surgical approaches to treat cervical spondylotic myelopathy: outcomes of the prospective multicenter AOSpine North America CSM study in 264 patients. Spine 2013;38(26):2247–2252

93. Du W, Wang L, Shen Y, Zhang Y, Ding W, Ren L. Long-term impacts of different posterior operations on curvature, neurological recovery and axial symptoms for multilevel cervical degenerative myelopathy. Eur Spine J 2013;22(7):1594–1602

94. Ahn DK, Park HS, Kim TW, et al. The degree of bacterial contamination while performing spine surgery. Asian Spine J 2013;7(1): 8–13

95. Fang A, Hu SS, Endres N, Bradford DS. Risk factors for infection after spinal surgery. Spine 2005;30(12):1460–1465

96. Shiraishi T. Skip laminectomy—a new treatment for cervical spondylotic myelopathy, preserving bilateral muscular attachments to the spinous processes: a preliminary report. Spine J 2002;2(2):108–115

97. Yukawa Y, Kato F, Ito K, et al. Laminoplasty and skip laminectomy for cervical compressive myelopathy: range of motion, postoperative neck pain, and surgical outcomes in a randomized prospective study. Spine 2007;32(18):1980–1985

98. Sivaraman A, Bhadra AK, Altaf F, et al. Skip laminectomy and laminoplasty for cervical spondylotic myelopathy: a prospective study of clinical and radiologic outcomes. J Spinal Disord Tech 2010;23(2):96–100

99. Yuan W, Zhu Y, Liu X, Zhou X, Cui C. Laminoplasty versus skip laminectomy for the treatment of multilevel cervical spondylotic myelopathy: a systematic review. Arch Orthop Trauma Surg 2014; 134(1):1–7

100. Traynelis VC, Arnold PM, Fourney DR, Bransford RJ, Fischer DJ, Skelly AC. Alternative procedures for the treatment of cervical spondylotic myelopathy: arthroplasty, oblique corpectomy, skip laminectomy: evaluation of comparative effectiveness and safety. Spine 2013; 38(22, Suppl 1):S210–S231

101. Robins JMW, Luo L, Mallalah F, et al. Skip laminectomy versus cervical laminectomy, an analysis of patient reported outcomes, spinal alignment and re-operation rates: The Leeds spinal unit experience (2008–2016). Interdisc Neurosurg 2019;16:44–50

17 Posterior Cervical Fixation Techniques after Laminectomy

Jutty Parthiban, Maurizio Fornari, Umesh Srikantha, Francesco Costa, and Carla D. Anania

Introduction

Cervical laminectomy is a standard procedure applied to decompress the spinal cord in cervical spondylotic myelopathy (CSM) and ossified posterior longitudinal ligament (OPLL). Since the paraspinal muscles are dissected extensively from their attachments, the tension band that maintains the classical lordosis is lost and that leads to loss of lordosis and progresses to kyphosis in the long run, especially in young patients and in upper spinal segments. This can lead to progression of neurological deficit, due to ventral cord compression and loss of biomechanical stability of subaxial cervical spine. This is more complex when the muscles attached to the spinous process of axis C2 are detached, leading to loss of rotational component at craniocervical junction. To avoid and prevent such complications to occur, laminoplasties and muscle-sparing techniques were developed. In spite of all these developments, laminectomy still holds a key place in the surgeon's choice. However, to prevent loss of lordosis and progression of kyphosis, posterior instrumentations are now popularly added, following laminectomy in select cases. Since spinal laminectomy has already been done, the available bony structures are lateral masses and facet joints and adjacent nonexcised laminae. Subsequent to invention of screw techniques, the following are now in practice to stabilize cervical spine following laminectomy: C1 atlas lateral mass screw, C2 axis pedicle and pars screw, C3–6 lateral mass and pedicle screw, and C7 pedicle screw. Polyaxial screws secured in these bony structures are coupled with rods to stabilize the cervical spine. These posterior fixation techniques need surgical expertise and are elegant and effective. The authors like to call this group of fixations as posterior lateral fixation techniques.

In this chapter, we will describe the history, indications, and background of each technique separately, the screw entry points with relevant important anatomical relations, screw insertions and fixation, art of avoiding complications, along with case examples.

Indications for Posterior Lateral Cervical Fixations

In recent times, posterior instrumentation following long-segment laminectomies for cervical OPLL has become a norm in many centers. However, in degenerative spondylotic myelopathy, instrumentations are judiciously used. In rigid, fused, and elderly degenerative spine, laminectomies are done as standalone procedures with good results. However, progression in degeneration leads to loss of lordosis and progression of kyphosis in younger patients. Hence, the requirement for instrumentation needs to be analyzed critically. Serial roentgenogram of cervical spine demonstrating progressive loss of lordosis, progression of kyphosis, segmental instability and multilevel listhesis, neck pain, restriction of range of movements, pain, paresthesia, and buckling in upper and lower limbs, following flexion and extension movements of neck, indicate the need for instrumentation following decompressive laminectomy. Posterior fixations are also done in conjunction with anterior decompressions in select complex cases, wherein segmental anterior cord compressions need to be decompressed and fixed anteriorly and posteriorly to achieve satisfactory stabilization. Apart from radiological evidence of fusion, per operative observation of solid fusion at facet joints contraindicates posterior instrumentation, especially in short segments. Finally, it is the experience of the surgeon that stands first in the judgement of instrumentation following cervical laminectomy.

Background and History

Atlantoaxial (C1–C2) Fixation

In 1994, Goel and Laheri described the C1 lateral mass and C2 pars screws joined together with a plate as a novel technique of C1–C2 stabilization.[1] This was later modified by Harms and Melcher in 2001, wherein the screws were joined with a rod.[2] This technique has become increasingly popular, both because of its biomechanical stability, and the versatile nature of pathological conditions where it can be applied. Minimally invasive atlantoaxial fixation techniques have also been described in recent times.[3,4] Atlantoaxial fusion can also be included as part of occipitocervical fixations or as an extension of subaxial cervical spine fixations whenever needed.

Subaxial (C3–6) Lateral Mass Fixation

The major advancement in this field has been the development of the osteosynthetic lateral mass (articular pillar) plate and screw system introduced by Roy Camille, a French orthopaedic surgeon in the 1970s who popularized this technique. This dynamic fixator functions as a tension band and resists flexion and rotational movements most efficiently. Magerl modified the technique with changes in the screw trajectory, using longer screw and gaining bicortical purchase of the lateral mass, and claimed biomechanical superiority. In 1987, Cooper introduced the lateral mass plate and screw fixation technique in North America using the Roy Camille vitallium plates.[5,6] The modified Magerl technique was introduced by An, in 1991, and was

followed successfully by Haid and Traynelis.[7] Jeanneret, in 1996, introduced the rod system called "Cervi Fix," a versatile system with improvised specific angulations required for the lateral masses, pedicles, and the occipital bone as well.

Subaxial (C3–7) Pedicle Screw Fixation

Placing pedicle screws in cervical spine were restricted to C2 and C7 for a long time until Abumi, in 1994, described and popularized its usage at all levels in the subaxial cervical spine.[8–10] Ebraheim in 1997 described the free hand technique later.[11] Very recently, Zhang et al in 2020 described free hand technique using a universal entry point and trajectory in all cervical, thoracic, and lumbar spine.[12]

Cervical pedicle screw, in view of its purchase into all three vertebral columns, provides the strongest construct among all screws that can be inserted into the subaxial cervical spine. Since cervical pedicle screws are technically demanding and have the potential to cause serious neurovascular injuries, their use remains restricted as compared to easier alternatives (lateral mass screws, facet screws) that are available for rigid fixation in the subaxial cervical spine. A majority of surgeons who routinely place pedicle screws into C2 and C7 still prefer to combine it with lateral mass screws in C3 to C6 vertebra.[13]

Technique of Screw Placement and Fixation

In this section, the authors will describe the related anatomy, screw entry point, and trajectory of screwing.

Atlantoaxial (C1–C2) Screw Fixation

C1 Lateral Mass Screw

Inserting a C1 lateral mass screw is easy and straightforward once adequate exposure is obtained. The C1 lateral mass is like a cuboid when seen from posterior aspect, and once the lateral and medial margins are known, the screw entry point lies at the center. Three slightly different methods have been described to insert C1 lateral mass screws: (a) the sublaminar (direct); (b) translaminar and (c) notching technique (**Fig. 17.1**). The sublaminar (direct insertion) was described by Goel, wherein the entry point lies under the posterior arch of C1, mediolaterally at the middle of the lateral mass, with the screw being directed superiorly (10–15°) and medially (10–15°) (**Fig. 17.1a–c**).[1] This technique requires a good exposure of the C1 lateral mass, more dissection, and often sacrifice of the C2 root for adequate exposure to the entry point. To minimize the venous plexus dissection and preserve C2 nerve root, Tan described a technique of inserting a C1 lateral

mass screw through the lamina, with hardly any medial (0–5°) or superior (0–5°) angulation (**Fig. 17.1d–f**).[14] Concerns with this technique would include the thin nature of lamina (which may lead to fracture) and any inadvertent superior breach, which could potentially damage the vertebral artery. The notching technique described by Lee in 2006 is essentially a compromise between the other two, wherein a notch is created at the inferior border of the posterior arch of C1 which, in turn, will lead to the lateral mass of C1 (**Fig. 17.1g–i**) (**Table 17.1**).[15] The screw in this situation is inserted with an intermediate medial (10°) and superior (5–10°) angulation as compared to the other two techniques. Bicortical purchase for C1 lateral mass screws has been described for improving pull-out strengths; however, it carries with it an increased risk of injury to carotid artery and

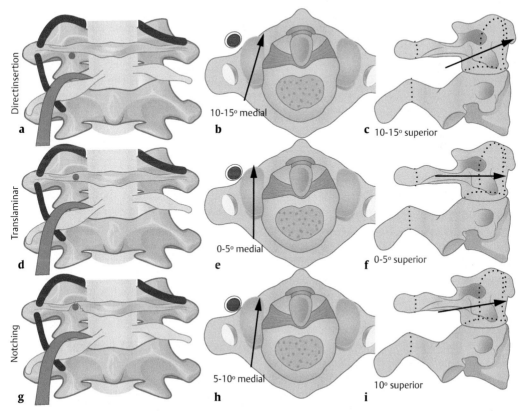

Fig. 17.1 C1 Lateral mass screw techniques. Diagram showing various techniques, namely, direct insertion, translaminar, and notching.

Table 17.1 Anatomical references for C1 lateral mass screw positioning

Author	Entry point	Axial trajectory	Sagittal trajectory
Goel and Laheri (sublaminar)[1]	Under the posterior arch, mediolaterally at the center of lateral mass	10°–15° medially	10°–15° superiorly
Tan (translaminar)[14]	Through lamina at mid lateral mass	0°–5° medially	0°–5° superiorly
Lee (notching technique)[15]	Notch at inferior border of arch at mid lateral mass	10° medially	5°–10° superiorly

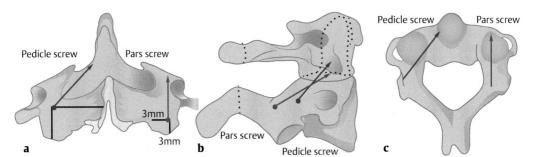

Fig. 17.2 C2 pars and pedicle screw techniques. Diagram showing pars and pedicle screw insertion and trajectory. Dorsal (**a**), lateral (**b**), axial (**c**) views.

hypoglossal nerve, both of which lie within 2 to 3 mm of the anterior aspect of C1 lateral mass.[16,17]

C2 Fixation Options

The axis (C2) provides the maximum number of options to insert a screw, more than any other single vertebral bone in the human body. This section will discuss the two posterior fixation points at C2 pars screw and pedicle screw. Each of these screws can be connected via a rod to the C1 lateral mass screw to achieve a comprehensive atlanto-axial fixation.

The C2 pars screw (**Fig. 17.2**) has a relatively straighter course with the entry point around 3 mm superior to the inferior border and 3 mm lateral to the medial border of the inferior facet of C2, being directed 20° superiorly and 10° medially.[18] Identifying the medial border of the pars as it curves superiorly and medially can be an easy guide to the

direction of the screw. The C2 pedicle screw (**Fig. 17.2**) has a relatively more oblique angle, the entry point being situated at the junction of a vertical line bisecting C2 inferior articular surface and a horizontal line at junction of upper 1/3rd and lower 2/3rd of lamina, being directed 30° medially and 20 to 30° superiorly. In comparison to the pars screw, the pedicle screw has a superior and lateral entry point (closer to the vertebral foramen) and a more medial and superior angulation, so that the screw tip lies closer to the base of dens medial to the superior facet of C2, while the screw tip in a pars screw lies under the superior facet of C2 (**Table 17.2**).[19,20]

Subaxial (C3 to C6) Lateral Mass Screw Fixation

Surgical Anatomy of Lateral Mass

Understanding of the anatomical relationships of the lateral masses of the cervical

Table 17.2 Anatomical references for C2 fixations:

Entry point		Axial trajectory	Sagittal trajectory
Pars screw	3 mm superior to inferior border and 3 mm lateral to medial border of inferior facet	10° medially	20° superiorly
Pedicle screw	Junction of vertical line bisecting C2 inferior articular surface and a horizontal line at upper 1/3 and lower 2/3 of lamina	30° medially	20°–30° superiorly

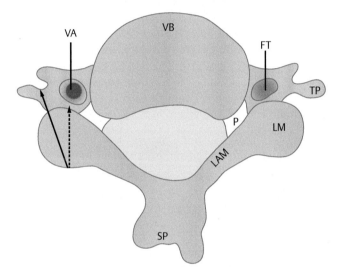

Fig. 17.3 Surgical anatomy of lateral mass of subaxial cervical spine axial view: VA: vertebral artery, VB: vertebral body, FT: foramen transversarium, TP: transverse process, P: pedicle, LM: lateral mass, LAM: lamina, SP: spinous process. Arrows show the direction of screws in lateral mass.

spine is very important to achieve proper screw placement. Since the surgeon visualizes only the posterior aspect of these masses, those structures that are immediately anterior to them are of prime concern when screws are placed. The lateral mass (articular pillar) is the bulky lateral extension of the lamina and is connected to the vertebral body through the pedicles in an anteromedial direction. The transverse process, which harbors the foramen transversarium in its medial part, is connected to the vertebral body through a thin strut. It is also connected to the lateral mass through a relatively thicker bony portion (**Fig. 17.3**). The lateral masses are called articular pillars, since the superior and the inferior articular processes are formed from these masses.

The three superior facets are usually not seen from posterior. The lateral masses of the C7 vertebra are relatively thinner than the other cervical vertebrae. The margin of the lateral mass is defined superiorly and inferiorly by the facet joints, laterally by the extreme edge of the mass, and medially by the lateral margin of the lamina. The center point of the mass (hillock) is the highest point and coincides with the summit of the facet. The vital structures, the vertebral artery travelling through foramen transversarium and the cervical nerve root emerging from the spinal canal through the intervertebral foramen, are placed anterior to the lateral masses and are not seen from behind.

Cadaver studies by Pait et al described the surgical anatomy of lateral mass in detail.[21,22] The lateral mass, which is square-shaped when viewed from posterior approach, is divided into four quadrants, namely, superolateral, inferolateral, superomedial and inferomedial, using the following bony landmarks: 1) lateral facet line (LFL), a line from one facet joint to the next facet joint along the posterolateral border of the lateral mass; 2) medical facet line (MFL), a line from one facet joint to the next facet joint at the junction of the lamina and the lateral mass; 3) rostrocaudal line (RCL), a line on the posterior surface of the pillar in the rostrocaudal direction dividing the mass into two vertical halves; and 4) intrafacet line (IFL), a line extending mediolaterally through the center of the mass perpendicular to the above lines (**Fig. 17.4**). The vertebral artery courses under the superomedial and inferomedial quadrants along the MFL. The cervical nerve root, on emerging from the neural foramina, travel in a lateral, oblique, forward and downward direction from the superomedial to the inferolateral quadrant. During their course, the nerve roots lie dorsal to the vertebral artery. The superolateral quadrant, under which vital neurovascular structures do not lie, is the

safe quadrant and is considered ideal for the placement of lateral mass screws (**Fig. 17.5**).

In addition to the basic surgical anatomy, a few critical points have to be borne in mind for proper screw placement. Cadaver studies have demonstrated variation in the measurement of the landmark lines from one lateral mass to the other and at different levels. The distance between the dorsal surface of the lateral mass peek and underlying vertebral artery is of clinical importance. The average distance is between 14 and 15 mm. Hence, a screw passed from hillock straight ahead should be of 14 mm length or less to avoid vertebral artery injury. Anomalies of the vertebral artery should be kept in mind. The position of the foramen transversarium may vary in relation to each lateral mass and at

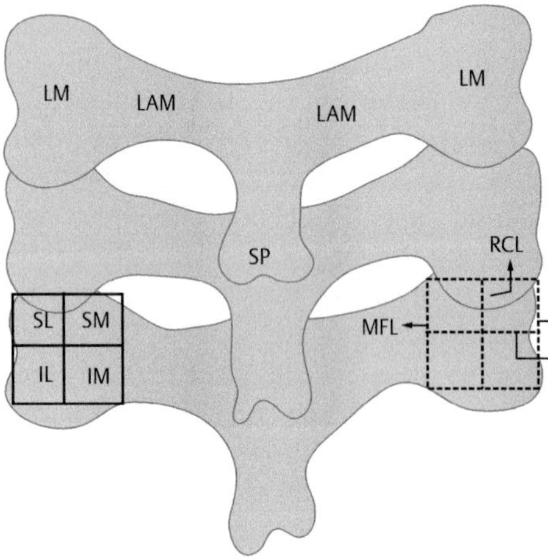

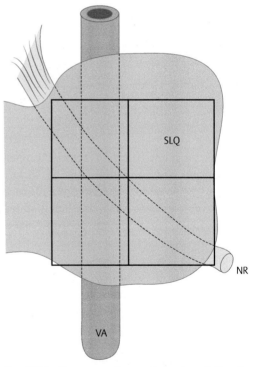

Fig. 17.4 Four quadrants of lateral mass. Quadrants: SM: superomedial, IM: inferomedial, IL: inferolateral, SL: superolateral. Lines: LFL: lateral facet line, MFL: medial facet line. RCL: rostrocaudal line, IFL: intrafacet line. Screw entry point is marked 1 mm medial to the center of the lateral mass.

Fig. 17.5 Neurovascular anatomy in relation to lateral mass. The vertebral artery (VA) is anterior in relation to superior and inferior medial quadrants. The nerve root (NR) traverses anteriorly from superomedial to inferolateral in relation to lateral mass. SLQ: superolateral quadrant.

different level. Axial cut of the CT/MRI scans will help in determining the exact lateral angulation required to enable safe placement of the screws. The lateral masses are irregularly oval in the axial cut and squarish dome-shaped in the posterior. This knowledge is important in selecting the entry point of the screw to gain maximum purchase of the lateral mass.

Standard Screw Trajectories

There are many trajectories described in the literature with regard to screw placement. **Table 17.3** shows the different angulations and the screw entry points followed by the different authors.[23] The site of entry is either at the center or medial to the center of the lateral mass in order to gain the maximum purchase. Universally, each author has advocated placing the screws in the superior lateral quadrant. However, lateral angulation varies from 10° to 30° and the direction of screws in the sagittal plane varies from the perpendicular of the long axis of the spine (straight ahead) to 40° cephalad (parallel to the facet joints). Each author claims excellent results using their respective trajectories.[5,6,24–32] Heller comparing the Roy Camille and Magerl techniques and found that both were safe in experienced hands.[28] However, reported studies have shown the following:

- The more medial and cephalad the trajectory, the more likely a nerve root injury could occur.
- When the screws were directed using the Haid (An, Traynelis) method, the distance between the screw and the vertebral artery averaged 7 mm and the distance from the nerve root averaged 5 mm.[27]
- Risks of facet joint violation and incorporation of the adjacent motion segment are higher when screws were directed strictly anteriorly.

Table 17.3 Anatomical references for subaxial cervical spine lateral mass screw positioning

Author	Site of entry (relation to midpoint of lateral mass)	Direction	
		Sagittal plane angulation	Lateral
Camille	Center	Perpendicular (straight ahead)	10°
Magerl[27]	1 to 2 mm medial and rostral	40° cephalad to facet joint	25°
Anderson et al[34]	1 mm medial	Parallel to facet joint	10°
Cooper[7]	1 mm medial	Perpendicular to the long axis of the spine	10°
Sawin and Traynelis[51]	1 mm medial	15° cephalad	10°–20°
Haid et al[25]	1 mm medial	10°–20° cephalad	30°
Nazarian and Louis[31]	At the intersection of a vertical line 5 mm medial to lateral edge of facet joint, and a horizontal line 3 mm below the inferior edge of facet joint line above	Straight ahead, 90° to the surface of lateral mass	No lateral angulation
Riew et al[23]	1 mm medial and 1 mm caudal to the center of lateral mass	Aim towards upper and outer corner of lateral mass	Aim towards upper and outer corner of lateral mass

- Various studies, including cadaveric, were undertaken to study the efficacy of different screw trajectories in use.

Gill and Montessano, from their research, found that bicortical screws had the highest mean of stiffness as compared to unicortical screws and, hence, were biomechanically superior.[33,34]

Drilling the Lateral Mass

The trajectory at each level is planned from the preoperative radiological study. Authors have used different trajectories at different levels with satisfactory results. Minor adjustments may have to be made preoperatively. The aim is to place the screws in the superolateral quadrant of the lateral mass.

Each lateral mass must be inspected carefully. The central point of the lateral mass, which usually corresponds to the highest point of the lateral mass, is marked. The screw entry point is selected 1 mm medial to the central point of the lateral mass. Using a 2.7 mm diameter diamond drill bit fitted into a long, angled handle, the outer cortex is pierced gently at a slow speed. The drill is angled laterally by about 25 degrees and usually about 15 degrees rostrally in the trajectory of eventual screw placement (**Fig. 17.6**). As the trajectory is directed away from the foramen transversarium, vertebral artery injury should not occur. The trajectory can be monitored using fluoroscopy. Torque movement during drilling should be avoided to

prevent a wide proximal cortical opening. Steady and precise drilling is performed until the inner cortex is pierced, which will be felt by a "give away" sensation. This step is important to get bicortical purchase. While removing the drill bit, the trajectory should not be changed. Blood may ooze profusely from the hole, which can be stopped by applying bone wax over the entry point. The same procedure is performed in all the lateral masses selected for fixation. An appropriate tap is used to tap the other cortex only and bone wax is reapplied if the oozing continues. In this way, the lateral masses from C3 to C6 can be drilled.

Cervical Pedicle Fixation C3 to C7

Identifying Entry Point

Pedicles in the cervical region present a high variability in width and orientation, making it difficult to use a standard screw entry point and trajectory. A careful analysis of preoperative CT scan is mandatory to determine width, length, and orientation of the screws. In the modern era, this can be overcome by the use of image guided systems coupled with navigation systems.[4,5,35,36] Usually, the width of the screw varies from 3 to 4 mm, and it is proven to be a good compromise between screw size and pull out resistance.

Identifying the correct entry point is a critical step in placement of subaxial cervical pedicle screws. The lateral vertebral

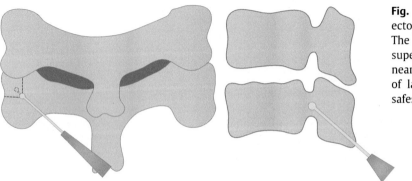

Fig. 17.6 Screw trajectory in lateral mass. The screw directed superolaterally from near the center point of lateral mass is the safest trajectory.

notch is a reliable landmark to identify the entry point, and is relatively unaltered even in severe degenerative changes.[37,38] From C3–C6, the notch is located at the exact same level as the pedicles and is at a slightly lower level than the pedicle at C7. Hence, the entry point at C3–C6 can be at the level of the notch and slightly higher than the notch at C7 (**Fig. 17.7**). Using these surface landmarks, a cervical pedicle screw will actually traverse through three portions: the lateral mass, pedicle, and the vertebral body. Using surface landmarks alone also minimizes the margin of error, since the pedicle is not directly visualized (**Fig. 17.8**). Hence, for better accuracy, Abumi technique recommends to drill lateral and upper half of the lateral mass, in order to directly identify the cancellous bone leading into the pedicle (**Fig. 17.9a**).

In the "key-slot" technique, only a small portion of the medial lateral mass has to be drilled to identify the cancellous bone leading to the pedicle (**Fig. 17.9b**).[39] This is, in essence, a modification of the Abumi technique to minimize bone loss within the lateral mass. Ebraheim et al described pedicle screw entry and trajectory from dry bone studies in 1997 (**Table 17.4**).[11]

Identifying and Traversing the Pedicle

Once the pedicle entry point is identified, sequential curettage of the pedicle is done (similar to funnel technique used in thoracic spine) with a 1 mm cup curette, a medial angulation of 35 to 45°, and the curette being directed toward the medial pedicle wall for the reasons mentioned above. Sometimes, if there is significant resistance, a small burr attached to a high-speed burr can be used. However, one should be confident of the trajectory before using the burr. Whenever in doubt, it is better to open a small area of the lamina medial to the pedicle (laminoforaminotomy) to directly visualize and palpate the medial wall of the pedicle, which would give a good estimate of the direction of the screw (**Fig. 17.9c**).

Assessing Screw Accuracy

The most ideal way to assess screw accuracy is by doing a postoperative CT scan. Neo et al

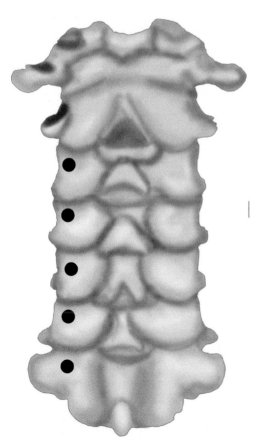

Fig. 17.7 Pedicle screw entry point in subaxial cervical spine.

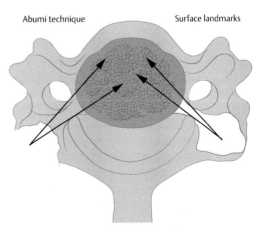

Fig. 17.8 Pedicle screw trajectory.

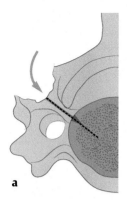 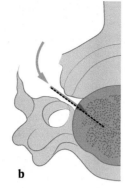 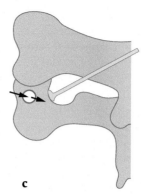

a   b   c

Fig. 17.9 Technique of entering pedicle. **(a)** Drill lateral and upper half of the lateral mass. **(b)** Identify the cancellous bone leading to the pedicle. **(c)** Palpate the medial wall of the pedicle.

Table 17.4   Anatomical references for pedicle screw positioning in cervical spine

Technique	Entry point	Axial trajectory	Sagittal trajectory
Abumi et al[8]	Lateral to the center of the facet/lateral mass and close to the inferior margin of the superior articular surface	25° to 45° medial to the midline in the horizontal plane	Parallel to the endplate of the vertebral body for C5 to C7 and slightly cranially inclined for C2 to C4
Ebraheim et al[11]	Superior and lateral corner of the lateral mass	45° medially for C3 to C6 and 35% medially for C7	10° caudally inclined for C3 and C4 1° cranially inclined for C6 and vertically for C5

classified the vertebral foraminal breach into four grades (**Fig. 17.10a–d**): grade I: within pedicle; grade IIa: perforation < 25% and no contact with neurovascular structures; grade IIb: perforation < 25% and contact; grade III: perforation > 25%.[40] Apart from this, medial wall breach can also be divided into four grades (**Fig. 17.10e–h**): grade 0: no perforation; grade 1: < 25%; grade 2: 20% to 50%; grade 3: > 50% of the screw diameter violation into the canal. One newer way of intraoperative accuracy assessment is by doing an intraoperative 3D imaging (3D C-arm or O-arm), wherein corrective measures can be taken in case of grade 3 breach before closing the wound. In situations where a CT scan was not available for assessment, Lee et al considered the position of the screw head and screw tip on plain radiographs/C-arm to get a reasonable accuracy information about the integrity of pedicle screw. As per them, a screw head that is located at the lateral margin of the lateral mass with the tip located medial to uncovertebral joint is considered safe.[41]

Rod Fixation and Fusion

Appropriate diameter titanium rods are selected, contoured to required lordosis, and fixed with the screw heads before completing final tightening.

Since laminectomy has been done, bony fusion can be achieved at facet joints. The facet joint capsules removed, cartilaginous surface drilled out, and existing joint space packed with corticocancellous bones obtained from laminectomy. Fusion procedure can be done before securing the rods over the screw heads. Illustrative cases showing all these techniques are in **Figs. 17.11** and **17.12**.

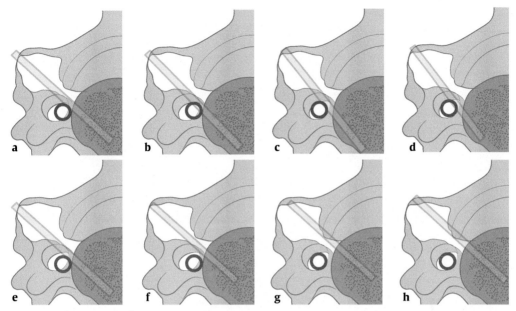

Fig. 17.10 Assessment of screw accuracy.

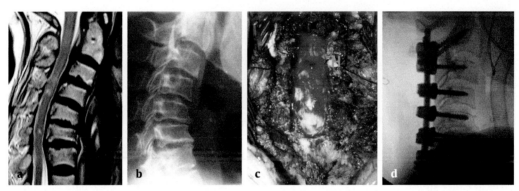

Fig. 17.11 Illustrative clinical case example C2–7 cervical pedicle screw fixation. Preoperative sagittal T2W MR image **(a)** and a lateral plain radiograph **(b)** showing a fixed kyphotic deformity in the cervical spine with intrinsic cord signal changes. Intraoperative view after laminectomy and preparation for pedicle screw insertion **(c)**. Intraoperative image after insertion of pedicle screws from C2–C7 with correction of the kyphotic deformity **(d)**.

Recent Advances

Intraoperative 3D imaging (CT based/O-arm based) combined with navigation has been extremely helpful in identifying exact entry points and trajectory for subaxial pedicle screws, even in presence of severe degeneration and other instances where surface and anatomical landmarks are distorted or deformed (**Fig. 17.13**). Intraoperative 3D imaging can also assess screw integrity on the operating table, so that any major breaches can be detected and corrective measures, if needed, can be taken before closing the wound. In addition, robotic assisted surgery and impedance measuring probes are helpful in reducing the risks involved in pedicle screw placement. Recent literature claims

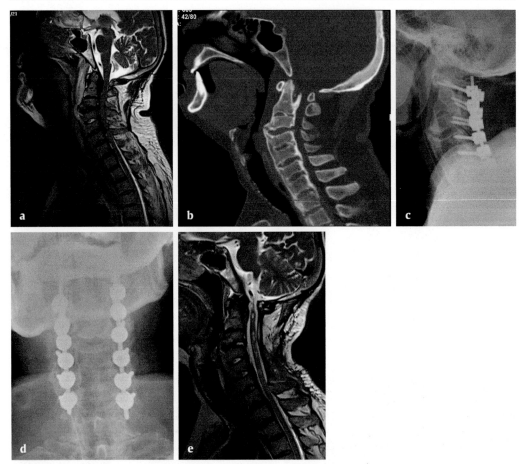

Fig. 17.12 Illustrative clinical case example of C1 lateral mass, C2 pars, and C3–6 lateral mass fixation. Preoperative sagittal MR image of a progressive spastic quadriparetic patient shows canal stenosis and cord compression from C1 to C6 due to segmental ossified posterior longitudinal ligament (OPLL) **(a)**. Sagittal CT showing OPLL significant at C2 crocodile calcification and cervical canal stenosis **(b)**. X-ray lateral view **(c)** showing C1 lateral mass, C2 pars and C3–6 lateral mass screws, and contoured rod fixation. X-ray AP view **(d)** showing C1–C6 posterior lateral fixation. Note the lateral mass screws at C3–6 are laterally and superiorly directed. Note C1 posterior arch excision and C2–C6 laminectomy. Postoperative sagittal MRI **(e)** showing the decompressed spinal cord from C1 to C6.

these technological advances reduce complications significantly.[36,42,43]

Complications

Complications at C1–C2 Fixations

One of the most feared, yet less common complications of a C1–C2 procedure is vertebral artery injury. This can happen during exposure if dissection is carried out too laterally at the superior aspect of both C1 and C2, a vertebral artery anomaly is not recognized, or during screw placement, due to vertebral foraminal breach.[44,45] Risk of vertebral artery injury is higher in case of high riding vertebral artery. A pars screw is the best choice in this situation.

Paresthesia along the C2 nerve distribution, mostly as a result of inappropriate

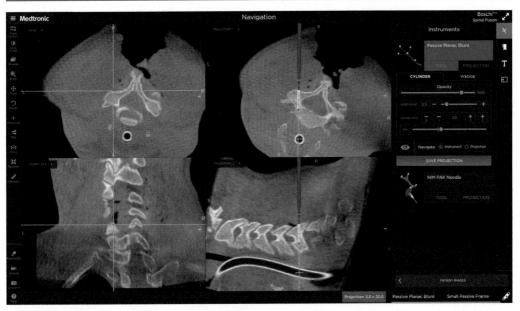

Fig. 17.13 Intraoperative neuronavigation guidance for pedicle screw fixation.

handling of the C2 ganglion in order to over-zealously preserve the C2 root, is common, albeit innocuous. C2 neuralgia has also been reported in a significant proportion of cases with C2 nerve root transection, although recent evidence suggests that sharply dividing the C2 ganglion in its middle overlying the C1–C2 joint is safe and does not result in postoperative neuralgia.[46–50]

Complications at Lateral Mass Fixations

Violation of the facet joint with ankylosis of an additional segment, screw loosening, and screw pull out are reported complications. Vertebral artery damage, directly related to screw placement is rare. Clinically, nerve root injury in the form of radiculopathy ranges between 0 to 0.6%. Redirection of the screws helps in treating this problem. Although anatomical and cadaveric studies predicted 3.6% nerve root injury, this is not so in clinical practice. Currently, studies are being undertaken to assess nerve root involvement after drilling and the subsequent placement of screws

using evoked electromyography (EMG) and electrophysiological studies with intraoperative neuromonitoring (IONM).[51] These studies may be useful in redirecting the screws in the event of the nerve being involved.

Complications at Pedicle Screw Fixations

Apart from the fact that cervical pedicle screws are technically demanding, one of the major concerns is injury to neurovascular structures in the event of a misplaced screw. Literature reports around 4 to 12% of major (grade IIb and III) and 9 to 30% of overall perforations with more than 3/4th of the perforations being on the lateral pedicle wall.[52,53] Among the vertebral levels, the incidence of major breach was higher in C3 and C4 and almost nil in C7. Despite high rates of lateral pedicle wall breach, incidence of "symptomatic" vertebral artery injury is considerably less in cervical pedicle screw as compared to C2 pedicle and transarticular screw, with the overall rate being 23% of cases having intraoperative vertebral artery injury.[54]

The higher rates of lateral wall breach can be attributed to the thinner lateral wall and impedance from the paravertebral muscle to attain a sufficiently medial trajectory. In such cases, a separate stab incision can be placed, and a transmuscular route can be followed to obtain the required medial trajectory.[55]

Screw loosening and pull out, implant failure, infections, dural tears, pseudo arthrosis, loss of reduction and corrections can be expected in all procedures.

Biomechanics of Posterior Cervical Fixations

Studies indicate that, in isolation, C1 lateral mass–C2 pedicle screw constructs are more stable than other constructs (transarticular screw or C2 pars screws).[56] When laminectomy is already done, the question of interlaminar wires does not arise here. However, in normal situations, a three-point fixation is biomechanically superior; hence, addition of Gallies fusion was recommended along with other lateral fixations at C1–2. In subaxial spine, lateral mass screws are easier to apply but pedicle screws are biomechanically superior to them, since the pedicle screws address all three columns of the spine. Kothe et al demonstrated higher early stability as well as during cyclic loading in multilevel human models with instability.[57] Many other studies also demonstrated their effectiveness in stabilizing all the three columns of the spine.[58]

Pedicle screws at C2 and C7 are particularly strong at where muscles are inserted at junctional regions, especially at cervicothoracic region. Noninclusion of C2 in subaxial upper level stabilization can increase stress load at C2–3 level; hence, it is advisable to include C2 in fixation (**Fig. 17.14a–c**). Similarly, extending fixation to upper thoracic level is advisable in lower cervical level. The pull-out strengths of pedicle screws are higher than lateral mass screws and lateral mass screws are weak in osteoporotic spines. The complications are relatively less with lateral mass screws in comparison with pedicle screws. Finally, despite the cited complications related to pedicle screw insertion in cervical spine large cohort studies demonstrated lower incidences of these complications, demonstrating that the safety margin is larger than hypothesized.

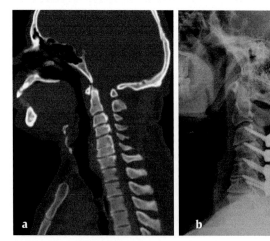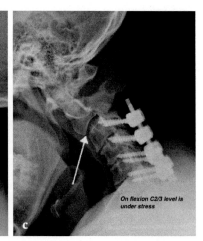

Fig. 17.14 Illustrative case example on stress at C2 and C3. CT sagittal view showing ossified posterior longitudinal ligament (OPLL) segmental C3–C6 (**a**). X-ray lateral neutral view (**b**) showing lateral mass screw fixation C3–C6. X-ray lateral flexion view (**c**) showing biomechanical stress at C2–C3 level (*white arrow*).

Conclusion

Posterior lateral cervical instrumentations following long-segment laminectomies provide excellent biomechanical stability to the cervical spine and prevent loss of lordosis and progressive kyphosis, thus preventing worsening of neurological deficits.

Complications of hardware application can be avoided with experience in surgical technique, good case selection, and proper screw placements and fixations. Spine surgeons should be familiar with all the above techniques and should select them judiciously as required.

Take-home Points

- Posterior cervical instrumentation following laminectomy provides biomechanical stability and makes sense.

- C1 lateral mass screw placement is simple and straightforward.

- C2 pars screw is easier to place than pedicle screw. Inclusion of C2 in fixation prevents adjacent segment strain.

- In subaxial spine, pedicle screws are biomechanically superior to lateral mass screws.

- Lateral mass screw placement is simple and elegant.

- Surgical experience and use of image guidance reduce complications.

References

1. Goel A, Laheri V. Plate and screw fixation for atlanto-axial subluxation. Acta Neurochir (Wien) 1994;129(1-2):47–53
2. Harms J, Melcher RP. Posterior C1-C2 fusion with polyaxial screw and rod fixation. Spine 2001;26(22):2467–2471
3. Srikantha U, Khanapure KS, Jagannatha AT, Joshi KC, Varma RG, Hegde AS. Minimally invasive atlantoaxial fusion: cadaveric study and report of 5 clinical cases. J Neurosurg Spine 2016;25(6):675–680
4. Holly LT, Isaacs RE, Frempong-Boadu AK. Minimally invasive atlantoaxial fusion. Neurosurgery 2010; 66(3, Suppl):193–197
5. An HS, Gordin R, Renner K. Anatomic considerations for plate-screw fixation of the cervical spine. Spine 1991; 16(10, Suppl): S548–S551
6. Cooper PR, Cohen A, Rosiello A, Koslow M. Posterior stabilization of cervical spine fractures and subluxations using plates and screws. Neurosurgery 1988;23(3):300–306
7. Cooper PR. Posterior stabilization of the cervical spine. Clin Neurosurg 1993;40:286–320
8. Abumi K, Itoh H, Taneichi H, Kaneda K. Transpedicular screw fixation for traumatic lesions of the middle and lower cervical spine: description of the techniques and preliminary report. J Spinal Disord 1994; 7(1):19–28
9. Abumi K. Cervical spondylotic myelopathy: posterior decompression and pedicle screw fixation. Eur Spine J 2015; 24(2, Suppl 2): 186–196
10. Abumi K, Shono Y, Taneichi H, Ito M, Kaneda K. Correction of cervical kyphosis using pedicle screw fixation systems. Spine 1999;24(22):2389–2396
11. Ebraheim NA, Xu R, Knight T, Yeasting RA. Morphometric evaluation of lower cervical pedicle and its projection. Spine 1997;22(1):1–6
12. Zhang ZF. Freehand pedicle screw placement using a universal entry point and sagittal and axial trajectory for all subaxial cervical, thoracic and lumbosacral spines. Orthop Surg 2020;12(1):141–152
13. Abumi K, Shono Y, Ito M, Taneichi H, Kotani Y, Kaneda K. Complications of pedicle screw fixation in reconstructive surgery of the cervical spine. Spine 2000;25(8):962–969
14. Tan M, Wang H, Wang Y, et al. Morphometric evaluation of screw fixation in atlas via posterior arch and lateral mass. Spine 2003; 28(9):888–895
15. Lee MJ, Cassinelli E, Riew KD. The feasibility of inserting atlas lateral mass screws via the posterior arch. Spine 2006;31(24): 2798–2801
16. Eck JC, Walker MP, Currier BL, Chen Q, Yaszemski MJ, An K-N. Biomechanical comparison of unicortical versus bicortical

C1 lateral mass screw fixation. J Spinal Disord Tech 2007;20(7):505–508

17. Seybold EA, Baker JA, Criscitiello AA, Ordway NR, Park CK, Connolly PJ. Characteristics of unicortical and bicortical lateral mass screws in the cervical spine. Spine 1999; 24(22):2397–2403

18. Schleicher P, Onal MB, Hemberger F, Scholz M, Kandziora F. The C2-pars interarticularis screw as an alternative in atlanto-axial stabilization. A biomechanical comparison of established techniques. Turk Neurosurg 2018;28(6):995–1004

19. Chin KR, Mills MV, Seale J, Cumming V. Ideal starting point and trajectory for C2 pedicle screw placement: a 3D computed tomography analysis using perioperative measurements. Spine J 2014;14(4):615–618

20. Clifton W, Vlasak A, Damon A, Dove C, Pichelmann M. Freehand c2 pedicle screw placement: surgical anatomy and operative technique. World Neurosurg 2019;132:113

21. Pait TG, McAllister PV, Kaufman HH. Quadrant anatomy of the articular pillars (lateral cervical mass) of the cervical spine. J Neurosurg 1995;82(6):1011–1014

22. Pait TG, Borba LAB. Stabilization of the cervical spine (C3–7 with articular mass (Lateral mass) plate and screws. Neurosurgical operative atlas. The Americal Association of Neurological Sciences 1996;5:91–100

23. Parthiban JKBC. Posterior stabilisation of the sub axial cervical spine. In: Ramamurhi B, Tandon PN, eds. Textbook of Operative Neurosurgery. New Delhi: BI Publications Pvt Ltd; 2005:1057–1068

24. Borne G, Bedou G, Pinaudeau M, el Omeiri S, Cristino G. Treatment of severe lesions of the lower cervical spine (C3-C7). A clinical study and technical considerations in 102 cases. Neurochirurgia (Stuttg) 1988;31(1):1–13

25. Haid RW Jr, Padadopoulous SM, Sonntag VKH, et al. Posterior cervical stabilization with lateral mass osteosynthetic plate technique. In: Jacksonville FL, ed. Levtech Technical Bulletin. Levtech Inc.; 1991

26. Heller JG, Carlson GD, Abitbol JJ, Garfin SR. Anatomic comparison of the Roy-Camille and Magerl techniques for screw placement in the lower cervical spine. Spine 1991; 16(10, Suppl):S552–S557

27. Magerl F, Grob D, Seeman D. Stable dorsal fusion of the Cervical Spine (C2-Th1) using hook plates. In: Kehr P, Weidner A, eds. Cervical Spine I. Springer- Verlag; 1987:217–21

28. Roy Cammile R, Sailant G, Berteaux D, et al. Early management of spinal injuries. In: Mc Kibbon B, ed. Recent Advances in Orthopedics. Churchill Livingstone; 1997:57–87

29. Roy-Camile R, Sailant G, Maxzel C. Internal fixation of the unstable cervical spine by posterior osteosynthesis with plates and screws. In: The Cervical Spine Research Society Editorial Committee, ed. The Cervical Spine. Lippincott Co.; 1989:390–404

30. Weidner A. Internal fixation with metal plates and screws. In: The Cervical Spine Research Society Editorial Committee, ed. The Cervical Spine. Lippincott Co.; 1989:404–21

31. Nazarian SM, Louis RP. Posterior internal fixation with screw plates in traumatic lesions of the cervical spine. Spine 1991; 16(3, Suppl):S64–S71

32. Joaquim AF, Mudo ML, Tan LA, Riew KD. Posterior subaxial cervical spine screw fixation: a review of techniques. Global Spine J 2018;8(7):751–760

33. Gill K, Paschal S, Corin J, Ashman R, Bucholz RW. Posterior plating of the cervical spine. A biomechanical comparison of different posterior fusion techniques. Spine 1988; 13(7):813–816

34. Montesano PX, Juach EC, Anderson PA, Benson DR, Hanson PB. Biomechanics of cervical spine internal fixation. Spine 1991; 16(3, Suppl):S10–S16

35. Jones EL, Heller JG, Silcox DH, Hutton WC. Cervical pedicle screws versus lateral mass screws. Anatomic feasibility and biomechanical comparison. Spine 1997;22(9): 977–982

36. Ishikawa Y, Kanemura T, Yoshida G, et al. Intraoperative, full-rotation, three-dimensional image (O-arm)-based navigation system for cervical pedicle screw insertion. J Neurosurg Spine 2011;15(5): 472–478

37. Karaikovic EE, Kunakornsawat S, Daubs MD, Madsen TW, Gaines RW Jr. Surgical anatomy of the cervical pedicles: landmarks for posterior cervical pedicle entrance localization. J Spinal Disord 2000;13(1):63–72

38. Pan Z, Zhong J, Xie S, et al. Accuracy and safety of lateral vertebral notch-referred technique used in subaxial cervical pedicle screw

placement. Oper Neurosurg (Hagerstown) 2019;17(1):52–60

39. Lee S-H, Kim K-T, Abumi K, Suk K-S, Lee J-H, Park K-J. Cervical pedicle screw placement using the "key slot technique": the feasibility and learning curve. J Spinal Disord Tech 2012;25(8):415–421

40. Neo M, Sakamoto T, Fujibayashi S, Nakamura T. The clinical risk of vertebral artery injury from cervical pedicle screws inserted in degenerative vertebrae. Spine 2005;30(24):2800–2805

41. Lee S-H, Kim K-T, Suk K-S, et al. Assessment of pedicle perforation by the cervical pedicle screw placement using plain radiographs: a comparison with computed tomography. Spine 2012;37(4):280–285

42. Theologis AA, Burch S. Safety and efficacy of reconstruction of complex cervical spine pathology using pedicle screws inserted with stealth navigation and 3D image-guided (O-arm) technology. Spine 2015; 40(18):1397–1406

43. Takahata M, Yamada K, Akira I, et al. A novel technique of cervical pedicle screw placement with a pilot screw under the guidance of intraoperative 3D imaging from C-arm cone-beam CT without navigation for safe and accurate insertion. Eur Spine J 2018;27(11):2754–2762

44. Schroeder GD, Hsu WK. Vertebral artery injuries in cervical spine surgery. Surg Neurol Int 2013;4(Suppl 5):S362–S367

45. Yeom JS, Buchowski JM, Kim H-J, Chang B-S, Lee C-K, Riew KD. Risk of vertebral artery injury: comparison between C1-C2 transarticular and C2 pedicle screws. Spine J 2013;13(7):775–785

46. Dewan MC, Godil SS, Mendenhall SK, Devin CJ, McGirt MJ. C2 nerve root transection during C1 lateral mass screw fixation: does it affect functionality and quality of life? Neurosurgery 2014;74(5):475–480, discussion 480–481

47. Yeom JS, Buchowski JM, Kim H-J, Chang B-S, Lee C-K, Riew KD. Postoperative occipital neuralgia with and without C2 nerve root transection during atlantoaxial screw fixation: a post-hoc comparative outcome study of prospectively collected data. Spine J 2013;13(7):786–795

48. Florman JE, Cushing DA, England EC, White E. How to transect the C2 root for C1 lateral mass screw placement: case series and review of an underappreciated variable in outcome. World Neurosurg 2019;127:e1210–e1214

49. Elliott RE, Kang MM, Smith ML, Frempong-Boadu A. C2 nerve root sectioning in posterior atlantoaxial instrumented fusions: a structured review of literature. World Neurosurg 2012;78(6):697–708

50. Schroeder GD, Hsu WK. Vertebral artery injuries in cervical spine surgery. Surg Neurol Int 2013; 4(5, Suppl 5):S362–S367

51. Sawin PD, Traynelis VC. Posterior articular mass plate fixation of the subaxial cervical spine. In: Menezes AH, Sonntag VKH, eds. Principles of Spinal Surgery. McGraw Hill; 1996;1081–1104

52. Uehara M, Takahashi J, Ikegami S, et al. Screw perforation features in 129 consecutive patients performed computer-guided cervical pedicle screw insertion. Eur Spine J 2014;23(10):2189–2195

53. Wang Y, Xie J, Yang Z, et al. Computed tomography assessment of lateral pedicle wall perforation by free-hand subaxial cervical pedicle screw placement. Arch Orthop Trauma Surg 2013;133(7):901–909

54. Lee C-H, Hong JT, Kang DH, et al. Epidemiology of iatrogenic vertebral artery injury in cervical spine surgery: 21 multicenter studies. World Neurosurg 2019;126:e1050–e1054

55. Uehara M, Takahashi J, Hirabayashi H, et al. Perforation rates of cervical pedicle screw insertion by disease and vertebral level. Open Orthop J 2010;4(1):142–146

56. Chun DH, Yoon DH, Kim KN, Yi S, Shin DA, Ha Y. biomechanical comparison of four different atlantoaxial posterior fixation constructs in adults: a finite element study. Spine 2018;43(15):E891–E897

57. Kothe R, Rüther W, Schneider E, Linke B. Biomechanical analysis of transpedicular screw fixation in the subaxial cervical spine. Spine 2004;29(17):1869–1875

58. Nagashima K, Koda M, Abe T, et al. Implant failure of pedicle screws in long-segment posterior cervical fusion is likely to occur at C7 and is avoidable by concomitant C6 or T1 buttress pedicle screws. J Clin Neurosci 2019;63:106–109

18 Anterior versus Posterior Approach for Spinal Canal Decompression: Indications for Patients with Cervical Myelopathy

Nikolay Konovalov, Stanislav Kaprovoy, and Vasiliy Korolishin

Introduction

Degenerative changes that take place in the cervical spine represent a common and ubiquitous process in the adult population. These processes cause the bony and ligamentous structures of the cervical spine to deteriorate and are a natural consequence of aging. Typically, cervical degenerative pathology is asymptomatic in the majority of the population, but it tends to get worse over time.[1]

Radiographically, degenerative changes can be found in up to 10% of the population by the age of 25 and in nearly 95% by the age of 65 and older. Generally, patients over 40 years of age present with symptomatic cervical degenerative diseases in need of surgical treatment.[2–4]

Degenerative diseases at the level of the cervical spine or cervical spondylosis are a mixed group of pathologic processes involving the vertebral column, intervertebral discs and joints, ligaments of the spine and occur due to natural processes of aging or secondary to trauma. The term cervical spondylosis was coined by Brain in 1952.[2,5]

Cervical spondylosis management is divided into conservative and surgical, and is critically dependent on the underlying pathology. The main treatment goals are to alleviate pain, improve neurologic deficit and functional limitations, and prevent further neurologic deterioration.[5]

The decision between anterior versus posterior surgical approach continues to be an ongoing debate. Some authors advocate that the choice of operative technique is somewhat on the verge of art and science. Depending on the underlining pathology, a group of patients can be better suited for either an anterior or posterior approach, whereas in many cases, the pathology can be treated with either approach.[6]

In their study, Cole et al reported an overall 30-day complication rate in the anterior approach group lower than posterior group, except for dysphagia complications (6.4% in anterior, 1.6% in posterior). The complication rate for anterior approaches, excluding dysphagia, was 12.3% in comparison with 17.8% for posterior approaches. Anterior approaches resulted in shorter hospital stay (1.5 nights) and lower 30-day readmission rate.[5,7]

Selection of optimal surgical approach must be based on a number of crucial factors. When deciding on anterior versus posterior versus combined approach, the surgeon should take into account the site of cord compression, number of levels involved, sagittal alignment, and spinal stability. Axial neck pain, risk of pseudarthrosis, and other patient comorbidities should also be taken into account. The above-mentioned variables are frequently ambiguous, which leads to surgeon training and patient preference becoming the deciding factors in selecting the surgical approach.[8]

General Considerations

The most frequent cause for cervical spondylotic myelopathy is spinal canal stenosis of various etiologies. Surgical treatment is aimed to expand the spinal canal and decompress the spinal cord. Approaches to the cervical spine are typically divided into two groups: anterior approach group, which consists of anterior cervical discectomy and fusion (ACDF), anterior corpectomy and fusion and cervical disc arthroplasty as an alternative method, and posterior approach group, consisting of laminectomy and laminoplasty.[9]

In cases of cervical myelopathy, the choice of approach is not always obvious and this problem was thoroughly investigated for the past couple of decades. Generally, it is considered that when addressing 1 or 2 level pathology, an anterior approach is preferable and allows for direct decompression of anteriorly located pathologies– osteophytes, posterior longitudinal ligament ossification, and disc herniation. It also offers lower postoperative pain, lower infection rates, cervical kyphosis correction, and treatment of radiculopathy.[10] **Fig. 18.1** presents a case of two-level anterior cervical discectomy and fusion for cervical stenosis.

In cases of primarily dorsal spinal cord compression over multiple spinal segments and preserved cervical lordosis, posterior surgical approaches have been preferred. In cases of focal kyphosis and posteriorly located pathology, a combined approach can be discussed. Posterior approaches allow for a wider spinal cord decompression, but depend on the cord drifting away from the lesion. It is imperative to preoperatively assess the sagittal alignment of the cervical spine, since the cord may not drift posteriorly with significant cervical kyphosis.[10,11] **Fig. 18.2** presents a case of posterior cervical discectomy and fusion for cervical stenosis. The advantages and disadvantages of either approaches are summarized in **Table 18.1**.

Single Level versus Multiple Level CSM

When selecting the appropriate surgical approach for cervical spondylotic myelopathy (CSM), the first question the surgeon faces is the number of vertebral levels needed to treat. Some authors state that choosing the appropriate surgical approach should depend on the underlining pathology, patient's preferences, and surgeon's experience. Many authors advocate the number of involved vertebral levels as the most important factor in selecting the appropriate approach.[12,13]

Traditionally, anterior surgical approaches were preferred for one- or two-level pathology. Posterior methods, on the other hand, were selected in cases spanning more than two vertebral levels (multisegmental pathology). In recent years, anterior and posterior surgical approaches have been progressively used for multisegmental diseases with similar clinical outcomes.[14]

In patients with a preserved cervical lordosis, the general idea is that a 1 to 3 segmental ACDF is an effective and safe procedure for spinal cord decompression. In cases of a straight spine, when performing ACDF, appropriate placement of the interbody graft or device can add a minimum of 5 degrees of lordosis per operated level, resulting in a more physiologic lordotic curvature and overall sagittal balance correction. Extensive posterior decompression is generally not advocated in the setting of a straight cervical spine, but it should also be noted that a multisegmental ACDF (more than 3 segments) can often result in graft extrusion or subsidence, vertebral body fracture, and pseudoarthrosis. In patients with multilevel CSM and a straightened cervical spine, dynamic cervical radiography is recommended to assess preoperative stability. If instability is present, other surgical options should be considered, such as posterior decompression and fusion.[12]

To sum up the above stated, when selecting the optimal surgical approach, it is recommended that patients are divided into three categories: patients with normal cervical lordosis, patients with a straightened spine, and patients with kyphotic deformity. In cases with normal cervical lordosis, the number of involved vertebral levels is the main parameter when selecting the optimal surgical intervention. With less than three

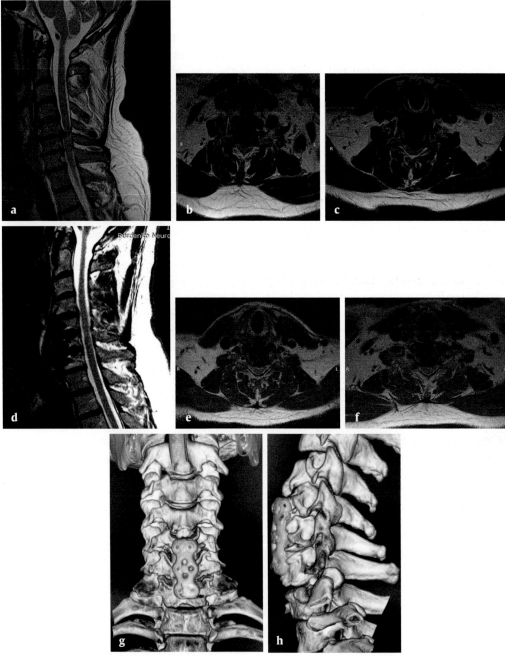

Fig. 18.1 This is a 54-year-old male patient with 6 months' symptom duration and Japanese Orthopaedic Association (JOA) score of 13. Preoperative sagittal **(a)** MRI of the cervical spine with signs of spinal cord compression at the level of C5–C6 **(b)** and C6–C7 **(c)**. A two-level anterior cervical discectomy and fusion (ACDF) and anterior plating was performed. Postoperative MRI of the cervical spine **(d, e, f)** shows no spinal cord compression at operated levels. Postoperative CT scans **(g, h)** show good preservation of the lordosis. He improved postoperatively and JOA score after 2 months was 16.

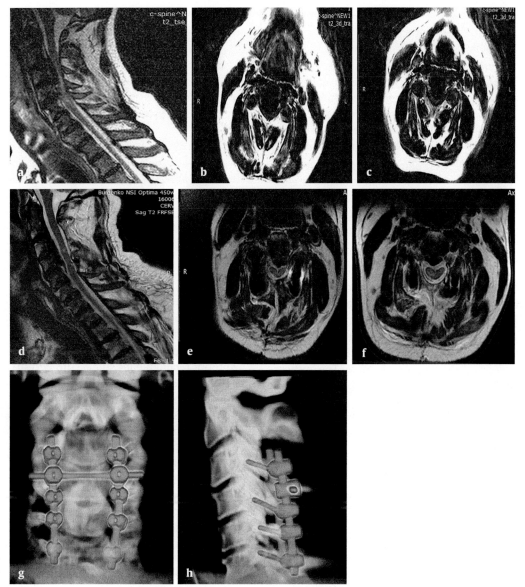

Fig. 18.2 This is a 69-year-old patient. Symptom duration was 2 months and Japanese Orthopaedic Association (JOA) score was 6. Preoperative sagittal **(a)** MRI of the cervical spine with signs of spinal cord compression at the level of C3–C4 **(b)** and C4–C5 **(c)**. A three-level laminectomy and lateral mass screw fixation was performed. Postoperative MRI of the cervical spine **(d, e, f)** shows no spinal cord compression at operated levels. Postoperative CT scans **(g, h)** show good preservation of the lordosis. Postoperative JOA score 3 months after surgery improved to 12.

involved levels, ACDF or arthroplasty are considered beneficial and the methods of choice. Patients with three or more vertebral levels require laminectomy or laminoplasty. In cases with a straightened spine, the number of levels is a primary factor for selection of appropriate approach. For patients with three or less levels involved, ACDF with anterior cervical plate fixation is considered adequate, however, in those with more than three involved levels and presence of spinal instability, posterior decompression and fusion is

Table 18.1   The advantages and disadvantages of anterior and posterior approaches

	Advantages	Disadvantages
Anterior approach	Complete foraminal decompression Better postoperative alignment Direct decompression of anterior elements (disc, PLL and osteophyte) Indirect decompression by stretching of LF through disc height restoration	Adjacent segment degeneration Possible dysphagia/hoarseness Visible scar in the front Possible pseudarthrosis
Posterior approach	Ease of multilevel decompression Direct decompression of posterior elements (LF) Indirect decompression by posterior drift of spinal cord away from anterior compression	Inadequate decompression for severe anterior compression or kyphosis Extensive loss of ROM Postoperative axial neck pain Possible C5 palsy

Abbreviations: LF, ligamentum flavum; PLL, posterior longitudinal ligament; ROM, range of motion.

considered the method of choice. Irreducible cervical kyphosis with less than two vertebral levels is treated by ACDF, and in cases with more than two level pathology, anterior cervical corpectomy and fusion (ACCF) is deemed the method of choice. The authors would like to emphasize that patient's cervical MRI should be evaluated on spinal canal patency and characteristics of subarachnoid space (SAS).[12]

Sagittal Alignment Effect to Choice the Approach

Surgical outcomes in patients with CSM also depend on sagittal alignment of the cervical spine. Growing evidence suggests a strong correlation between sagittal alignment and quality of life (QOL) and disability in the aging population.[15–17]

One of the most common reasons for surgery in the elderly is spinal deformity. Majority of cases include myelopathy with deformities in level of worse angle curve or upper/below one. Some authors suggest that correction of cervical balance is the main task of surgery and osteotomy is necessary for rigid kyphosis only.[18]

Certainly, for sagittal balance correction, posterior osteotomy with pedicle subtraction osteotomy (PSO) or Smith–Peterson

method is the best choice, but this condition is very rarely associated with multilevel spinal stenosis. The goal of cervical osteotomy is generally to correct sagittal balance of cervical–thoracic junction.

Anterior technique for spinal cord decompression and sagittal balance correction is considered the method of choice and associated with corpectomy or multiple level discectomy. Cases with kyphotic deformity were more likely to be treated by anterior approach, as many surgeons believed it to be ideal.

Flexible kyphotic deformities can be treated by posterior decompressions and fusion, but more rigid kyphotic deformities will typically require an anterior or combined approach.[19–21]

Surgical strategy in cases of CSM with a kyphotic cervical spine remains debatable. In a study by Uchida et al, the outcomes of ACDF for CSM with local kyphosis (angle of 10° or more) were equal to those of laminoplasty alone at follow-up in their series of 43 patients. In the ACDF group, correction of kyphosis was somewhat mild at follow-up, remaining a mean of 9.2°. The Japanese Orthopedic Association scores were acceptable for both groups.[18]

Chiba et al reported an acceptable clinical outcome after laminoplasty alone in several patients with cervical kyphosis. The authors speculated that dorsal displacement of the spinal cord after laminoplasty, especially in cases with multiple level disc height reduction, is sufficient for acceptable recovery. On the other hand, several authors contradicted this idea. In a study, Baba et al reported significantly poorer neurological improvement in patients with preoperative kyphosis (mean angle of 11.7°). Moreover, Suda et al showed poorer outcomes in a group of patients treated for CSM with laminoplasty in the context of local kyphosis with an angle exceeding 13° (with myelomalacia) and 5° (without myelomalacia) compared to a group with CSM and no kyphosis.[22-24]

For patients with multiple-level CSM along with kyphosis and spinal cord stretched over anterior osteophytes, a combined approach as well as posterior decompression and fusion, may be acceptable.[25,26]

The main part of patients with symptomatic CSM is due to cervical hyperlordosis, which is associated with sagittal imbalance and thoracic hyperkyphosis. Buell et al recommend utilization of "the cervical spinal deformity classification system" for detecting curvature point with future planning of alignment changing.[27]

In cases with multiple level CSM, associated with a straight cervical spine and instability, posterior surgical approach with decompression and fusion is considered the method of choice. Lawrence et al proposed an individualized approach to patients with CSM, taking into account pathological and anatomical differences (ventral vs. dorsal, focal vs. diffuse, sagittal or dynamic instability). Authors found analogous outcomes between surgical approaches with regard to effectiveness and patient safety.[28]

Preoperative analysis of cervical sagittal alignment should be considered as a crucial step in selecting the optimal surgical approach in the setting of CSM. In cases with multiple-level CSM along with preservation of cervical lordosis, the posterior approach is considered to be the method of choice.[29]

Many publications state that laminoplasty is safer, faster, and associated with better prognosis than laminectomy without fusion. All authors noted that laminectomy is associated with long-term complications in comparison with laminoplasty.[30]

Ossification of the Posterior Longitudinal Ligament

Toshikazu et al in their study reported that anterior decompression for multiple-level ossified posterior longitudinal ligament (OPLL) is safer than laminoplasty. On the other hand, Subodh et al reported no significant difference in outcome and short-term recovery rate between two groups of patients with multiple level OPLL and recommended posterior approach as the method of choice.[31]

It is suggested that anterior decompression and fusion for OPLL with an occupying ratio of more than 60% is better as compared with laminoplasty, since ACDF proved better recovery rate at long-term follow-up. Due to a deficit of comprehensive high-level studies comparing outcomes of both approaches, the optimal treatment strategy remains controversial.[31]

Feng et al performed a meta-analysis selecting Japanese Orthopaedic Association (JOA) scores, complications, blood loss, and surgical time as end points for clinical outcome evaluation of anterior versus posterior surgical approaches. The meta-analysis showed no statistical difference in preoperative JOA score between two groups, with postoperative JOA score and overall recovery rate higher in the anterior group. In cases with a canal-occupying ratio between 50 to 60%, anterior surgical approach resulted with significantly higher postoperative JOA score and recovery rate, whereas for cases with canal-occupying ratio lower than 50 to 60%, the postoperative JOA score and recovery were similar for both groups.[31]

Authors also report significantly higher postoperative complication rates in the anterior surgery group, such as implant failure rate, blood loss, and surgical time. C5 nerve palsy, axial pain, and radiculopathy were notably higher in the posterior group.[31]

Axial Neck Pain

A meta-analysis by Liu et al comparing anterior versus posterior surgical approach for axial neck pain found no difference in outcomes. The authors noted that few studies actually reported pain outcomes– only two of the ten studies reviewed. Cunningham et al reported higher postoperative neck pain after laminoplasty, but they reviewed older studies, where bracing, prolonged immobilization, and opening the C7 lamina were standard practice.[32,33]

Although not well described in the literature, the amount of preoperative neck pain plays a role into selection of surgical approach. Patients with CSM usually present with notable spondylosis and spinal cord compression. The source of axial neck pain remains unclear, and in cases with moderate or severe neck pain and substantial degenerative changes, decompression and fusion, rather than just a decompression such as laminoplasty, is recommended.[10]

Patient Comorbidities

Surgical approaches to the cervical spine can be associated with numerous complications, associated with quality and direction of approach. Age and comorbidities such as arterial hypertension, lung disease, diabetes, and obesity play an important role in selecting an appropriate surgical approach. Boakye et al in their study reported age is the most important outcome factor in patients with CSM undergoing ACDF.[34]

Macagno et al stated that comorbid factors such as anemia, rheumatoid arthritis, chronic pulmonary disease, chronic blood loss, anemia, congestive heart failure, coagulopathy, diabetes, hypertension, liver disease, electrolyte imbalance, neurological disorders, obesity, peripheral vascular disease, pulmonary circulation disorders, renal failure, cardiac valvular disorder, and pathologic weight loss play a huge role in development of perioperative complications.[8]

In anterior surgical approaches, severe osteoporosis can become an issue due to long strut graft settling and nuances of achieving a stable fixation. This potential complication should be considered when selecting posterior laminoplasty if other factors make that a reasonable surgical option.[35]

Meyer et al stated that multiple segments stenosis with sever osteoporosis requires a posterior approach for safe spinal cord decompression and adequate fusion. Most surgeons cautiously approach patients with severe osteoporosis. Low-bone quality reduces pull-out strength of pedicle screw and can cause delayed bone fusion. It is recommended to treat osteoporosis prior to performing spinal fusion, using effective strategies to increase bone quality. Perioperative strategies in osteoporotic patients which may affect the radiological and clinical outcomes include antiresorptive and anabolic agents, proper instrumentation, and BMA.[36,37]

Other medical comorbidities that play a major role in making surgical treatment less desirable and drastically increasing the risk of surgical site infection are diabetes and smoking. In patients with diabetes, good glucose control is crucial; this can have significant impact on postoperative outcomes. Diabetes is a risk factor for developing surgical site infection in patients with posterior spinal fusion. A retrospective study of 124 patients reported higher rates of postoperative surgical site infection and prolonged hospitalization in the diabetic patients group, although no statistical comparison with patients without diabetes was presented.[38]

In another study of 273 patients after spine surgery with and without infection, diabetes was reported as the highest risk factor for surgical site infection. Chen et al stated that the patients with diabetes should participate in shared decision-making process prior to surgery and receive specific counseling on the risks of surgical site infection in the informed consent process.[39,40]

Based on the analyzed data, we formulated an algorithm to aid the decision process concerning the surgical approach (**Flowchart 18.1**).

Conclusion

Cervical myelopathy is one of the main causes of disability, especially in the elderly population. Understanding this condition is essential for early diagnosis and treatment. Success of surgical and conservative treatment options is multifactorial, and high-quality comprehensive studies are lacking. The controversy in selecting the optimum surgical approach is still relevant, and depends on the location of the spinal cord compression, number of cervical levels involved, sagittal alignment and

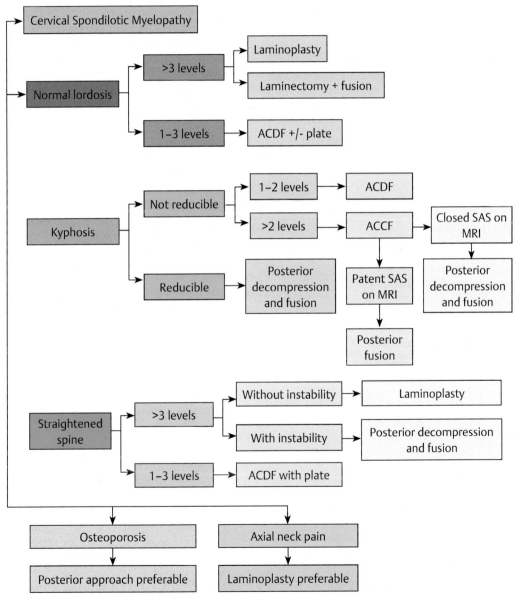

Flowchart 18.1 Algorithm for decision of surgical approach in cervical spondylotic myelopathy (CSM) patients. ACCF: anterior cervical corpectomy and fusion; ACDF: anterior cervical discectomy and fusion; SAS: subarachnoid space.

instability, associated axial neck pain, risks of pseudarthrosis and patient comorbidities.

The goal of surgery is spinal cord decompression with expansion of the vertebral canal while correcting cervical lordosis and stabilizing the spine, if the risk of kyphosis is high. Further high-quality studies with long-term follow-up are necessary to further define the natural history of this condition and help predict the most efficient surgical strategy.

Take-home Points

- In spite of many difficulties degenerative cervical spine stenosis associated with SCM requires surgery.
- But every case needs individual and informed decision-making considering all parameters and nuances of patient's condition.

References

1. Herkowitz HN, Rothman RH, Simeone FA. Rothman-Simeone, The Spine. 6th ed. Philadelphia: Saunders Elsevier; 2011
2. Benzel EC, Francis TB. Spine Surgery: Techniques, Complication Avoidance, and Management. 3rd ed. Philadelphia, PA: Elsevier/Saunders; 2012
3. Herkowitz HN, Rothman RH, Simeone FA. The Spine. 5th ed. Philadelphia: Saunders Elsevier; 2006
4. Oglesby M, Fineberg SJ, Patel AA, Pelton MA, Singh K. Epidemiological trends in cervical spine surgery for degenerative diseases between 2002 and 2009. Spine 2013;38(14):1226–1232
5. Boos N, Aebi M. Spinal Disorders: Fundamentals of Diagnosis and Treatment. Berlin; New York: Springer; 2008
6. Emery SE. Anterior approaches for cervical spondylotic myelopathy: which? When? How? Eur Spine J 2015;24(Suppl 2):150–159
7. Sugawara T. Anterior cervical spine surgery for degenerative disease: a review. Neurol Med Chir (Tokyo) 2015;55(7):540–546
8. Macagno A, Liu S, Marascalchi BJ, et al. Perioperative risks associated with cervical spondylotic myelopathy based on surgical treatment strategies. Int J Spine Surg 2015;9:24
9. Chen Z, Liu B, Dong J, et al. A comparison of the anterior approach and the posterior approach in treating multilevel cervical myelopathy: a meta-analysis. Clin Spine Surg 2017;30(2):65–76
10. Bakhsheshian J, Mehta VA, Liu JC. Current diagnosis and management of cervical spondylotic myelopathy. Global Spine J 2017; 7(6):572–586
11. Wilson JR, Tetreault LA, Kim J, et al. State of the art in degenerative cervical myelopathy: an update on current clinical evidence. Neurosurgery 2017;80(3S):S33–S45
12. Farrokhi MR, Ghaffarpasand F, Khani M, Gholami M. An evidence-based stepwise surgical approach to cervical spondylotic myelopathy: a narrative review of the current literature. World Neurosurg 2016;94:97–110
13. Jeon HC, Kim CS, Kim SC, et al. Posterior cervical microscopic foraminotomy and discectomy with laser for unilateral radiculopathy. Chonnam Med J 2015;51(3):129–134
14. Lebl DR, Bono CM. Update on the diagnosis and management of cervical spondylotic myelopathy. J Am Acad Orthop Surg 2015;23(11):648–660
15. Gum JL, Glassman SD, Douglas LR, Carreon LY. Correlation between cervical spine sagittal alignment and clinical outcome after anterior cervical discectomy and fusion. Am J Orthop 2012;41(6):E81–E84
16. Ahn PG, Kim KN, Moon SW, Kim KS. Changes in cervical range of motion and sagittal alignment in early and late phases after total disc replacement: radiographic follow-up exceeding 2 years. J Neurosurg Spine 2009; 11(6):688–695
17. Glassman SD, Bridwell K, Dimar JR, Horton W, Berven S, Schwab F. The impact of positive sagittal balance in adult spinal deformity. Spine 2005;30(18):2024–2029
18. Uchida K, Nakajima H, Sato R, et al. Cervical spondylotic myelopathy associated with kyphosis or sagittal sigmoid alignment: outcome after anterior or posterior decompression. J Neurosurg Spine 2009; 11(5):521–528
19. Lin Q, Zhou X, Wang X, Cao P, Tsai N, Yuan W. A comparison of anterior cervical discectomy and corpectomy in patients with multilevel cervical spondylotic myelopathy. Eur Spine J 2012;21(3):474–481

20. O'Shaughnessy BA, Liu JC, Hsieh PC, Koski TR, Ganju A, Ondra SL. Surgical treatment of fixed cervical kyphosis with myelopathy. Spine 2008;33(7):771–778

21. Shamji MF, Mohanty C, Massicotte EM, Fehlings MG. The association of cervical spine alignment with neurologic recovery in a prospective cohort of patients with surgical myelopathy: analysis of a series of 124 cases. World Neurosurg 2016;86:112–119

22. Chiba K, Toyama Y, Watanabe M, Maruiwa H, Matsumoto M, Hirabayashi K. Impact of longitudinal distance of the cervical spine on the results of expansive open-door laminoplasty. Spine 2000;25(22):2893–2898

23. Baba H, Maezawa Y, Furusawa N, Imura S, Tomita K. Flexibility and alignment of the cervical spine after laminoplasty for spondylotic myelopathy. A radiographic study. Int Orthop 1995;19(2):116–121

24. Suda K, Abumi K, Ito M, Shono Y, Kaneda K, Fujiya M. Local kyphosis reduces surgical outcomes of expansive open-door laminoplasty for cervical spondylotic myelopathy. Spine 2003;28(12):1258–1262

25. Fehlings MG, Barry S, Kopjar B, et al. Anterior versus posterior surgical approaches to treat cervical spondylotic myelopathy: outcomes of the prospective multicenter AOSpine North America CSM study in 264 patients. Spine 2013;38(26):2247–2252

26. Sun Y, Li L, Zhao J, Gu R. Comparison between anterior approaches and posterior approaches for the treatment of multilevel cervical spondylotic myelopathy: A meta-analysis. Clin Neurol Neurosurg 2015;134:28–36

27. Buell TJ, Buchholz AL, Quinn JC, Shaffrey CI, Smith JS. Importance of sagittal alignment of the cervical spine in the management of degenerative cervical myelopathy. Neurosurg Clin N Am 2018;29(1):69–82

28. Lawrence BD, Jacobs WB, Norvell DC, Hermsmeyer JT, Chapman JR, Brodke DS. Anterior versus posterior approach for treatment of cervical spondylotic myelopathy: a systematic review. Spine 2013;38(22, Suppl 1)S173–S182

29. Geck MJ, Eismont FJ. Surgical options for the treatment of cervical spondylotic myelopathy. Orthop Clin North Am 2002;33(2):329–348

30. Kiely PD, Quinn JC, Du JY, Lebl DR. Posterior surgical treatment of cervical spondylotic myelopathy: review article. HSS J 2015;11(1):36–42

31. Feng F, Ruan W, Liu Z, Li Y, Cai L. Anterior versus posterior approach for the treatment of cervical compressive myelopathy due to ossification of the posterior longitudinal ligament: A systematic review and meta-analysis. Int J Surg 2016;27:26–33

32. Liu T, Xu W, Cheng T, Yang HL. Anterior versus posterior surgery for multilevel cervical myelopathy, which one is better? A systematic review. Eur Spine J 2011;20(2):224–235

33. Cunningham MR, Hershman S, Bendo J. Systematic review of cohort studies comparing surgical treatments for cervical spondylotic myelopathy. Spine 2010;35(5):537–543

34. Boakye M, Patil CG, Santarelli J, Ho C, Tian W, Lad SP. Cervical spondylotic myelopathy: complications and outcomes after spinal fusion. Neurosurgery 2008;62(2):455–461, discussion 461–462

35. Hughes SS, Pringle T, Phillips F, Emery S. Settling of fibula strut grafts following multilevel anterior cervical corpectomy: a radiographic evaluation. Spine 2006;31(17):1911–1915

36. Meyer F, Börm W, Thomé C. Degenerative cervical spinal stenosis: current strategies in diagnosis and treatment. Dtsch Arztebl Int 2008;105(20):366–372

37. Park SB, Chung CK. Strategies of spinal fusion on osteoporotic spine. J Korean Neurosurg Soc 2011;49(6):317–322

38. Simpson JM, Silveri CP, Balderston RA, Simeone FA, An HS. The results of operations on the lumbar spine in patients who have diabetes mellitus. J Bone Joint Surg Am 1993;75(12):1823–1829

39. Olsen MA, Nepple JJ, Riew KD, et al. Risk factors for surgical site infection following orthopaedic spinal operations. J Bone Joint Surg Am 2008;90(1):62–69

40. Chen S, Anderson MV, Cheng WK, Wongworawat MD. Diabetes associated with increased surgical site infections in spinal arthrodesis. Clin Orthop Relat Res 2009;467(7):1670–1673

19 Complications of Anterior Cervical Discectomy and Fusion

Nicholas Ahye, Joel Passer, Anand Kaul, Scott C. Robertson, Francesco Costa, and Bong-Soo Kim

Introduction

Anterior cervical discectomy and fusion (ACDF) is one of the most common procedures performed by spine surgeons. It has repeatedly been demonstrated to be an effective method for decompression and fusion of the cervical spine. There are a variety of indications for the procedure, including trauma, degenerative disease, infection, and oncological processes. As an essential and versatile procedure, it is important for surgeons to be aware of potential procedure-related complications, techniques to avoid them, and appropriate management if they occur. Improving the safety and reliability of this operation involves careful analysis of factors and techniques that affect outcome measures such as fusion rates and postoperative pain and neurological status, and reduce procedure-related complications. While these outcome measures are generally favorable when using standard techniques, differences in intraoperative technique and postoperative management may impact patient outcomes.

As a common procedure, it is simple to generate a large study population and analyze how frequently complications occur and how they affect patient outcomes. These complications can occur during or after surgery and can appear in either an early or delayed fashion (**Table 19.1**). The appropriate treatment for ACDF-related complications is guided by some larger randomized controlled trials, retrospective and cohort studies, or case reports for those that occur more infrequently. In this chapter, both intraoperative and postoperative complications will be reviewed. Their incidence, management, expected outcomes, and techniques of avoidance are highlighted.

Intraoperative Complications

Durotomy and Cerebrospinal Fluid Leak

Techniques of dissection in spinal surgery have a focus on avoiding an unintentional durotomy. This complication of spinal surgery can alter the surgical plan, complicate the postoperative course, and prolong the hospital stay. Additional surgical procedures may also be required to successfully treat a persistent cerebrospinal fluid (CSF) leak. The intraoperative and postoperative decision-making to manage an unintentional durotomy in anterior cervical spine surgery requires an understanding of available options. Overall, the risk of unintentional durotomy in anterior cervical spine surgery is low, and retrospective reviews of ACDF series have shown rates of intraoperative CSF leak ranging from 0.5 to 1%.[4–6] Especially in cases where only a discectomy is being performed, the narrow surgical corridor may preclude the opportunity to perform a primary dural repair. Careful preoperative planning and meticulous technique can help to avoid this complication.

Techniques to Avoid Cerebrospinal Fluid Leak

Working within the disc space requires efficiency and precision of movement, to avoid unintentional plunging of an instrument, which can cause either a durotomy or spinal cord injury. Performing the discectomy begins with an annulotomy, which is often done with sharp dissection. This is executed in a very controlled manner, with only shallow use of any sharp instruments in the

Table 19.1 List of complications associated with ACDF

Complication	Rate
Dysphagia	10–82%[1–3]
Intraoperative CSF leak	0.5–1%[4–6]
RLN palsy	0.1–21%[7,8]
Esophageal perforation	0.3–5%[5,9,10]
ASD	3% (1 year)[11] 13.6% (3 years)[11] 25% (5 years)[11]
Pseudarthrosis (single-level ACDF)	3.7%[12]
Subsidence (overall)	21%[13]
Postoperative hematoma	6%[14] 0.4% required return to OR
Postoperative infection	0.07–1.6%[6,9,15]
Postoperative neurologic deficit	0–3.3%[16–19]
Vertebral artery injury	0.3%[10,20]
Horner's syndrome	0.06–0.62%[21,22]
Thoracic duct injury	0.02%[23]

Abbreviations: ACDF, anterior cervical discectomy and fusion; ASD, adjacent segment disease; CSF, cerebrospinal fluid; RLN, recurrent laryngeal nerve.

disc space. A number of instruments can be used to perform the disc removal, including a Kerrison punch, curettes, or a pituitary rongeur. Soft discs are usually easily removed, however desiccated and calcified discs may require more dissection and manipulation. When the posterior longitudinal ligament (PLL) is reached, a decision must be made whether to release the ligament. Doing so can improve the extent of decompression and may allow for better deformity correction. However, dissecting the PLL carries a risk of violating the dura, due to their proximity and the possible presence of adhesions, especially with a calcified PLL.

A calcified PLL tends to be more adherent to the ventral dura, which leads to an increased risk of CSF leak during PLL dissection. Presence of ossification of the posterior longitudinal ligament (OPLL) is known to have an increased risk of durotomy during ACDF.[4,24] In OPLL, the ligament can

be difficult to distinguish from the dura. Identification of the longitudinal fibers of PLL, which usually contrasts with the smoother appearance of dura, should always be done carefully. The visual appearance will not always be a reliable way to make this critical distinction, especially in advanced degenerative disease. In cases where it is difficult to confidently distinguish the PLL from dura, it is prudent to avoid further dissection, as the theoretical benefit would be outweighed by a high risk of durotomy. If more ventral decompression is required in this scenario, a corpectomy should be considered.

Reoperation on the cervical spine for an anterior approach may be indicated in cases of ventral compression from adjacent segment disease or progression of other pathology. A reoperation on the ventral cervical spine will involve dissection of scar tissue and adhesions, which can make identification of anatomical structures more difficult.

Reoperation has been shown to be associated with an increased risk of durotomy.[4] Removal of old hardware and establishing of planes of dissection should be performed with caution. The surgeon should be mindful of any structures that may be adherent to dura.

Intraoperative Repair Techniques

If a durotomy does occur, identification of the dural defect should be attempted. Due to the limited dural exposure in an ACDF, it may not be possible to expose it entirely. Initially, the intradural pressure will likely cause CSF to fill the field, requiring aspiration until the rate of fluid accumulation is slowed. This maneuver will also decrease intradural pressure, which may help to prevent fistula formation after the repair is made. The exposed dura should be explored to see if the opening can be identified. At this point, a decision must be made about how to repair it.

When possible, primary closure of the defect should be attempted. A 6-0 Prolene suture (Ethicon, NJ) or other nonresorbable suture can be used to perform closure of the durotomy. Nonpenetrating titanium dural clips may also be utilized to perform a primary closure, which have been used with success.[25] They theoretically offer the advantage of avoiding CSF leakage through the holes where the dura is pierced by the suture needle. Oftentimes, the narrow surgical corridor and limited dural exposure during a discectomy may not make it technically possible to perform a primary closure. In these cases, or in cases where a primary closure is to be augmented, there are several options to close the dural defect.

A local muscle graft can be harvested and placed over the durotomy. This layer of nonvascularized tissue can help to obstruct further outflow of CSF. A dural substitute or Gelfoam (Pfizer, NY) can also be laid over the defect to reestablish a barrier against CSF outflow.[26] These overlay grafts, or a primary closure, can be further augmented with a fibrin glue or other polymerizing dural sealant.[26] Mass effect from these sealants can contribute to spinal cord compression, so the amount that is used should be limited, and leave room to accommodate the interbody graft. Avoidance of placing a drain in the wound may avoid negative pressure, reopening a CSF pathway, and increasing risk of a postoperative CSF leak.

At this point, consideration should be made as to whether the remainder of the operation should be completed, or if the surgical plan needs to be modified. The surgeon may not want to proceed with operating on other levels, especially if factors exist that could increase the risk of durotomy at another level. During surgical planning, in higher risk patients, there should be consideration to perform a discectomy on the most critical level first, so that in case a CSF leak occurs, the level with the greatest compression or instability has been corrected.

Postoperative Management

Close monitoring of the operative site after surgery is required. Leakage of CSF from the incision or swelling of the neck needs to be detected as early as possible to avoid complications of a persistent CSF leak. The patient's head should be elevated 30 to 45 degrees at all times to reduce the CSF pressure at the site of the durotomy. Signs of intracranial hypotension should raise suspicion for an active CSF leak, especially a positional headache. Neck swelling can be evaluated with a CT of the neck to identify a fluid collection. If there is concern for potential airway compromise, the patient should be considered for intensive care unit observation or bedside reopening of the incision and emergent return to the OR.

If there is evidence of a persistent CSF leak postoperatively, there should be consideration for lumbar drain placement. Drainage of CSF 10 to 15 mL an hour can be attempted for 72 hours before clamping to see if the leak will stop. When a lumbar drain fails to stop a persistent CSF leak, the patient should be considered for reexploration of the wound.[5] This surgery should focus on another attempted closure of the durotomy using the previously described techniques. Intraoperative salvage techniques, including rotating a vascularized muscle flap over the defect, have been described.[27] If this is not successful, the patient may require permanent CSF diversion with a ventriculoperitoneal or lumboperitoneal shunt.

Outcomes

Several studies have evaluated outcomes after repair of ACDF durotomies. In one series, a cohort of patients who underwent an ACDF had a 1% intraoperative CSF leak rate.[5] In 9 of the 13 patients with a CSF leak, primary closure was achieved without the need for further intervention. Of the remaining cases, three required wound reexploration and one required shunt placement. Another series with an intraoperative leak rate of 0.5% had complete resolution of all leaks with lumbar drainage that failed primary intraoperative repair.[6] The overall rate of persistent CSF leak after primary intraoperative repair remains low. There have previously been questions raised as to whether a CSF leak affects fusion rate; however, a small series showed a 100% fusion rate.[28] The rarity of this complication makes larger, more definitive studies on management difficult to design. However, for such a common procedure, it is imperative to know the effective strategies to manage this complication.

Neurologic Complications

Perioperative Spinal Cord Injury

Injury to the spinal cord or nerve roots due to anterior cervical spine surgery is a feared complication that can carry significant morbidity. The overall risk of spinal cord injury (SCI) from anterior cervical spine surgery has been reported as 0 to 3.3%.[16–19] This series also showed that severe motor weakness occurred in only three of 1,000 cervical spine cases. There are multiple possible causes for a new neurologic deficit after anterior cervical spine surgery, some of which remain theoretical. Nerve and spinal cord trauma during surgery can be related to thermal injury from cautery. Blunt injury from the drill burr or hardware placement can also cause neurological

damage. Change in the position of the spinal cord or nerve roots has been studied for an association with new weakness after surgery, as these structures can be subjected to new tension if they are displaced after the decompression or deformity correction.[29,30] Spinal cord shift after surgery, as measured on MRI, has been shown to be associated with new deficit.[30]

Several risk factors for SCI in anterior cervical spine surgery have been established. Patients with existing stenosis and myelopathy, more advanced age, and those undergoing multilevel corpectomy are at greater risk.[18,19] A wider corpectomy was also shown to have a higher association with a postoperative C5 palsy, leading some surgeons to perform more narrow decompressions.[31] Recognition of these higher risk scenarios may cause the surgeon to enlist more rigorous precautions for a safer outcome.

Preparation for surgery should incorporate several techniques that can help reduce the risk of a surgery related SCI. During induction of general anesthesia and endotracheal tube (ETT) placement, use of video laryngoscopy can reduce or eliminate the need for neck manipulation to secure the airway. This is especially important for cases with critical spinal stenosis, in which hyperextension of the neck could potentially cause cord injury.[18] If there is a grossly unstable fracture, a fiberoptic intubation while the patient remains in a rigid cervical collar needs to be considered. Neurophysiological monitoring with somatosensory-evoked potentials (SSEPs) and/or motor-evoked potentials (MEPs) is commonly used during spinal surgery. Its use for anterior cervical spine surgery is variable, may be decreasing over time, and the impact on outcomes remains controversial.[32,33] It can alert the surgeon to impaired neurologic function while a patient is under general anesthesia, which may prompt an intervention to prevent a lasting deficit. This often relies on information from transcranial electrical stimulation, spontaneous electromyography (EMG) activity, and continuous SSEPs. Neurophysiologic monitoring should always establish baseline recordings prior to patient positioning, so that any changes can be detected. If there is a change in nerve responses after patient is positioned, they should be returned to a neutral position until the responses recover, and if they do not, a wake up should be considered before deciding if to proceed. Patients who have critical spinal stenosis and spinal cord compression are also at risk for ischemia during surgery. Blood pressure monitoring with an arterial line to maintain a mean arterial pressure (MAP) greater than 80 mmHg throughout the case ensures spinal cord perfusion and can guard against a vascular insult.[18,34]

During surgery, changes in neurophysiological monitoring responses can occur for a number of reasons. A decrease in amplitude of 50% or more should always be taken seriously and prompt the surgeon to evaluate for sources of injury to the cord or nerve roots. The operative field should be assessed for any sources of compression, including retractors, hardware, or any packing that was placed for hemostasis. The patient's physiological parameters need to be evaluated, especially temperature and MAP, which can cause changes in nerve responses. Fluoroscopy can be used to make changes to spinal alignment if that is felt to be a reason for compression. The affected extremities should be checked to make sure they are in a neutral position and are not at risk for a compression neuropathy. If correction of all these elements does not result in restoration of amplitudes, the surgeon may consider a wake up test, adjusting the surgical plan or shortening the procedure to more quickly assess whether the changes are translating into a true neurological deficit.

Patients who develop a postoperative neurologic deficit should immediately have imaging of the area that was operated upon. Malpositioning of hardware and epidural hematoma can be ruled out promptly. Although rare, with a reported incidence of 0.1%, a postoperative epidural hematoma needs to be evacuated quickly to improve chances of good recovery.[35] Patients who have SCI following anterior cervical spine surgery can be treated with a protocol that involves raising MAPs to 85 to 90 mm Hg for a period of 5 to 7 days.[18,36] This MAP goal can be accomplished with vasopressors or intravenous (IV) fluid administration. Dopamine and norepinephrine are commonly used agents, which avoid too much alpha receptor activation that could reduce spinal cord perfusion by causing vasospasm.

Postoperative C5 Palsy

C5 nerve root palsy is a well-known complication of cervical spine surgery, more often associated with posterior procedures. It also occurs in anterior cervical spine surgery at a rate of 5 to 12%.[29,37] The patient will experience significant deltoid weakness, which does not have innervation from other roots, as well as some biceps weakness, which does receive dual innervation. There are several possible causes for this complication which have been debated in the literature. Greater spinal cord shift after a decompression has been shown to have an increased rate of C5 palsy, possibly due to increased tension on the nerve root.[30] Neurophysiological monitoring has been shown to be helpful in avoiding a C5 palsy. One study showed a reduction in rate of C5 palsy when surgical technique was modified after EMG activity of C5 was detected.[32] Transcranial MEPs may be a more useful modality, as they were shown to have 100% sensitivity and 99% specificity in predicting a C5 palsy for anterior cervical spine surgery.[38]

Recovery from a C5 palsy tends to correlate with severity of the motor weakness, with the more severe deficits having lower recovery rates.[29] Data has shown a mean recovery time of 4 months, and a 67% full recovery rate without any further interventions.[16,37] There has not been any evidence of other treatments, such as IV steroids, providing any benefit to recovery time or rates. As neuromonitoring changes do not correlate with severity of postoperative deficit, the initial postoperative physical examination remains an important predictor of recovery.[29,38]

Vascular Injury

Large vessels in the neck are susceptible to injury during an ACDF. The operative corridor requires lateral retraction of the carotid artery, which is contained within the carotid sheath along with the internal jugular vein. The vertebral artery, although not visualized during the procedure, can sustain damage during the decompressive stage of the operation when working near the uncovertebral junction and neural foramen. Besides the risk of sharp injury, there is potential for thrombosis of vessels due to prolonged retraction. While evaluating imaging studies preoperatively, identifying an anomalous course of the carotid or vertebral arteries might help in preventing an intraoperative injury.

If vascular injury does occur, the first maneuver is to attempt intraoperative control. Brisk bleeding that quickly fills the field may require large caliber suction to identify the source of bleeding. If the vessel injury can be clearly identified, a primary repair can be attempted. Ligation can also be performed, which could carry a risk of posterior circulation stroke in some patients.[20] Neurologic sequelae from vertebral artery injury during an ACDF could be as high as 17.9%.[39] However, if the bleed is too brisk to be identified, or the vessel is not well-visualized in the surgical field, as is the case with the vertebral artery, there should be consideration for packing of the wound temporarily to tamponade the bleeding. Rapid wound closure may be warranted, so that the patient can be taken for an immediate angiogram, which can diagnose the location and type of injury as well as offer therapeutic interventions. Patients who had only tamponade of the hemorrhage experienced a 45% rate of delayed vascular complications.[39] Pseudoaneurysm and fistula formation can also occur, causing delayed bleeding with significant morbidity.[40] Endovascular treatment of the vessel injury may offer definitive treatment for this complication.

Vertebral artery injury during an ACDF has a reported incidence of 0.3%, making it a rare complication.[9,20] This is most likely to occur during the discectomy. ACDF technique limits lateral decompression to the medial aspect of the uncovertebral junction, as putting instruments past it can put the vertebral artery at risk. Intraoperative repair of a vertebral artery injury has also been described as a way of managing this very rare complication.[41]

Thrombosis of the internal jugular vein after ACDF is a rare but recognized complication.[42,43] It may present as postoperative neck swelling for which a complete workup, including imaging studies, such as duplex ultrasonography, should be performed. Internal jugular thrombosis does carry a 2 to 3% risk of pulmonary embolism and should therefore be diagnosed and treated promptly. This rare complication has been treated with anticoagulation, or in some appropriate cases, thrombectomy.[44]

Horner's Syndrome

Horner's syndrome is a rare but well-known complication of an ACDF. It occurs as a result of damage to the cervical sympathetic chain, which courses ventrolaterally to the vertebral column and within the longus colli muscle. Characteristic findings due to the loss of sympathetic innervation include pupillary miosis, ptosis, and facial anhidrosis. Reported rates of postoperative Horner's syndrome range from 0.06 to 0.62%.[21,22] Damage to the sympathetic chain can happen due to excessive dissection, cauterization, or sectioning of the longus colli. Studies on this rare complication have shown it most commonly occurs when operating at the C5 and C6 levels.[45] This correlates with anatomical studies, demonstrating that the sympathetic chain is located 1 cm lateral to the medial border of the longus colli at the level of C6, whereas it is closer to 2 cm lateral to the medial border of the longus colli at more superior levels.[46,47]

Outcomes and Prevention of Horner's Syndrome

A published case series identified 30 cases of Horner's syndrome after ACDF and evaluated the postoperative courses.[22] In all cases, Horner's syndrome was immediately identified postoperatively. C5–6 was the level operated upon in 64% of the cases. Within 1 year, 82% had at least partial resolution of symptoms, and 61% of the entire cohort had complete recovery. Knowledge of the sympathetic chain anatomy is essential in understanding the intraoperative techniques to prevent a Horner's syndrome. Dissection of the longus colli is the step in which most of the risk is incurred. After dividing the longus colli in the midline, dissection should proceed in a lateral dissection within the subperiosteal plane. Blunt dissection should be performed with Kittner or Peanut sponges. Sharp dissection and cautery are avoided in this step. Retractors need to be placed underneath the longus colli not only to avoid damage but also to achieve stable retractor position and improve visualization of the operative field.

Esophageal Perforation Injury

Injury to hollow viscus during ACDF, including the esophagus, larynx and pharynx, is an uncommon and avoidable complication. However, without early recognition, it can portend to rates of morbidity and mortality as high as 50%.[9] Rates of esophageal perforation injury (EPI) during an ACDF range from 0.3% to 5% in the literature.[6,9,10] Signs and symptoms of EPI include significant postoperative dysphagia, pneumonia, fevers, odynophagia, food intolerance, hoarseness, neck crepitus, a tender or erythematous neck, and leakage from the incision with early septicemia. Development of a retropharyngeal abscess or mediastinitis after an ACDF is also a warning sign, and these findings in particular are associated with significant morbidity and mortality. They are considered surgical emergencies in this setting and require emergent return to the OR for esophageal repair and washout.

These red flag symptoms should be worked up with imaging such as X-rays, CT, or MRI. Plain X-rays may be useful in identifying air within the prevertebral space, subcutaneous emphysema, or widening of the retropharyngeal space indicative of a possible mediastinitis. Oral contrast agents may help identify the location of an injury; however, this method is associated with false negative rates as high as 10%.[48,49] CT and MRI have higher anatomical resolution that allows identification of soft-tissue injury and cervical hardware malpositioning, migration, or loosening. Finally, an intraoperative flexible endoscopic examination of the oropharynx and esophagus will give direct visualization of viscus injury and is preferred over rigid and/ or direct laryngoscopy, which has increased potential to exacerbate existing EPI.

Management of Esophageal Perforation Injury

There is currently no standard algorithm for management of ACDF-related esophageal injuries. Involvement of other specialties with experience in repairing an injury will be required. Most discussion of EPI and related management in the literature is limited to review of case reports or small case series. There is a proposed systematic classification of ACDF-related EPI, based on their time to recognition from surgery as well as a proposed algorithm of injury repair according to the timing of injury, size, and mechanism.[10] It also classifies early injuries to the esophagus as those which are identified intraoperatively or within the first 30 days of surgery. Delayed injuries are those diagnosed beyond 30 days after surgery.

Early EPI most commonly occurs during the surgical approach from excessive retraction of the midline structures or sharp dissection when attempting to expose the longus colli muscles and underlying vertebral column.[6] Patients who have a history of head and neck surgery, malignancy, or radiation are at a higher risk for EPI, due to obscured tissue planes and scar tissue or adhesions. Early recognition of EPI is paramount in avoiding a serious complication. There should be a low threshold to investigate the possibility of an EPI if it is suspected, which may include pausing the surgery and requesting intraoperative consultation. Delayed EPI has been reported to occur as far as 18 years post-operatively. The mechanism of delayed injury is thought to be a consequence of chronic irritation of the esophagus by anterior cervical hardware, leading to inflammation, ischemia, and subsequent necrosis.[10,50,51] The posterior esophageal mucosa within the cricopharyngeal region is only covered with a thin fascial layer; therefore, it is the region most at risk for perforation by screw back-out, implant loosening, or migration.[52]

Intraoperative management of perforation requires early recognition of perforation and intraoperative consultation with subspecialty service such as otolaryngology, thoracic, and/or general surgery for evaluation and possible primary closure with absorbable suture. Proactive inspection of the soft-tissue surface of the hollow viscus is imperative to confirm no violation occurred. Placement of an orogastric tube by anesthesia prior to the start of surgery helps to identify the esophagus not only for the approach surgeon but also for the consultant who may need to repair an injury intraoperatively.

Conservative management of an EPI is reserved for injuries noted outside the operating room that are small, usually less than 1 cm. These small injuries will likely heal without surgical intervention, provided the patient is devoid of any of the red flag symptoms such as septicemia or mediastinitis that require emergent surgical intervention. Management involves bowel rest with parenteral nutrition and coverage with broad-spectrum antibiotics.[53] If the patient will require more than 2 weeks of bowel rest, gastrostomy tube placement for nutrition is recommended.[6,10,54,55] Larger EPIs, measuring greater than 1 cm, require primary surgical repair. The use of rotational muscle flaps can close the defect and help protect the esophagus from future compressive friction.[56–58] In the setting of an infection, hardware should be considered for removal if it appears involved, in order to ensure source control.

The following case describes diagnosis and management of a delayed esophageal perforation following anterior cervical spine surgery. This patient was a 40 year-old female who underwent a C4–7 ACDF and a C6 corpectomy with fibular allograft at an outside hospital several years prior. The original surgery was complicated by malalignment of hardware requiring revision surgery on the same day. She presented to the gastroenterologist with worsening of a chronic dysphagia. Barium swallow evaluation demonstrated a large diverticulum in the cervical esophagus measuring 7.8 × 5.9 × 1.9 cm (**Fig. 19.1**). She was evaluated by neurosurgery, thoracic surgery, and plastic surgery. Preoperative imaging showed presence of proper bony fusion. A plan was made to remove the cervical hardware and repair the esophagus. The patient underwent anterior neck exploration. There were adhesions of the esophagus to the anterior cervical plate. All hardware was removed without difficulty and a 7 cm perforation of the esophagus was noted. The perforation was primarily closed and covered with a supraclavicular artery island flap.

Recurrent and Superior Laryngeal Nerve Injury

Multiple sensitive nerve structures are vulnerable to injury during the ACDF approach. While these nerves are not always visualized, a detailed knowledge of their anatomy is invaluable to reducing the chance of nerve injury. The recurrent laryngeal nerve (RLN) and superior laryngeal nerve (SLN) have vital functions innervating muscles of the larynx. Injury of either nerve can occur due to stretch injury from retraction, tissue manipulation, and intubation, or from inadvertent division during the approach if it is not recognized. Damage to these nerves can cause vocal cord paralysis and voice hoarseness, both of which can be either transient or permanent. Patients with prior neck surgery or pathology should always be evaluated for vocal cord function preoperatively, as damage to the single working vocal cord can lead to airway obstruction upon extubation, and the patient may require emergent cricothyroidotomy and permanent tracheostomy.

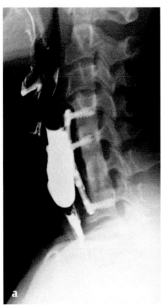
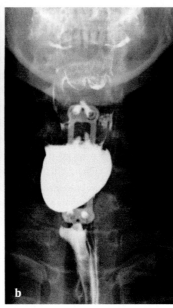

Fig. 19.1 AP and lateral X-ray of the neck performed during barium swallow evaluation. Bony fusion from C4–7 is seen. There is a large diverticulum in the posterior esophagus at the level of the hardware measuring 7.8 × 5.9 × 1.9 cm.

The RLN originates from the vagus nerve. After exiting the skull base at the jugular foramen, the fibers travel with the vagus nerve, and branch off in the chest (**Fig. 19.2**). This pattern of traveling downward and then returning to the neck is why the nerve is described as recurrent. There are well-described anatomic studies on the nerve, which have shown that on the right side, it loops under the subclavian, and then travels obliquely in the sagittal plane toward the tracheoesophageal groove where it ascends.[59] On the left side, the nerve branches under the aortic arch before ascending. Historically, anatomical studies suggested that the course of the right RLN had less redundancy, and was therefore more susceptible to stretch injury.[60] However, updated studies have refuted this previously held notion, showing that the course of the RLN in the neck does not have as much variation as once thought.[59,61] In addition, studies of RLN injury incidence have not shown any difference between a right- and left-sided approach.[61]

The SLN is also a branch of the vagus nerve, which provides both motor and sensory innervation to the larynx. It descends

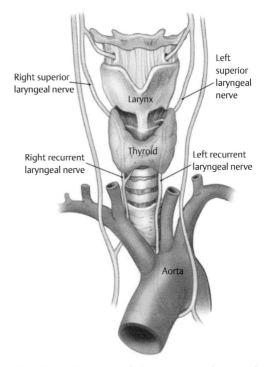

Fig. 19.2 Anatomy of the recurrent laryngeal nerve in the cervical and thoracic regions. Reprinted from: *Atlas of Neurosurgical Techniques. Spine and Peripheral Nerves* (p. 187) by R Fessler, L Sekhar, 2016, Thieme. Copyright 2016.

posterior and then medial to the carotid artery, at the level of the pharynx, before branching into an internal and external branch. The external branch is responsible for innervating the cricothyroid muscles, which serve to tense the vocal cords.[62] Loss of this motor function can cause a change in voice pitch, which may be permanent. In addition, the paralyzed position of the innervated muscles, or loss of sensory function in this area, can increase the risk of aspiration. The superior and recurrent laryngeal nerves are not routinely identified during the ACDF approach. However, the knowledge of their anatomy and function can be used to improve surgical technique to reduce risk of injury.

Incidence

Clinical findings in a patient with an RLN injury can include dysphonia or respiratory distress. There is wide variation in the literature regarding rates of RLN injury, ranging from less than 0.1 to 21%.[7,8] Differences in definition, screening, and method of detection for RLN injury are likely responsible for this wide range. In addition, subtle voice changes may not be detected postoperatively or are attributed to something other than nerve injury. It is becoming accepted that this complication is likely more common than once thought. In the majority of patients, RLN injury will be transient with mild symptoms. One study showed that 16% of patients had partial resolution with residual symptoms of RLN injury after ACDF.[1] Of this cohort, 73.7% had complete resolution, and the remainder were lost to follow-up. While it is not common to have a persistent RLN injury, it can have a significant impact on quality of life, especially if the patient has persistent hoarseness, voice change, or respiratory difficulty.

SLN injury is often considered even more rare than RLN injury. Studies for ACDF have shown SLN injury rates of 0.125 to 1.1%.[63,64] Some authors have argued that perhaps it is an unrecognized cause of postoperative dysphonia or dysphagia. When clinically significant, it can be responsible for significant voice change, causing problems with voice pitch or a decreased cough reflex, which increases aspiration risk. Most of the reported cases in these studies showed that the nerve injury was only transient.

Overall, the incidence of RLN injury is likely more common than previously thought. The majority of patients only experience a transient voice change, however there is potential for this to become permanent. Vocal cord paralysis secondary to RLN injury can have dangerous consequences if not managed appropriately. Understanding the anatomy of the nerve and utilizing techniques to avoid injuring it are essential to reducing the risk of injury.

Techniques for Avoiding RLN and SLN Injury

A patient who has undergone prior surgery, radiation, or has a known malignancy of the neck, needs to have laryngoscopy for evaluation for assessment of vocal cord function prior to surgery. Repeat anterior cervical spine surgery is one of the highest risk factors for RLN injury, possibly due to presence of adhesions or scar tissue, making the nerve to be less able to tolerate stretch.[7,8,65] If a patient only has vocal cord function on one side, and the other side is injured, after extubation, they will have an airway obstruction that will require emergent cricothyroidotomy. In these cases, where there is a paralyzed vocal cord, reconsideration of the approach, or only operating on the affected side, can reduce the risk of this disastrous complication. Reduction of ETT cuff pressures, after retractors are put in place, should be performed routinely during the operation.[66] The nerve will usually be located in a space between the retractor and ETT cuff, and it is therefore subjected to pressure from both. More severe symptoms have been correlated with higher ETT cuff pressures.[67] Minimizing tissue retraction when able, and also being familiar with nerve anatomy, can also help reduce this risk.

Management of RLN Injury

Patients with persistent symptoms after a RLN injury may require additional medical management. Consultation with an otolaryngologist is appropriate when the patient has severe symptoms or fails to improve. Patient with voice changes can undergo speech therapy and exercises that can increase vocal cord motion. Injection augmentation of the vocal cords can help to restore swallowing and voice function, although this may not be a permanent solution.[68] Other surgical procedures, such as medialization laryngoplasty or cricothyroid subluxation, can modify the muscles and vocal cord tissues to improve function.[68] Reinnervation procedures, using ansa cervicalis or supraclavicular nerve as a graft, can also be attempted as a salvage therapy to restore function.[69]

Thoracic Duct Injury

Thoracic duct injury during an ACDF is a rare but feared complication. It is most often encountered during exposure of the lower subaxial cervical spine from a left-sided approach. A recent systematic review reported an incidence of 0.02%.[23] The thoracic duct can be identified dorsal to the subclavian vein and should be carefully protected during surgical approach. Chronic chyle loss leads to fluid, electrolyte, and protein depletion. Metabolic derangements, peripheral lymphocytopenia, and poor immunity can all result. Uncorrected chyle loss can also cause progressive weakness, dehydration and peripheral edema, and reported mortality up to 50% when untreated.[70] When a thoracic duct injury is identified intraoperatively, suture ligation has been used successfully to avoid future complications.[23,71] In addition to previously mentioned findings, there is potential for formation of a fistula from the thoracic duct to the subcutaneous space which could present as overlying erythema and edema.[71,72] Chyle leak into the intrathoracic space and chylothorax can be managed conservatively if the patient is minimally symptomatic.

Conservative options may include diet modifications and somatostatin and octreotide management.[73,74] However, if symptomatic, chest tube drainage or surgical ligation of the thoracic duct is recommended.[75,76]

Early Postoperative Complications

Dysphagia

Dysphagia is one of the most common complications following anterior cervical spine surgery. It manifests as pain or difficulty with swallowing, which could be accompanied by the sensation of food sticking in the throat or even choking. Swallowing is a complex function, requiring the coordination of numerous muscles innervated by multiple branched nerves.[77] Anterior cervical spine approaches involve retraction of tissues which can cause stretch injury of superior laryngeal, recurrent laryngeal, vagus, and glossopharyngeal nerves, depending on the level. In addition, the esophagus and other muscles associated with swallowing may also need to be retracted during these surgeries. Dysfunction in any part of the process can easily cause swallowing problems.

For many patients who experience postoperative dysphagia, it is transient and not prohibitive of a regular oral diet. Other patients may have to adhere to a modified diet to reduce risk of aspiration if their swallowing function is truly impaired. At its most severe, a chronic postoperative dysphagia can prevent patients from tolerating a diet by mouth for an extended period of time, possibly requiring even enteral tube feedings until it improves.

A variety of studies have evaluated patients with postoperative dysphagia to understand which factors increase risk. Not all studies are comparable, due to differences in technique and institutional protocols for the procedure itself and postoperative care, but it is a common finding overall. Postoperative rates of reported dysphagia vary widely, often due to differences in definition of dysphagia and method of assessment. Studies have shown that 10 to 82% of patients experience dysphagia.[1-3] There are a number of factors that are associated with an increased risk of dysphagia, including age, duration of preoperative symptoms, higher cervical level, reoperation, and multilevel surgeries.[1,2,77,78] Other studies have evaluated the rates over time after surgery. One such analysis showed that among the patients who developed dysphagia within the first 6 months after surgery, 88% still had symptoms by 6 weeks, 29.6% by 3 months, and 7.4% at 6 months.[79] Interestingly, in this study, all patients had complete resolution by 12 months.

Strategies to Prevent Dysphagia

Several strategies have been described to reduce the tissue injury and swelling that lead to the development of dysphagia. Decreasing the endotracheal cuff pressure after retractors are put in place is a commonly used strategy to reduce pressure on the midline structures and is routinely recommended.[66] Minimizing the amount of retraction and tissue manipulation when able can also lessen postoperative swelling.

Steroid administration has been used and studied as a method to reduce postoperative tissue and airway edema. Preoperative, intraoperative, and postoperative administration have all been utilized.[80-83] Steroids also have theoretical adverse effects of potentially increasing wound complications or infections. Regardless, steroid administration for an ACDF remains commonplace at many institutions. Reduced rates of dysphagia and even length of hospital stay have been shown in multiple studies.[80,83,84] However, other studies have demonstrated no benefit to intraoperative steroid administration, so it is possible that there is no advantage.[82] While there are generally no increase in wound complications, fusion appears to be delayed, with decreased 6 month rates but equivalent at 2 years.[81,82]There is substantial variation among these studies with the type of steroid, route of administration, timing and dose, according to

surgeon preference or institutional protocols, making comparison of the data difficult. One randomized trial used a steroid protocol in which they administered one intraoperative dose of IV dexamethasone at 0.06 mg/kg, followed by four additional doses over the first 24 hours of the postoperative period.[82] These patients did not have any increase in wound complications. Lateral neck X-rays can also be performed to monitor improvement in the edema. A speech therapy evaluation should also be performed to ensure the patient is not at risk of aspiration.

The presence of an anterior cervical plate has also been theorized to contribute to postoperative dysphagia, due to its mass effect on the midline structures. Proximity of the esophagus to cervical hardware makes it vulnerable to irritation from the instrumentation. Proper surgical technique involves making the plate sit as flat against the vertebral bodies as possible. This often requires drilling of osteophytes. A lateral view intraoperative X-ray might be able to visualize the hardware's position. To combat this effect, newer anterior cervical instrumentation devices that have a lower or even "zero" profile are being used. They have been studied to investigate whether this will help reduce dysphagia rates. A mix of results, with some demonstrating improvement in dysphagia rates and others with no change, have been seen in these studies, indicating that more work in this area is needed.[85,86] Other strategies, such as disc arthroplasty instead of fusion, in appropriate patients, have been shown to be possibly lowering the rates of dysphagia as well.[87]

Postoperative Hematomas (POH)

POH are uncommon after ACDF, with a reported incidence up to 6%.[14] Clinically significant POHs are even more rare and most commonly secondary to inadequate intraoperative hemostasis. A large database review included 37,361 ACDFs and found that the incidence of POH requiring return to OR was 0.4%.[88] As much as 37% of these hematomas were diagnosed after discharge. Symptoms of postoperative hematoma can include neck swelling, stridor, or significant dysphonia, which may indicate early airway compromise. In severe cases, tracheal deviation is noted. These critical findings necessitate emergent return to OR for exploration of the wound. Factors found to be associated with clinically significant POH included multilevel procedures > 3 levels, preoperative international normalized ratio >1.2, body mass index (BMI) < 24, American Society of Anesthesiologists (ASA) classification 3, and male sex.[88] Patients in this same series who required reoperation had longer length of stay and were at higher risk for reintubation, prolonged mechanical ventilation, deep wound infections, and ventilator-associated pneumonia.

The use of a surgical site drain after ACDF is usually done with the intention of reducing the risk of POH. This practice remains controversial and is often surgeon-dependent. There are no studies that have demonstrated any significantly decreased risk of POH with use of drain.[89–91] Risk factors for having elevated drain output have been identified, such as age greater than 50 years, smoking history, and ACDF with two or more levels, however there was no evidence that less drain output reduced risk of repeat surgery.[89]

Postoperative Infection (POI)

The reported incidence of POI is 0.07 to 1.6%.[6,9,15] Most POI are superficial and often present with erythema and swelling localized to the incision, with or without purulent drainage. In the rare occurrence of a more serious infection such as those from an esophageal perforation injury (EPI), retropharyngeal abscess or mediastinitis can occur due to spread of infection along deep fascial planes in the craniocaudal direction. These subsequently present with symptoms as described previously in this chapter. The most common infectious organisms noted include Gram-positive cocci such as *Staphylococcus aureus*, *Staphylococcus epidermidis*, and beta-hemolytic streptococci. Gram-negative infections

from *Escherichia coli*, or species of Klebsiella, Pseudomonas, Aerobacter, and Proteus, are commonly present in IV drug users.[92,93] Indolent, low virulence skin flora such as Propionibacterium and Diphtheroids have been associated with delayed soft-tissue surgical site-related POI.[52] Common organisms involved with EPI-related infections include both streptococcus and staphylococcus species as well as Pseudomonas, Bacteroides, anaerobic Gram-positive cocci and *Candida albicans*.[94]

Superficial infections are often successfully managed conservatively with a combination of IV and oral antibiotics, whereas deeper infections will require surgical debridement and washout with a prolonged course of IV antibiotics. The use of vancomycin powder in the anterior cervical incision has been shown to reduce rates of surgical site POI and may be favored by some surgeons.[95]

Delayed Postoperative Complications

Pseudarthrosis

Pseudarthrosis is typically defined as lack of bone growth across the disc space at one or more years of radiographic follow-up after the index operation. Pseudarthrosis rates after ACDF have a wide reported variance. This variation is likely related to differences in technique, type of interbody device used, number of levels operated upon, and plating technique. A large meta-analysis showed a 3.7% overall pseudarthrosis rate in one-level ACDF, with rates differing between autograft (0.9%) and allograft use (4.8%).[12] A more recent large single institution retrospective study reported radiographic pseudarthrosis rates of 42% in three-level and 56% in a four-level ACDF.[96] Recent comparison between allograft and polyetheretherketone (PEEK) has shown mixed results, with some studies showing a five to six-fold increased rate of pseudarthrosis with PEEK use, compared to allograft, in both single and multilevel ACDF.[97,98] Another study also examined this but showed no difference.[99] A recent literature review demonstrated that the use of titanium cages, carbon cages, and zero-profile/stand-alone cages protect against the development of pseudarthrosis, while the use of PEEK, polymethyl methacrylate (PMMA) and trabecular metal cages are risk factors that contribute toward the development of pseudarthrosis.[100] Other patient-specific risk factors for development of pseudarthrosis include younger age, use of specific medications such as proton-pump inhibitors, smoking, or angiotensin-converting enzyme (ACE) inhibitors.[101–104]

A novel prediction tool has been proposed to assess the risk of pseudarthrosis preoperatively. N-terminal telopeptide is a fragment of type I collagen and has been shown to be a reliable marker of bony turnover. A single study recently showed that preoperative serum N-terminal telopeptide levels were higher in patients who had successful fusion compared to those without fusion at both 6 months and 1 year postoperatively.[105]

Diagnosis

Diagnosis of pseudarthrosis can be made using several radiographic modalities.[106] Typical static AP and lateral plain film X-rays may demonstrate pseudarthrosis when absence of osseous bridging is noted, however this has been shown to have poor correlation to intraoperative findings. Dynamic flexion-extension lateral X-rays have been shown to have a much stronger correlation. This involves measurement of the interspinous movement at the fused level or the Cobb angle. A difference of < 1 mm difference in interspinous distance between flexion and extension confirms fusion, while a difference > 1 mm is typical of pseudarthrosis. In unclear circumstances, CT of the cervical spine can be obtained to evaluate for formation of bridging bone outside of the graft; however, interpretation of this is subjective.

Over time, as many as 2/3 of all patients with pseudarthrosis can become symptomatic.[103] However, a separate study showed that up to 70% of patients with non-symptomatic pseudarthrosis at 1 year postoperatively will demonstrate fusion at 2 years postoperatively. It may be reasonable, therefore, to observe asymptomatic patients.[107] Additionally, those patients with symptomatic pseudarthrosis have been shown to have poorer mental health and pain disability outcomes than those patients who do not have nonunion. Finally, pseudoarthrosis is associated with increased direct costs, postoperative costs, and total costs compared to those with fusion.[108]

Adjacent Segment Disease (ASD)

Adjacent segment pathology can be divided into two categories. Adjacent segment degeneration is defined as new radiographic degenerative findings at an adjacent level to a surgically treated level which has no clinical correlation. ASD is defined as the same radiographic changes but with clinical correlation such as worsened neck pain and radicular or myelopathic symptoms.[104] ASD is thought to develop due to increased biomechanical stress on adjacent spinal segments.[109] Risk factors for ASD include preexisting degeneration prior to index surgery, the failure to restore or maintain cervical lordosis, as well as excessive disc space distraction during surgery.[110,111] Rates of ASD have been shown to be approximately 3% at 1 year, 13.6% at 5 years, and 25% at 10 years.[11] A more recent meta-analysis estimated the incidence of reoperation for ASD at 0.8% per year.[112]

The major alternative proposed procedure to reduce development of ASD is cervical disc arthroplasty. This procedure has been shown in biomechanical studies to preserve motion at adjacent segments, but clinical data has not been as clear.[113] A meta-analysis of several prospective trials investigating cervical disc arthroplasty compared to ACDF has shown minimal clinically significant differences between the two procedures.[114] However, more recently published data with longer follow-up of 7 and 10 years have shown a trend toward decreased symptomatic ASD.[114-116]

Subsidence and Fusion Failure

Subsidence is a frequent phenomenon after ACDF. It is generally defined as a > 3 mm loss of intervertebral height comparing immediate postoperative films to most recent follow-up. A large literature review demonstrated an overall subsidence rate of 21% in 4,784 studied patients who underwent ACDF with PEEK, PMMA, or titanium grafts.[13] Several studies have shown that rates of subsidence increase when operating more caudally in the cervical spine, with the highest rates observed at C5–6 and C6–7.[117-119] Several strategies for decreasing rates of subsidence have been proposed. The use of anterior plates has been shown to decrease the rate of subsidence for allografts that is comparable to use of autograft alone.[13,120,121] Placement of interbody devices more than 3 mm posterior to the anterior margin of the vertebral body has also been shown to increase rates of subsidence; however, the clinical outcomes between those with and without subsidence were not statistically significant.[122] Additionally, use of interbody devices > 5.5 mm in height has been shown to increase the rate of subsidence.[123] A separate single center study recently reported no differences in pseudarthrosis, subsidence, and revision surgery rate in PEEK versus structural allograft for one- or two-level ACDF in patients with a minimum of 2 years follow-up after index surgery.[99] Despite all of these findings, most clinical literature supports no significant correlation between subsidence and clinical symptoms.[13]

Regardless of the cause of one of these long-term complications, management is similar for all three of these conditions. Patients without symptoms are conservatively managed with physical therapy, anti-inflammatory medication, and injections. Symptomatic patients with neck pain, radicular, or myelopathic symptoms can be managed with either revision anterior surgery or posterior fusion (**Fig. 19.3**). Revision anterior surgery carries an increased risk of postoperative dysphagia, hoarseness and esophageal, tracheal or vascular injury, due to scar tissue. Rates of dysphagia at 2 years after surgery are significantly higher in revision surgery (27.7%) versus index surgery (11.3%).[124] Preoperative evaluation by an otolaryngologist is advised to rule out undiagnosed unilateral vocal cord paralysis. A recent meta-analysis showed 97.1% fusion rates in the posterior fusion groups versus 86.4% fusion rates in revision anterior surgery.[125] Additionally, up to 44% of anterior revision surgery patients have required a second revision surgery for persistent nonunion.[126]

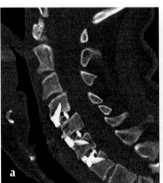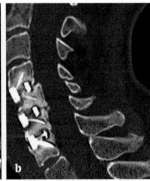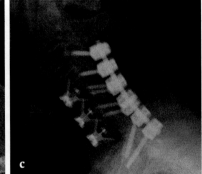

Fig. 19.3 A 78-year-old female who underwent C4–7 anterior cervical discectomy and fusion (ACDF) with standalone cages (**a**). 14-month follow-up CT shows subsidence at all levels and screw loosening (**b**). Cervical X-ray after posterior decompression and fusion, performed 15 months after the original surgery (**c**).

Conclusion

The ACDF is a commonly performed, versatile, and effective surgery. Performing it with appropriate technique often results in successful fusion and good patient outcomes, but the risk of a complication always remains. From the rare to the common, being aware of the possible complications with this procedure is essential to being able to perform it properly. Many of the considerations for this surgery with regard to preoperative, postoperative, and intraoperative decision-making can be guided by an understanding of how to increase the chances of a successful operation.

While the management of these complications may not always be straightforward, this chapter has gathered some of the best available evidence and reports of how to treat them. The described surgical strategies can help to avoid nerve and vessel injury and increase the chance of a successful fusion. Techniques for dealing with minor to potentially fatal clinical situations should be committed to the spine surgeon's skill set, so that this procedure can continue to be performed safely and with expertise.

Take-home Points

- CSF leak from an unintentional durotomy can be repaired intraoperatively, and it is rare that they require additional surgery.

- Vascular injuries can be avoided with intimate knowledge of the anatomy. Endovascular management may be required in some situations.

- Esophageal perforation injury is uncommon, however morbidity is high especially if it is not discovered and managed in a timely fashion. Small perforations are amenable to conservative treatment, but most will require a multidisciplinary approach for diagnosis and repair.

- Clinically significant postoperative hematomas are very rare; however, risk factors for POH include multilevel procedures > 3 levels, preoperative international normalized ratio > 1.2, BMI < 24, ASA classification 3, and male sex.

- Most postoperative infections are superficial and can be managed with antibiotics, unless there is evidence of wound dehiscence or involvement of cervical hardware which would warrant reexploration.

- Dysphagia and RLN and SLN injury occur at lower rates with reduced endotracheal cuff pressures. Steroids can also be used without an increase in wound complications.

- Long-term complications such as pseudarthrosis, ASD, and subsidence are not uncommon. Typically, these issues can be managed conservatively. However, patients can become symptomatic with neck pain, radicular pain, or with myelopathy. When symptomatic, surgical options include revision anterior surgery or posterior fusion.

References

1. Gokaslan ZL, Bydon M, De la Garza-Ramos R, et al. Recurrent laryngeal nerve palsy after cervical spine surgery: a multicenter AOSpine clinical research network study. Global Spine J 2017; 7(1, Suppl):53S–57S

2. Riley LH III, Skolasky RL, Albert TJ, Vaccaro AR, Heller JG. Dysphagia after anterior cervical decompression and fusion: prevalence and risk factors from a longitudinal cohort study. Spine 2005;30(22):2564–2569

3. Rihn JA, Kane J, Albert TJ, Vaccaro AR, Hilibrand AS. What is the incidence and severity of dysphagia after anterior cervical surgery? Clin Orthop Relat Res 2011;469(3):658–665

4. Hannallah D, Lee J, Khan M, Donaldson WF, Kang JD. Cerebrospinal fluid leaks following cervical spine surgery. J Bone Joint Surg Am 2008;90(5):1101–1105

5. Syre P, Bohman L-E, Baltuch G, Le Roux P, Welch WC. Cerebrospinal fluid leaks and their management after anterior cervical discectomy and fusion: a report of 13 cases and a review of the literature. Spine 2014; 39(16):E936–E943

6. Fountas KN, Kapsalaki EZ, Nikolakakos LG, et al. Anterior cervical discectomy and fusion associated complications. Spine 2007;32(21):2310–2317

7. Erwood MS, Hadley MN, Gordon AS, Carroll WR, Agee BS, Walters BC. Recurrent laryngeal nerve injury following reoperative anterior cervical discectomy and fusion: a meta-analysis. J Neurosurg Spine 2016; 25(2):198–204

8. Beutler WJ, Sweeney CA, Connolly PJ. Recurrent laryngeal nerve injury with anterior cervical spine surgery risk with laterality of surgical approach. Spine 2001; 26(12):1337–1342

9. Taylor BA, Vaccaro AR, Albert TJ. Complications of anterior and posterior surgical approaches in the treatment of cervical degenerative disc disease. In: Seminars in Spine Surgery. WB Saunders Company; 1999:337–46

10. Harman F, Kaptanoglu E, Hasturk AE. Esophageal perforation after anterior cervical surgery: a review of the literature for over half a century with a demonstrative case and a proposed novel algorithm. Eur Spine J 2016;25(7):2037–2049

11. Hilibrand AS, Carlson GD, Palumbo MA, Jones PK, Bohlman HH. Radiculopathy and myelopathy at segments adjacent to the site of a previous anterior cervical arthrodesis. J Bone Joint Surg Am 1999;81(4):519–528

12. Shriver MF, Lewis DJ, Kshettry VR, Rosenbaum BP, Benzel EC, Mroz TE. Pseudoarthrosis rates in anterior cervical discectomy and fusion: a meta-analysis. Spine J 2015;15(9):2016–2027

13. Noordhoek I, Koning MT, Jacobs WCH, Vleggeert-Lankamp CLA. Incidence and clinical relevance of cage subsidence in anterior cervical discectomy and fusion: a systematic review. Acta Neurochir (Wien) 2018;160(4):873–880

14. Jandial R, McCormick PBP. Core Techniques in Operative Neurosurgery. E-Book: Expert Consult - Online. Elsevier Health Sciences; 2011

15. Ghobrial GM, Harrop JS, Sasso RC, et al. Anterior cervical infection: presentation and incidence of an uncommon postoperative complication. Global Spine J 2017; 7(1, Suppl):12S–16S

16. Currier BL. Neurological complications of cervical spine surgery: C5 palsy and intraoperative monitoring. Spine 2012;37(5):E328–E334

17. Flynn TB. Neurologic complications of anterior cervical interbody fusion. Spine 1982;7(6):536–539

18. Ahn H, Fehlings MG. Prevention, identification, and treatment of perioperative spinal cord injury. Neurosurg Focus 2008; 25(5):E15

19. Bertalanffy H, Eggert H-R. Complications of anterior cervical discectomy without fusion in 450 consecutive patients. Acta Neurochir (Wien) 1989;99(1-2):41–50

20. Burke JP, Gerszten PC, Welch WC. Iatrogenic vertebral artery injury during anterior cervical spine surgery. Spine J 2005;5(5):508–514, discussion 514

21. Traynelis VC, Malone HR, Smith ZA, et al. Rare complications of cervical spine surgery: Horner's syndrome. Global Spine J 2017; 7(1, Suppl):103S–108S

22. Lubelski D, Pennington Z, Sciubba DM, Theodore N, Bydon A. Horner syndrome after anterior cervical discectomy and fusion: case series and systematic review. World Neurosurg 2020;133:e68–e75

23. Derakhshan A, Lubelski D, Steinmetz MP, et al. Thoracic duct injury following cervical spine surgery: a multicenter retrospective review. Global Spine J 2017; 7(1, Suppl):115S–119S

24. Yeh K-T, Chen H, Yu T-C, Peng C-H, Liu K-L, Wu W-T. Management and outcome of cerebrospinal fluid leakage during anterior cervical fusion for an ossified posterior longitudinal ligament. Tzu-Chi Med J 2013;25(4):249–252

25. Song D, Park P. Primary closure of inadvertent durotomies utilizing the U-Clip in minimally invasive spinal surgery. Spine 2011;36(26):E1753–E1757

26. Mitchell BD, Verla T, Reddy D, Winnegan L, Omeis I. Reliable intraoperative repair nuances of cerebrospinal fluid leak in anterior cervical spine surgery and review of the literature. World Neurosurg 2016;88:252–259

27. Lien JR, Patel RD, Graziano GP. Sternocleidomastoid muscular flap: treatment of persistent cerebrospinal fluid leak after anterior cervical spine surgery. J Spinal Disord Tech 2013;26(8):449–453

28. Elder BD, Theodros D, Sankey EW, et al. Management of cerebrospinal fluid leakage during anterior cervical discectomy and fusion and its effect on spinal fusion. World Neurosurg 2016;89:636–640

29. Pennington Z, Lubelski D, Westbroek EM, et al. Time to recovery predicted by the severity of postoperative C5 palsy. J Neurosurg Spine 2019;32(2):191–199

30. Takase H, Murata H, Sato M, et al. Delayed C5 palsy after anterior cervical decompression surgery: preoperative foraminal stenosis and postoperative spinal cord shift increase the risk of palsy. World Neurosurg 2018;120:e1107–e1119

31. Saunders RL. On the pathogenesis of the radiculopathy complicating multilevel corpectomy. Neurosurgery 1995;37(3):408–412, discussion 412–413

32. Jimenez JC, Sani S, Braverman B, Deutsch H, Ratliff JK. Palsies of the fifth cervical nerve root after cervical decompression: prevention using continuous intraoperative electromyography monitoring. J Neurosurg Spine 2005;3(2):92–97

33. Ajiboye RM, D'Oro A, Ashana AO, et al. Routine use of intraoperative neuromonitoring during ACDFs for the treatment of spondylotic myelopathy and radiculopathy is questionable. Spine 2017;42(1):14–19

34. Braly BA, Lunardini D, Cornett C, Donaldson WF. Operative treatment of cervical myelopathy: cervical laminoplasty. Adv Orthop 2012;2012:508534

35. Lawton MT, Porter RW, Heiserman JE, Jacobowitz R, Sonntag VKH, Dickman CA. Surgical management of spinal epidural hematoma: relationship between surgical timing and neurological outcome. J Neurosurg 1995;83(1):1–7

36. Saadeh YS, Smith BW, Joseph JR, et al. The impact of blood pressure management after spinal cord injury: a systematic review of the literature. Neurosurg Focus 2017;43(5):E20

37. Imagama S, Matsuyama Y, Yukawa Y, et al; Nagoya Spine Group. C5 palsy after cervical laminoplasty: a multicentre study. J Bone Joint Surg Br 2010;92(3):393–400

38. Bhalodia VM, Schwartz DM, Sestokas AK, et al. Efficacy of intraoperative monitoring of transcranial electrical stimulation-induced motor evoked potentials and spontaneous electromyography activity to identify acute- versus delayed-onset C-5 nerve root palsy during cervical spine surgery: clinical article. J Neurosurg Spine 2013;19(4):395–402

39. Park H-K, Jho H-D. The management of vertebral artery injury in anterior cervical spine operation: a systematic review of published cases. Eur Spine J 2012;21(12):2475–2485

40. Daentzer D, Deinsberger W, Böker D-K. Vertebral artery complications in anterior approaches to the cervical spine: report of two cases and review of literature. Surg Neurol 2003;59(4):300–309, discussion 309

41. Pfeifer BA, Freidberg SR, Jewell ER. Repair of injured vertebral artery in anterior cervical procedures. Spine 1994;19(13):1471–1474

42. Karim A, Knapp J, Nanda A. Internal jugular venous thrombosis as a complication after an elective anterior cervical discectomy: case report. Neurosurgery 2006;59(3):E705–E705, discussion E705

43. Wong TC, Lam JJ, Ko PS. Internal jugular venous thrombosis following anterior cervical spinal surgery. Orthopedics 2005;28(8):793–794

44. Tajima H, Murata S, Kumazaki T, Ichikawa K, Tajiri T, Yamamoto Y. Successful interventional treatment of acute internal jugular vein thrombosis. AJR Am J Roentgenol 2004;182(2):467–469

45. Yasumoto Y, Abe Y, Tsutsumi S, Kondo A, Nonaka S, Ito M. [Rare complication of anterior spinal surgery: Horner syndrome]. No Shinkei Geka 2008;36(10):911–914

46. Ebraheim NA, Lu J, Yang H, Heck BE, Yeasting RA. Vulnerability of the sympathetic trunk during the anterior approach to the lower cervical spine. Spine 2000;25(13):1603–1606

47. Saylam CY, Ozgiray E, Orhan M, Cagli S, Zileli M. Neuroanatomy of cervical sympathetic trunk: a cadaveric study. Clin Anat 2009;22(3):324–330

48. Brinster CJ, Singhal S, Lee L, Marshall MB, Kaiser LR, Kucharczuk JC. Evolving options in the management of esophageal perforation. Ann Thorac Surg 2004;77(4):1475–1483

49. Giménez A, Franquet T, Erasmus JJ, Martínez S, Estrada P. Thoracic complications of

esophageal disorders. Radiographics 2002; 22(Spec No):S247–S258

50. Dakwar E, Uribe JS, Padhya TA, Vale FL. Management of delayed esophageal perforations after anterior cervical spinal surgery. J Neurosurg Spine 2009;11(3):320–325

51. Almre I, Asser A, Laisaar T. Pharyngoesophageal diverticulum perforation 18 years after anterior cervical fixation. Interact Cardiovasc Thorac Surg 2014;18(2):240–241

52. Jones WG II, Ginsberg RJ. Esophageal perforation: a continuing challenge. Ann Thorac Surg 1992;53(3):534–543

53. Ardon H, Van Calenbergh F, Van Raemdonck D, et al. Oesophageal perforation after anterior cervical surgery: management in four patients. Acta Neurochir (Wien) 2009; 151(4):297–302, discussion 302

54. Altorjay A, Kiss J, Vörös A, Bohák A. Nonoperative management of esophageal perforations. Is it justified? Ann Surg 1997; 225(4):415–421

55. Geyer TE, Foy MA. Oral extrusion of a screw after anterior cervical spine plating. Spine 2001;26(16):1814–1816

56. Ahn S-H, Lee S-H, Kim ES, Eoh W. Successful repair of esophageal perforation after anterior cervical fusion for cervical spine fracture. J Clin Neurosci 2011;18(10):1374–1380

57. Pichler W, Maier A, Rappl T, Clement HG, Grechenig W. Delayed hypopharyngeal and esophageal perforation after anterior spinal fusion: primary repair reinforced by pedicled pectoralis major flap. Spine 2006;31(9):E268–E270

58. Reid RR, Dutra J, Conley DB, Ondra SL, Dumanian GA. Improved repair of cervical esophageal fistula complicating anterior spinal fusion: free omental flap compared with pectoralis major flap. Report of four cases. J Neurosurg 2004; 100(1, Suppl Spine):66–70

59. Haller JM, Iwanik M, Shen FH. Clinically relevant anatomy of recurrent laryngeal nerve. Spine 2012;37(2):97–100

60. Weisberg NK, Spengler DM, Netterville JL. Stretch-induced nerve injury as a cause of paralysis secondary to the anterior cervical approach. Otolaryngol Head Neck Surg 1997;116(3):317–326

61. Kilburg C, Sullivan HG, Mathiason MA. Effect of approach side during anterior cervical discectomy and fusion on the incidence of recurrent laryngeal nerve injury. J Neurosurg Spine 2006;4(4):273–277

62. Friedman M, LoSavio P, Ibrahim H. Superior laryngeal nerve identification and preservation in thyroidectomy. Arch Otolaryngol Head Neck Surg 2002;128(3):296–303

63. Tempel ZJ, Smith JS, Shaffrey C, et al. A multicenter review of superior laryngeal nerve injury following anterior cervical spine surgery. Global Spine J 2017; 7(1, Suppl):7S–11S

64. Zhao J, Quan Z, Ou Y, Jiang D. [Prevention and treatment of early postoperative complications of anterior cervical spinal surgery]. Zhongguo Xiu Fu Chong Jian Wai Ke Za Zhi 2008;22(8):901–904

65. Staartjes VE, de Wispelaere MP, Schröder ML. Recurrent laryngeal nerve palsy is more frequent after secondary than after primary anterior cervical discectomy and fusion: insights from a registry of 525 patients. World Neurosurg 2018;116:e1047–e1053

66. Ratnaraj J, Todorov A, McHugh T, Cheng MA, Lauryssen C. Effects of decreasing endotracheal tube cuff pressures during neck retraction for anterior cervical spine surgery. J Neurosurg 2002; 97(2, Suppl):176–179

67. Jellish WS, Jensen RL, Anderson DE, Shea JF. Intraoperative electromyographic assessment of recurrent laryngeal nerve stress and pharyngeal injury during anterior cervical spine surgery with Caspar instrumentation. J Neurosurg 1999; 91(2, Suppl):170–174

68. Lynch J, Parameswaran R. Management of unilateral recurrent laryngeal nerve injury after thyroid surgery: A review. Head Neck 2017;39(7):1470–1478

69. Miyauchi A, Ishikawa H, Matsusaka K, et al. [Treatment of recurrent laryngeal nerve paralysis by several types of nerve suture]. Nippon Geka Gakkai Zasshi 1993;94(6):550–555

70. Kumar S, Kumar A, Pawar DK. Thoracoscopic management of thoracic duct injury: Is there a place for conservatism? J Postgrad Med 2004;50(1):57–59

71. Hart AKE, Greinwald JH Jr, Shaffrey CI, Postma GN. Thoracic duct injury during anterior cervical discectomy: a rare complication. Case report. J Neurosurg 1998; 88(1):151–154

72. Warren PS, Hogan MJ, Shiels WE. Percutaneous transcervical thoracic duct embolization for treatment of a cervical lymphocele following anterior spinal fusion: a case report. J Vasc Interv Radiol 2013;24(12):1901–1905

73. Markham KM, Glover JL, Welsh RJ, Lucas RJ, Bendick PJ. Octreotide in the treatment of thoracic duct injuries. Am Surg 2000; 66(12):1165–1167

74. Collard J-M, Laterre P-F, Boemer F, Reynaert M, Ponlot R. Conservative treatment of postsurgical lymphatic leaks with somatostatin-14. Chest 2000;117(3): 902–905

75. Lapp GC, Brown DH, Gullane PJ, McKneally M. Thoracoscopic management of chylous fistulae. Am J Otolaryngol 1998;19(4): 257–262

76. Ross JK. A review of the surgery of the thoracic duct. Thorax 1961;16(1):12–21

77. Wu B, Song F, Zhu S. Reasons of dysphagia after operation of anterior cervical decompression and fusion. Clin Spine Surg 2017; 30(5):E554–E559

78. Baron EM, Soliman AMS, Gaughan JP, Simpson L, Young WF. Dysphagia, hoarseness, and unilateral true vocal fold motion impairment following anterior cervical discectomy and fusion. Ann Otol Rhinol Laryngol 2003; 112(11):921–926

79. Kalb S, Reis MT, Cowperthwaite MC, et al. Dysphagia after anterior cervical spine surgery: incidence and risk factors. World Neurosurg 2012;77(1):183–187

80. Siasios I, Fountas K, Dimopoulos V, Pollina J. The role of steroid administration in the management of dysphagia in anterior cervical procedures. Neurosurg Rev 2018; 41(1):47–53

81. Jeyamohan SB, Kenning TJ, Petronis KA, Feustel PJ, Drazin D, DiRisio DJ. Effect of steroid use in anterior cervical discectomy and fusion: a randomized controlled trial. J Neurosurg Spine 2015;23(2):137–143

82. Haws BE, Khechen B, Narain AS, et al. Impact of local steroid application on dysphagia following an anterior cervical discectomy and fusion: results of a prospective, randomized single-blind trial. J Neurosurg Spine 2018;29(1):10–17

83. Cancienne JM, Werner BC, Loeb AE, et al. The effect of local intraoperative steroid administration on the rate of postoperative dysphagia following ACDF: a study of 245, 754 patients. Spine 2016;41(13):1084–1088

84. Song K-J, Lee S-K, Ko J-H, Yoo M-J, Kim D-Y, Lee K-B. The clinical efficacy of short-term steroid treatment in multilevel anterior cervical arthrodesis. Spine J 2014; 14(12):2954–2958

85. Hofstetter CP, Kesavabhotla K, Boockvar JA. Zero-profile anchored spacer reduces rate of dysphagia compared with ACDF with anterior plating. J Spinal Disord Tech 2015;28(5):E284–E290

86. Yang H, Chen D, Wang X, Yang L, He H, Yuan W. Zero-profile integrated plate and spacer device reduces rate of adjacent-level ossification development and dysphagia compared to ACDF with plating and cage system. Arch Orthop Trauma Surg 2015; 135(6):781–787

87. Segebarth B, Datta JC, Darden B, et al. Incidence of dysphagia comparing cervical arthroplasty and ACDF. SAS J 2010;4(1):3–8

88. Bovonratwet P, Fu MC, Tyagi V, et al. Incidence, risk factors, and clinical implications of postoperative hematoma requiring reoperation following anterior cervical discectomy and fusion. Spine 2019; 44(8):543–549

89. Basques BA, Bohl DD, Golinvaux NS, Yacob A, Varthi AG, Grauer JN. Factors predictive of increased surgical drain output after anterior cervical discectomy and fusion. Spine 2014;39(9):728–735

90. Kogure K, Node Y, Tamaki T, Yamazaki M, Takumi I, Morita A. Indwelling drains are not necessary for patients undergoing one-level anterior cervical fixation surgery. J Nippon Med Sch 2015;82(3):124–129

91. Adogwa O, Khalid SI, Elsamadicy AA, et al. The use of subfascial drains after multi-level anterior cervical discectomy and fusion: does the data support its use? J Spine Surg 2018;4(2):227–232

92. Wimmer C, Gluch H, Franzreb M, Ogon M. Predisposing factors for infection in spine surgery: a survey of 850 spinal procedures. J Spinal Disord 1998;11(2):124–128

93. Levi ADO, Dickman CA, Sonntag VKH. Management of postoperative infections after spinal instrumentation. J Neurosurg 1997;86(6):975–980

94. Rueth N, Shaw D, Groth S, et al. Management of cervical esophageal injury after spinal surgery. Ann Thorac Surg 2010;90(4):1128–1133

95. Caroom C, Tullar JM, Benton EG Jr, Jones JR, Chaput CD. Intrawound vancomycin powder reduces surgical site infections in posterior cervical fusion. Spine 2013; 38(14):1183–1187

96. Wewel JT, Kasliwal MK, Adogwa O, Deutsch H, O'Toole JE, Traynelis VC. Fusion rate following three- and four-level ACDF using allograft and segmental instrumentation: A radiographic study. J Clin Neurosci 2019;62:142–146

97. Krause KL, Obayashi JT, Bridges KJ, Raslan AM, Than KD. Fivefold higher rate of pseudarthrosis with polyetheretherketone interbody device than with structural allograft used for 1-level anterior cervical discectomy and fusion. J Neurosurg Spine 2018;30(1):46–51

98. Teton ZE, Cheaney B, Obayashi JT, Than KD. PEEK interbody devices for multilevel anterior cervical discectomy and fusion: association with more than 6-fold higher rates of pseudarthrosis compared to structural allograft. J Neurosurg Spine 2020;1(aop):1–7

99. Wang M, Chou D, Chang C-C, et al. Anterior cervical discectomy and fusion performed using structural allograft or polyetheretherketone: pseudarthrosis and revision surgery rates with minimum 2-year follow-up. J Neurosurg Spine 2019; 1(aop):1–8

100. Iunes EA, Barletta EA, Barba Belsuzarri TA, Onishi FJ, Cavalheiro S, Joaquim AF. Correlation between different interbody grafts and pseudarthrosis after anterior cervical discectomy and fusion compared with control group: systematic review. World Neurosurg 2020;134:272–279

101. Perdomo-Pantoja A, Shamoun F, Holmes C, et al. A retrospective cohort analysis of the effects of renin-angiotensin system inhibitors on spinal fusion in ACDF patients. Spine J 2019;19(8):1354–1361

102. Mangan JJ III, Divi SN, McKenzie JC, et al. Proton pump inhibitor use affects pseudarthrosis rates and influences patient-reported outcomes. Glob Spine J 2019 (e-pub ahead of print). doi:10.1177/2192568219853222

103. Phillips FM, Carlson G, Emery SE, Bohlman HH. Anterior cervical pseudarthrosis. Natural history and treatment. Spine 1997; 22(14):1585–1589

104. Hilibrand AS, Fye MA, Emery SE, Palumbo MA, Bohlman HH. Impact of smoking on the outcome of anterior cervical arthrodesis with interbody or strut-grafting. J Bone Joint Surg Am 2001;83(5):668–673

105. Steinhaus ME, Hill PS, Yang J, et al. Urinary N-telopeptide can predict pseudarthrosis after anterior cervical decompression and fusion: a prospective study. Spine 2019; 44(11):770–776

106. Lin W, Ha A, Boddapati V, Yuan W, Riew KD. Diagnosing pseudoarthrosis after anterior cervical discectomy and fusion. Neurospine 2018;15(3):194–205

107. Lee D-H, Cho JH, Hwang CJ, et al. What is the fate of pseudarthrosis detected 1 year after anterior cervical discectomy and fusion? Spine 2018;43(1):E23–E28

108. Pennington Z, Mehta VA, Lubelski D, et al. Quality of life and cost implications of pseudarthrosis after anterior cervical discectomy and fusion and its subsequent revision surgery. World Neurosurg 2020;133:e592–e599

109. Eck JC, Humphreys SC, Lim T-H, et al. Biomechanical study on the effect of cervical spine fusion on adjacent-level intradiscal pressure and segmental motion. Spine 2002;27(22):2431–2434

110. Alhashash M, Shousha M, Boehm H. Adjacent segment disease after cervical spine fusion: evaluation of a 70 patient long-term follow-up. Spine 2018;43(9):605–609

111. Li J, Li Y, Kong F, Zhang D, Zhang Y, Shen Y. Adjacent segment degeneration after single-level anterior cervical decompression and fusion: disc space distraction and its impact on clinical outcomes. J Clin Neurosci 2015;22(3):566–569

112. Lawrence BD, Hilibrand AS, Brodt ED, Dettori JR, Brodke DS. Predicting the risk of adjacent segment pathology in the cervical

spine: a systematic review. Spine 2012; 37(22, Suppl)S52–S64

113. Gandhi AA, Kode S, DeVries NA, Grosland NM, Smucker JD, Fredericks DC. Biomechanical analysis of cervical disc replacement and fusion using single level, two level, and hybrid constructs. Spine 2015;40(20):1578–1585

114. Phillips FM, Geisler FH, Gilder KM, Reah C, Howell KM, McAfee PC. Long-term outcomes of the US FDA IDE prospective, randomized controlled clinical trial comparing PCM cervical disc arthroplasty with anterior cervical discectomy and fusion. Spine 2015; 40(10):674–683

115. Ghobrial GM, Lavelle WF, Florman JE, Riew KD, Levi AD. Symptomatic adjacent level disease requiring surgery: analysis of 10-year results from a prospective, randomized, clinical trial comparing cervical disc arthroplasty to anterior cervical fusion. Neurosurgery 2019;84(2):347–354

116. Janssen ME, Zigler JE, Spivak JM, Delamarter RB, Darden BV II, Kopjar B. ProDisc-C total disc replacement versus anterior cervical discectomy and fusion for single-level symptomatic cervical disc disease: seven-year follow-up of the prospective randomized US Food and Drug Administration Investigational Device Exemption Study. J Bone Joint Surg Am 2015;97(21):1738–1747

117. Yamagata T, Takami T, Uda T, et al. Outcomes of contemporary use of rectangular titanium stand-alone cages in anterior cervical discectomy and fusion: cage subsidence and cervical alignment. J Clin Neurosci 2012; 19(12):1673–1678

118. Schmieder K, Wolzik-Grossmann M, Pechlivanis I, Engelhardt M, Scholz M, Harders A. Subsidence of the wing titanium cage after anterior cervical interbody fusion: 2-year follow-up study. J Neurosurg Spine 2006;4(6):447–453

119. Yson SC, Sembrano JN, Santos ERG. Comparison of allograft and polyetheretherketone (PEEK) cage subsidence rates in anterior cervical discectomy and fusion (ACDF). J Clin Neurosci 2017;38:118–121

120. Kaiser MG, Haid RW Jr, Subach BR, Barnes B, Rodts GE Jr. Anterior cervical plating enhances arthrodesis after discectomy and fusion with cortical allograft. Neurosurgery 2002;50(2):229–236, discussion 236–238

121. Samartzis D, Shen FH, Matthews DK, Yoon ST, Goldberg EJ, An HS. Comparison of allograft to autograft in multilevel anterior cervical discectomy and fusion with rigid plate fixation. Spine J 2003;3(6):451–459

122. Park J-Y, Choi K-Y, Moon BJ, Hur H, Jang J-W, Lee J-K. Subsidence after single-level anterior cervical fusion with a stand-alone cage. J Clin Neurosci 2016;33:83–88

123. Igarashi H, Hoshino M, Omori K, et al. Factors influencing interbody cage subsidence following anterior cervical discectomy and fusion. Clin Spine Surg 2019;32(7):297–302

124. Lee MJ, Bazaz R, Furey CG, Yoo J. Risk factors for dysphagia after anterior cervical spine surgery: a two-year prospective cohort study. Spine J 2007;7(2):141–147

125. McAnany SJ, Baird EO, Overley SC, Kim JS, Qureshi SA, Anderson PA. A meta-analysis of the clinical and fusion results following treatment of symptomatic cervical pseudarthrosis. Global Spine J 2015;5(2): 148–155

126. Carreon L, Glassman SD, Campbell MJ. Treatment of anterior cervical pseudoarthrosis: posterior fusion versus anterior revision. Spine J 2006;6(2):154–156

20 Complications of Posterior Cervical Spine Surgery

Ben Roitberg, Francesco Costa, and Se-Hoon Kim

Introduction and Background

Complications rate and avoidance of complications not only make up a key part of the management of surgical patients but also play a major role in surgical decision-making. The choice of surgical approach and even the decision to recommend operative treatment hinge on the balance between the chance of success, chance of failure, and risk of complications.

Complications can systematically be divided into local and systemic. The local can be further subdivided in various ways, for example, into neurological, those related to tissue healing, and those related to bleeding and infections. Operations with the use of hardware have additional issues related to hardware placement and stability. In this chapter, the authors will present an overview of the common complications in each area. The scope of the chapter does not permit a comprehensive review or a systematic review of the literature. Authors will attempt to be up to date with current opinion, and inevitably insert their own experience into the mix.

We are discussing complications—necessarily early and short-term adverse events taking place during the operation or in the immediate postoperative period. Long-term outcomes, durability, malunion, and long-term construct failure are also mentioned in the context of complications and related risk factors. A full discussion of long-term surgical outcomes is outside the scope of this chapter.

Systemic Complications of Posterior Cervical Spine Surgery

Some complications are specific to certain surgical procedures, and others are common to most procedures. To minimize their occurrence, the surgeon must have a keen understanding of the potential pitfalls common in each procedure.

Venous Thromboembolism and Pulmonary Embolism

Deep venous thrombosis (DVT) and the risk for subsequent pulmonary embolism (PE) are known complications of any surgical procedure, and the incidence of venous thromboembolism (VTE) in spinal surgery has been reported at 1.1%, with rates of 0.7% and 0.4% for DVT and PE, respectively.[1] Risk factors for VTE in the general population include long-term estrogen therapy, obesity, smoking, malignancy, trauma, pregnancy, older age (over 65), congenital conditions causing hypercoagulability, and immobilization/bed rest.[1] Factors specific to patients undergoing spine surgery include combined anterior/posterior surgical approach, prolonged operative time (more than 4 hours), and medical comorbid conditions such as chronic anemia, chronic venous insufficiency, diabetes, congestive heart failure, atrial fibrillation, and renal failure.[1,2] Yamada et al recently reported that female gender and rapidly progressive cervical myelopathy are high-risk factors that predict the development of DVT during the perioperative period of cervical spine surgery.[3]

Early diagnosis of DVT and PE is critical in order to initiate the appropriate therapeutic interventions and prevent potentially life-threatening complications. Signs of DVT include pain, warmth, swelling, and redness in an extremity. Venous Doppler ultrasonography should be ordered to confirm the presence of DVT in patients in whom the disease is suspected. D-dimer assays may also help establish the diagnosis of VTE.[1]

Signs of PE include dyspnea, oxygen desaturation, pleuritic chest pain, tachycardia, and tachypnea. In severe cases, hemodynamic instability, cyanosis, and right-sided heart failure may develop and lead to death. Diagnosis of PE relies on a fair degree of clinical suspicion, since symptoms are often vague and can be similar to normal postoperative complaints associated with surgical blood loss, recent intubation, and other situations. As with DVT, a positive result of a D-dimer assay may indicate presence of embolism but is not specific. The most accurate imaging modality for diagnosis is pulmonary angiography; CT studies have replaced conventional catheter angiography. Electrocardiography can help rule out other causes of chest pain and cardiac dysrhythmias and may reveal evidence of right-sided heart strain, with the most common findings being sinus tachycardia, right axis deviation, and right bundle branch block.[1]

The current standard of care for VTE and PE is to perform both mechanical and pharmacologic prophylaxis for all patients at risk. Although mechanical preventive tools such as early mobilization, compression stockings, and sequential compression devices are effective for the prevention of VTE, coadministration of chemical prophylaxis significantly decreases risk.[4] The North American Spine Society's clinical guidelines recommend mechanical prophylaxis for all patients in the perioperative and postoperative periods.[5]

Chemoprophylaxis may not be necessary in most elective spine surgery because many patients have low-risk profiles and return to normal ambulation soon after surgery. However, unfractionated heparin (UFH), low-molecular weight heparin (LMWH), or low-dose warfarin may be beneficial, as determined on a case-by-case basis, for more extensive procedures and for patients with higher risk profiles. No large-scale studies have determined safety regarding timing of chemoprophylaxis during or after surgery, but limited recommendations suggest that LMWH can be used even before elective surgery for patients at high risk.[1]

In general, treatment for VTE is continued for 3 to 6 months: 3 months for patients with first-time events or time-limited risk factors (i.e., surgery, immobilization, and trauma) and 6 months for recurrent or idiopathic DVT/PE.[6]

Ophthalmologic Complications: Vision Loss

Although a relatively uncommon complication in spinal surgery, postoperative visual loss (POVL) has been becoming increasingly recognized as a potential devastating complication and has been documented in many types of nonocular procedures.[7-9] Because of the poor outcome and paucity of treatment for POVL, every effort should be made to minimize this complication. To best prevent permanent ophthalmologic complications associated with prone positioning during posterior cervical spine surgery, surgeons should be aware of pathophysiology and related risks associated with spine surgery in the prone position, and initiate preventive measures and predictable treatment options.[8]

POVL includes four subtypes: ocular injury, central retinal artery occlusion (CRAO), cortical blindness, and ischemic optic neuropathy (ION).[1,10,11] Corneal abrasion, the most common ophthalmologic injury after spine surgery, is typically the result of positioning or physical trauma to the eye, and the symptoms are usually self-limiting and do not result in permanent visual deficits.[1,8,10,11] CRAO results in monocular blindness, often as a result of embolic events, but has also been associated with vasculopathies and poor positioning, with excessive pressure placed on the orbit in prone positioning.[1,7-11] Cortical blindness is thought to be associated with cardiovascular events and intraoperative hypoperfusion of cerebral tissue without any ocular pathology.[9,10] ION can be subdivided into anterior and posterior groups, according to the location of the ischemia.[9,10] Anterior ION is the result of injury just behind the optic disc, and posterior ION occurs in the midorbital region of the optic nerve and is the most common type of POVL in spine surgery. The incidence of POVL after spine surgery has been reported between 0.03% and 1.30%.[1,7,9-14] It has been reported that 1 case per 100 spine surgeons annually has a significant complication affecting vision.[10,12]

Important risk factors for developing POVL include positioning and complexity of surgery. Prone positioning without Mayfield pins was associated with higher incidences than anterior surgical approaches.[1,9,13-15] The incidence of POVL was three times higher for spinal fusion procedures than simple decompression.[1,9]

Apart from direct injury to the eye, several mechanisms have been proposed to explain the cause of POVL. Prone positioning is a significant risk factor by contributing to increased orbital pressure from the headrest or venous congestion to the dependent position of the orbit. Inadequate perfusion is also thought to play a role; intraoperative hypotension and high blood loss are common findings associated with POVL.[1,10,12-15] Other potential risk factors related to preexisting illnesses and known to affect circulation are as follows: hypertension, diabetes, coronary artery disease, cerebrovascular disease, and hyperlipidemia.[1,7,9,10,13,14]

To prevent POVL, preoperatively, the surgeon should review and optimize a patient's medical comorbid conditions, particularly diabetes mellitus and glaucoma.

Intraoperatively, the surgeon must place the patient's head in a rest or clamp that minimizes direct pressure on the orbits, such as a Mayfield head holder, in prone positioning. Positioning the head so that the orbits are above the level of the heart reduces venous congestion and intraocular pressure. If this position is not feasible for the intended procedure, it may be beneficial to employ rest periods during surgery to allow for elevation and adjustment of the position of the orbits. The surgeon could consider staging procedures if the duration of the surgery is expected to exceed 6 hours or the blood loss is anticipated to exceed 1 liter. Emerging evidence suggests that intraoperative intravascular volume replacement with colloidal solutions is preferable to using only crystalloid solutions.[1]

Neurological Complications of Posterior Cervical Spine Surgery

Spinal Cord Injury

The overall incidence of iatrogenic cervical spinal cord injuries is difficult to define or calculate due to the limited number of cases or series of occurrences, and the incidence of spinal cord injury resulting from cervical laminectomy varies from 0% to 10%.[16] Although iatrogenic spinal cord damage is most commonly attributed to direct mechanical trauma such as inadvertent cord manipulation, blunt forces directly onto the spinal cord, and introduction of an instrument under the lamina, vascular or ischemic factors such as intraoperative hypotension and over-distraction, may also contribute to neurologic compromise.[16] It is also notable that the hyperextension of neck required for intubation could cause compression of the spinal cord, resulting in a central cord injury in a patient with a severely stenotic cervical spinal canal.[17-19]

Injury to the spinal cord itself can result in variable and numerous clinical symptoms, ranging in severity from mild or no motor dysfunction, sensory dysfunction, or neuropathic symptoms to the most severe pattern of complete spinal cord injury.

Spinal cord or nerve root injuries can be caused by fracture of a hinge or loss of spinal canal enlargement after laminoplasty, resulting from insufficient fixation of the elevated laminae and the consequent migration of the lamina into the spinal canal. CT is useful for delineating the reconstructed laminae in such cases, and complete or partial removal of the migrated lamina is necessary. For prevention of the fracture of hinge in laminoplasty, the inner cortex of the lamina should be carefully thinned step-by-step until the surgeon is very familiar with the procedure. An immediate and rigid stabilization of the reconstructed laminae has been also proposed in a laminoplasty using titanium miniplates.[20,21]

Several cases of delayed dural damage and spinal cord compression from dislodged hydroxyapatite (HA) laminar spacers due to absorption of the tip of the spinous process have been reported following double-door laminoplasty.[22-24] The absorption of the tip of the spinous process has been reported to occur in approximately 10% of spinous process-splitting laminoplasty with the HA spacers and dislodgement of the HA spacer in approximately 3%.[22,23,25]

Nerve Root Palsy

Postoperative motor root deficits, typically involving the C5 root (C5 palsy), can vary from 5.5% to 15%, and are particularly more frequent after posterior procedures compared with anterior ones.[16,26] The incidence of C5 palsy from dorsal procedures has been reported to range from 0% to 30%, with an average of 4.6%.[27-33] In a recent meta-analysis on incidence of C5 palsy for patients after cervical surgery, the incidence after laminoplasty was 4.4% and the one after laminectomy and fusion was 12.2%.[34] Compared with anterior approaches, female patients and patients with cervical spondylotic myelopathy (CSM), posterior approaches, male

patients, and patients with ossification of posterior longitudinal ligament (OPLL) demonstrated a higher prevalence of C5 palsy.[34]

The postoperative nerve root palsy has been defined as postoperative upper extremity paresis, mainly the deltoid muscle and biceps brachii muscle, without concomitant deterioration of the underlying myelopathy symptoms.[33] C5 is by far the most frequently involved nerve root, followed by the sixth and seventh in order, and the eighth nerve root is rarely affected.[24] C5 palsy occurs unilaterally in the majority of patients, with approximately 8% of cases demonstrating bilateral involvement.[27,28] Approximately half of the patients are reported to have isolated muscle weakness, while half also report sensory deficits with/without pain in the C5 dermatome.[33]

Several investigations revealed that upper extremity palsy after laminoplasty developed in other cervical nerve roots (C6, C7, or C8), in isolation or combination, associated with high-signal intensity areas in the spinal cord on T2-weighted MR imaging.[24,35-37]

Time of onset of the postoperative C5 palsy is most often within the first week, but delayed presentation has been reported from 2 weeks to 6 weeks postoperatively.[27,31-33] The nerve root symptoms are variously attributed to direct manipulation or to indirect root traction associated with spontaneous migration after cord decompression and posterior decompression. Differing pathologic mechanisms have been proposed to explain the cause of C5 palsy, but no one mechanism adequately explains all occurrences. The unique short course of the C5 root increases its susceptibility to injury, but controversies still exist.[33] Unfortunately, there is no high-level evidence on which to base predictions of a given patient's vulnerability to postoperative C5 palsy. While myelopathic patients appear more vulnerable than radiculopathic patients, there does not appear to be strong correlations between underlying diagnosis, surgical approach, or preoperative MR images.[27,29,33] Sakaura et al have suggested five possible pathways that may contribute to the postoperative C5 palsy, and these include intraoperative inadvertent injury to the nerve root, traction or tethering of the nerve root from excessive dorsal shift of spinal cord after decompression, ischemia to the nerve root and spinal cord from decreased blood supply, segmental dysfunction of spinal cord, or reperfusion injury of the spinal cord.[27,33] The exact etiology of the postoperative nerve root palsy remains unclear, and each proposed mechanism for segmental motor palsy remains hypothetical.

Some reports have supported performing partial foraminotomy at one or more levels as a prophylactic measure during the posterior decompressive procedures, although the clinical benefit so far has not been proven.[33,38,39] While some reports have advised the role of intraoperative neurophysiologic monitoring (IONM) as a means of earlier detection of C5 nerve root irritation, the neurophysiologic techniques do not eliminate the risk of postoperative C5 palsy, and some prospectively reported instances of C5 palsy with no changes in the intraoperative spinal cord monitoring of transcranial electric motor-evoked potentials (MEPs).[33,40,41]

Once a nerve root palsy is identified, imaging studies should be performed to ensure that instrumentation, graft, or hematoma are not compressing the nerve root.[33,42,43] Conservative management such as use of steroids, cervical traction, muscle strengthening, low-frequency wave therapy, and exercising range of neck motion have been advocated for patients in whom no surgically treatable lesion is discovered, although no convincing evidence supports any of these interventions.[33]

Most nerve root palsies resolve spontaneously within 3 to 6 months postoperatively, sometimes within 2 years.[16,29,32] Patients with severe paralysis require significantly longer recovery times when compared to more mild cases.[27]

Since the exact etiology of the segmental motor palsy may be controversial and multifactorial and no preventive tools have been established yet, the potential risk of nerve root palsy after posterior cervical approaches should be described to the patients preoperatively.

Durotomy and CSF leakage

Incidental dural tears can occur while an electrocautery device is used during a posterior exposure, slipping between the lamina. Injury can occur with the high-speed drill or Kerrison rongeur, and while the lamina is elevated during a laminoplasty.[44] Durotomy and the resultant cerebrospinal fluid (CSF) leakage can be troublesome and lead to a pseudomeningocele, a cutaneous CSF fistula, poor wound healing, and meningitis.

The prevalence of cervical dural tears has been reported to range from 0.5% to 3%.[44–46] The combined complications rates of durotomy and nerve root injury in the posterior cervical laminoforaminotomy were between 2% and 5%.[47,48] Most durotomies are small, and the CSF leak is usually easily controlled with gelfoam tamponade and tight closure of the fascia.

Compared with the use of high-speed drill, applying an ultrasonic osteotome or ultrasonic bone curette in patients undergoing cervical laminoplasty could reduce the incidence of inadvertent durotomy.[49]

Vertebral Artery Injury

Vertebral artery (VA) injury is one of the most catastrophic iatrogenic complications of cervical spine surgery. Although VA injury during cervical spine procedures is rare, with incidence reported between 0.07% and 0.5% in the subaxial cervical spine,[50–53] it has serious consequences including fistulas, pseudoaneurysm, late-onset hemorrhage, thrombosis, embolism, cerebral ischemia, permanent neurologic deficits, and death.[50–54] It is therefore imperative to be familiar with the anatomy and the instrumentation techniques when performing anterior or posterior cervical spine surgeries.[55]

In a large survey comprising all cervical spine patients operated on by the members of the international Cervical Spine Research Society (CSRS), the overall incidence of VA injury during cervical spine surgery was 0.07%.[51] Posterior instrumentation of the upper cervical spine (32.4%), anterior corpectomy (23.4%), and posterior exposure of the cervical spine (11.7%) were the most common stages of the case to result in an injury to the VA. Less experienced surgeons had a higher rate of VA compared with their more experienced peers. The results of VA injury were highly variable, resulting in no permanent sequelae in 90% of patients; however, permanent neurologic injury or death occurred in 5.5% and 4.5% of cases, respectively.[51]

As with anterior procedures, preoperative planning and review of the cervical spine CT and MR images are essential in preventing VA injury. Preoperative CT angiography should be specifically reviewed to examine the course of the VAs and their relationship to the bony anatomy and surrounding structures, since anatomic variations of the VA can increase the risk of iatrogenic lacerations. The presence of an arcuate foramen and ponticulus posticus overlying the groove of the VA along the posterior arch of C1 can be identified by careful examination of preoperative lateral radiographs or reconstructed sagittal CT images. The prevalence of ponticulus posticus has been reported to be on average 16.7% (range, 1.3%– 68%), and ethnic variability was observed among different articles.[56–60]

Intraoperative imaging with fluoroscopy or CT may be beneficial in reducing the incidence of VA injury, especially in cases with unusual anatomy or prior surgery. Stereotactic guidance using computer navigation may also be helpful in avoiding inadvertent VA injury.[55]

Healing after Posterior Approach Operations on the Cervical Spine

Posterior approaches to the cervical spine have been associated with higher morbidity and, specifically, a higher rate of wound healing-related complications compared to anterior approaches.[61] More levels of fusion and posterior cervical fusions were associated with more complications and mortality than anterior fusion; medical comorbidities affected the outcome.[61] Some of the higher morbidity of the posterior approach is related to a higher revision rate due to wound healing problems in the posterior versus anterior approach. The revision rate correlated with the number of fused segments.[62] Wound dehiscence and postoperative infection were the most common causes of readmission after posterior cervical spinal fusion, with renal failure and anemia being notable risk factors.[63] These findings make intuitive sense; the posterior approach to the spine, including the cervical spine, often involves muscle and other tissue dissection, instrumentation, and graft placement. Any medical problem that impairs wound healing may result in lack of healing of the incision in posterior cervical spine operations. Much of the known literature is not specific to cervical spine but can be illuminating.

Factors Associated with Poor Wound Healing

Some of the worst outcomes associated with poor healing are seen in patients with severe renal failure and those with diabetes mellitus. Kidney disease and failure can cause healing problems and increased mortality.[64,65] Long-term follow up of surgical outcomes in patients with cervical disorders undergoing hemodialysis revealed a high complication rate—fatal infections 2/17, and progressive destructive bone changes at adjacent levels in 40% of those who had circumferential fusion.[66]

Not only diabetes status before surgery but also glucose level control after the operation during initial recovery were associated with the wound complication rate. Patients with both insulin-dependent diabetes mellitus (IDDM) and noninsulin-dependent diabetes mellitus (NIDDM) have a significantly increased risk of perioperative complications as compared with controls when treated by lumbar instrumentation and fusion.[67] Acute control of blood glucose helped improve outcome.[68]

Severe malnutrition has also been associated with poor wound healing. Some of the work has been done in lumbar and thoracic surgery, with relatively fewer publications directly describing the problems in the cervical spine. Protein malnutrition as well as specific deficiencies have been important. Preoperative nutrition assessment and optimization of nutritional parameters, including tight glucose control, normalization of serum albumin, and safe weight loss, may reduce the risk of perioperative complications such as infection.[69] Abnormally low weight body mass index (BMI) less than or equal to 20.39kg/m² was associated with higher risk of wound healing problems and surgical site infections after spinal instrumentation surgery.[70] Issues of wound healing are closely related to infection. Severe malnutrition and multiple comorbidities in the setting of spinal surgical wound infection will most likely result in a lack of effectiveness in eradicating the infecting pathogens.

General malnutrition, low weight, and protein deficiency are relatively easy to identify, but they are not the only important nutritional factors to affect wound healing. Particular attention needs to be directed at zinc, as deficiency of this essential mineral has been consistently associated with wound dehiscence and other healing problems,[71] whereas correction of the deficiency is helpful. The pathological effects of zinc deficiency include the occurrence of skin lesions, growth retardation, impaired immune function, and compromised would healing.[72] Zinc deficiency significantly increased the activity of matrix metalloproteinases (MMPs 2, 9, and 13), caused a reduced collagen type I/III ratio, and delayed cell proliferation and quality of intestinal wound healing.[73] Other minerals deficiency may also be a factor in wound healing. Adequate copper, magnesium, and manganese are needed for optimal strength of scar.[74] Isolated vitamin and

mineral deficiencies may occur in patients who are apparently well-nourished generally or obese, so a high index of suspicion for zinc deficiency must be maintained. Giving zinc beyond supplementation for deficiency appeared to improve bone fusion in the rat model.[75]

The influence of obesity on cervical spine wound healing is not clear. Higher morbidity, but not mortality, is seen in obese patients undergoing lumbar spine surgery.[76] In lumbar and thoracic spine operations, morbidity correlated with increased obesity, with superficial wound infection rates and pulmonary embolism rising even in mild obesity. In thoracolumbar spine surgery, obesity joined diabetes and smoking as significant risk factors.[77] The situation is somewhat different in cervical spine, where the role of obesity is not clear. Reports included increase in VTE but no increase in local complications for posterior cervical operations; also, high BMI did increase the risk of wound complications after posterior spinal fusion.[78,79] We can speculate that obesity does worsen the outcome, including wound healing after posterior approach to the cervical spine, but to a lesser degree than it does for thoracic and lumbar approaches.

Perioperative steroid use for spine patients, especially those with myelopathy, has been a source of controversy for years. We do not recommend the routine use of steroids in posterior approaches to the cervical spine, even for myelopathic patients. Intraoperative dexamethasone given to patients with cervical myelopathy increased the rate of wound complications, but did not improve neurological outcome.[80]

Factors that Apparently do not Specifically Increase the Risk of Poor Healing after Cervical Spine Operations

When considering posterior cervical spine operations, we should also recognize instances when risks are acceptable and sometimes lower than we might think. For example, Farshad et al[81] demonstrate that the risk of wound healing problems is not increased by preoperative use of corticosteroid injections in a large and well-organized outcome study. This is an important consideration, as we often use injections as a treatment option ahead of discectomy or other decompressive approaches.

With a wound complication rate of 6%, preoperative image-guided radiation therapy (IGRT), a highly conformal treatment, resulted in a very low rate of surgical wound complication.[82]

Although protein malnutrition is a risk factor for wound healing complications, it probably needs to be quite pronounced. Among adults undergoing elective spine surgery, the 30-day risk of complication was not associated with prealbumin or transferrin levels, when comparing upper to lower quartile in all operated patients in one study.[83] Apparently, there is a wide range where protein metabolism is adequate for wound healing in spine surgery.

Advanced age is associated with higher morbidity and mortality but not specifically due to wound healing problems. Although morbidity and mortality were higher in the oldest patients —above age 90 years— lack of healing was not the key issue.[84] Although age may be associated with poor nutrition.

Prevention and Treatment of Wound Healing Problems

The presence of risk factors does not have to preclude an operation if the indications are strong enough. Rather, we can take steps to mitigate risks by paying attention to medical optimization and surgical technique.

Placement of a drain when closing the incision may reduce wound "soakage" and possibly decrease the risk of dehiscence. However, not using closed surgical drains after multilevel posterior spinal surgery reduces postoperative blood loss and transfusion requirements.[85] Cervical muscle flap closure can be done prophylactically, with good

success for patients at high risk due to poor nutritional status.[86]

The choice of operation can also influence healing, both of bone and wound. For example, a laminoplasty without hardware may be more benign for cervical spine decompression without instability in patients with renal failure on hemodialysis.

When surgeons have some time before the intervention, they can consider and correct nutritional abnormalities, especially zinc and other essential minerals, and control diabetes both before the operation and during recovery. We should remember that nutritional deficiencies may be present in an obese patient, and patients may be malnourished or have a deficiency without obvious external signs, until the operation itself.

Despite careful optimization and choice of surgical approach, some patients will suffer wound dehiscence and healing problems. After dehiscence, options include wound packing and dressing changes, wound vacuum devices, surgical debridement, and various options of flap closure. Negative pressure devices are a relatively recent addition for wound dehiscence with infection. This treatment is effective and can be safe even for patients who have CSF leaks and related complications during previous surgery and comorbidities like diabetes.[87] More complex debridement with flap closure can be done with involvement of plastic surgery colleagues. For example, trapezius muscle flap or paraspinous muscle flap. [88,89]

Other Healing Problems

Wound dehiscence and healing problems are the key foci and relatively common major complications, but other types of healing affect the longer-term outcomes—bone fusion, muscle healing, maintenance of posture, and return to good function. Here, the same principles apply. Overall medical condition, comorbidities, and nutrition are key factors in bone fusion. Diabetes mellitus with poor preoperative glucose control results in less improvement in Nurick score after cervical spine surgery.[90] So not only wound healing but also overall neurological outcome can be affected by poorly controlled diabetes mellitus. Smoking, just like poor glycemic control, is associated with poor neurological healing not only wound healing.[91]

Muscle healing is affected by the number of levels operated due to obvious difference in amount of dissection. It is also affected by postoperative posture—the muscles are detached from the bone and reattach over the following 3 to 4 weeks. Maintenance of extended or straight posture during this time may allow the muscles to heal in a relatively short and well-aligned position. Kyphotic posture, as muscles are healing, can end up with healing in the bent position, with pain and difficulty extending along the neck. Therefore, in the authors' experience, using a hard collar for several weeks (3–4) after procedures like posterior laminectomy with or without fusion, and any type of laminoplasty, may help maintain good neck posture and decrease neck muscle pain even after the collar is removed.[92] On the other hand, bone morphogenic protein (BMP) does not help prevent nonunion in any spinal approaches when controlled for patients' characteristics.[93]

Bleeding

Postoperative spinal epidural hematoma (SEH) is a common radiological finding after posterior cervical surgery but only 0.1 to 2% of patients are symptomatic and require reintervention.

Established risk factors are multilevel surgical procedures, previous posterior cervical surgery, preoperative coagulopathy, and American Society of Anaesthesiologists (ASA) score. Risk factors that do not seem to be related to SEH in many studies are older age and use of preoperative nonsteroidal anti-inflammatory drugs (NSAIDs) or anticoagulant/antiplatelet drugs.

Time of onset of symptoms ranges from immediate postsurgery to 1 to 2 days (in such cases, symptoms appear days after surgery, but they represent limit cases). SEH can cause a wide range of symptoms from radiculopathy, hemi/paraparesis or plegia, sphincters dysfunction to, finally, death. The symptoms are not only related to the presence of blood but also to size and location, magnitude of spinal cord compression, and rapidity of development of the hematoma itself. Type of surgery (laminectomy versus laminoplasty versus instrumentation and fusion) does not seem to correlate with the development of SEH, while the use of drainage fails to demonstrate a protective role.

Immediate surgical evacuation minimizes the risk of postoperative neurologic compromise. A progressive and rapid neurological deterioration in the postoperative period is an important alarm sign. When the level of clinical suspicion is high, the radiological examinations are not necessary to confirm it.[94-96]

Patients undergoing posterior spine surgery are often aged and with many comorbidities and prevalent use of anticoagulant or antiplatelet drugs. The management of these therapies in spine surgery is still debated without a clear consensus. When it is advisable to stop it? When to restart? Is there an incremented risk of bleeding and postoperative hematoma?[97] Bono et al in 2009 NASS group stated that there is insufficient evidence to recommend the use of chemoprophylaxis in patients undergoing elective spine surgery.[5]

Perioperative hemorrhage risk in patients undergoing antithrombotic prophylaxis range from 0 to 4.3% in different studies.[98]

In particular, we should identify two different situations: 1) patients with a long-course use of anticoagulant/antiplatelet drugs for specific pathologies (such as cardiovascular pathologies) and 2) use of those drugs to prevent thrombosis in patients who underwent surgical procedures and consequent prothrombotic status because of temporary reduction of mobility with venous stasis. In the first case, different drugs can be used to prevent thrombotic events, and each one should be analyzed separately.

Vitamin K Antagonist (Warfarin)

Those drugs carry a higher risk of postoperative SEH. Rokito et al stated that the benefit of its use in VTE events is outweighed by the hemorrhagic risk, and the use of LMWH or UFH and stocking have a similar effect in prophylaxis.[99] For this reason, in case of moderate risk, last dose should be taken 5 days before surgery without bridging; otherwise, in case of elevated risk, the bridge with LMWH is necessary, with last dose from 4 to 24 hours before surgery, depending on the comorbidities. In case of high-risk situations and low-hemorrhage risk, it is possible to restart the therapy 24 hours after surgery; if it is not possible to restart the curative therapy, it is advisable to use temporary LMWH or UFH. The prophylactic protocol differs between surgeons, based on subjective criteria and personal experience. Generally, the introduction is between 24 and 48 hours after surgery.

The introduction of new anticoagulant drugs requires a revision of those protocols because of their short action time and faster effect. In emergency, to overcome the use of those drugs, it is possible to use coagulation factors II, VII, IX, and X.

Antiplatelet Drugs

Acetylsalicylic acid, clopidogrel, or ticlopidine have an irreversible effect for 7 to 10 days and they are not considered in the prophylaxis because of their postoperative bleeding risk. Their interruption is related to major arterial thrombotic accident (myocardial infarct, ischemic stroke). For this reason, general guidelines recommend not to interrupt the therapy preoperatively if the hemorrhage risk is low. The safety of this recommendation has not been confirmed for neurosurgery. If the interruption is necessary, it should be performed 5 days before surgery for clopidogrel and 3 days for acetylsalicylic acid. The use of LMWH and early resumption are mandatory to prevent major thrombotic events.

In addition, the introduction of new drugs requires revision of protocols. In emergency to overcome antiplatelet/antithrombotic drugs, it is advisable to perform a platelets transfusion.[98]

New Factor X Inhibitors

New factor X inhibitors such as rivaroxaban and apixaban offer efficacy equal to LMWH in VTE prevention, with similar incidence of postoperative hematoma in spine surgery.[100] Their reversal is very difficult. Andexxa (coagulation factor Xa [recombinant], inactivated-zhzo) received both US orphan drug and Food and Drug Administration (FDA) approval in 2018 for the reversal of factor X inhibitors. The new agent is extremely expensive and short-acting.

In case of postoperative prophylaxis, it should be noted that incidence of DVT or PE is respectively 0 to 0.6% and 0 to 0.2%, respectively. It depends on different factors such as comorbidities, preoperative and postoperative neurologic status, immobilization, and posterior cervical surgery with instrumentation. To reduce postoperative thrombosis risk, there are three strategies: pneumatic compression, pharmacological prevention with LMWH or UFH, or both. American guidelines in 2008 recommend no prophylaxis in moderate risk surgery, mechanic or pharmacological prophylaxis in case of minor risk factors, or combined prophylaxis in case of major risk factors.

In association with such therapies, another important preventing factor is early mobilization.

Low Molecular Weight Heparin (LMWH)

Different studies stated that its use does not relate with augmented hemorrhagic risk in patients who undergo spine surgery, the risk of epidural hematoma is very low, and its introduction within 36 hours is a safe procedure.

Proposed algorithm for the management of the different drugs is summarized in **Table 20.1**.[97,98]

Infection Rates

Surgical site infection (SSI) represents a common complication in spinal surgery. In particular, it represents the third case of readmission within 30 days from surgery and have important consequences, such as increment in hospitalization and disability, and lead to higher health care. Two recent meta-analyses estimate its incidence between 0.2% and 16.1%, depending on site and type of surgery: in cervical region, the overall incidence is about 3.4%.[101,102]

Surgical site infection can be divided into superficial, deep and organ space, depending on the anatomical structures involved; in instrumented surgery, infective process can involve implanted devices with or without osteomyelitis (**Fig. 20.1**). Common symptoms of SSI are wound dehiscence, purulent drainage, general signs of infection (from hyperthermia to septic shock) and, eventually, neurological signs due to compressive effect as well infective process (radiculitis, meningitis, etc.).

Risk factors can be divided into general (diabetes, obesity, hypertension, transfusion, urinary tract infections, duration of surgery) and spine surgery related (CSF leakage, posterior approach, open approach).

In details, the literature shows a higher incidence of SSI in cervical surgery in case of:

- Posterior approach that is double respect the anterior (5% vs. 2.3%).
- Instrumented surgery almost tripled with respect to noninstrumented surgery (4.4% vs. 1.4%).
- Open approach respect minimally invasive approach (3.8% vs. 1.5%).
- Duration of surgery more than 3 to 5 hours (depending on the studies) shows a triple risk factor (4.7% vs 1.3%).

However, it is necessary to specify that most of these data do not find a complete validation in literature among different studies.

CSF leakage seems to act with the help of a dual mechanism: on the one hand, incremented time of surgery to repair the dura; on the other hand, persistent fluid leakage affects wound healing. Similarly, factors such as age, BMI and other patient-related factors, and the need for blood transfusion are still debated; in fact, different studies reach opposite conclusions without any methodological superiority. In general, it is widely accepted that patients with multiple comorbidities have increased risk for SSI and healing problems as previously discussed in this chapter.[101,103–105]

Table 20.1 Proposed protocols for management of preoperative or prophylactic antithrombotic drugs

Drug	Risk of hemorrhage	Management protocol
VKA	High hemorrhagic risk	Stop: 5 days before surgery Restart: as soon as possible otherwise bridge with LMWH or UFH 24–48 hours after surgery
Antiplatelet drugs	High hemorrhagic risk	Stop: 3 to 5 days before surgery Restart: as soon as possible with bridge with LMWH or UFH
Factor X inhibitor	Low hemorrhagic risk	Stop: 1 to 2 days, proceed with surgical procedure after blood test dosage of the drugs (reference values depend on drug)
LMWH	Low hemorrhagic risk	Start: 24 to 36 hours after surgery

Abbreviations: LMWH, low-molecular weight heparin; UFH, unfractionated heparin; VKA, Vitamin K antagonists.

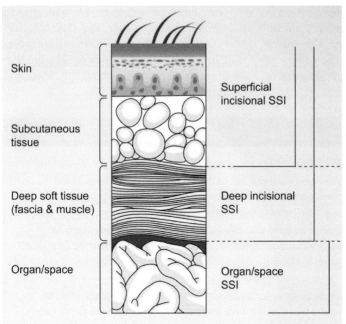

Fig. 20.1 Surgical site infection (SSI) can be classified in superficial, deep or organ space basing on the layer involved. In detail, a superficial site infection is limited to skin and subcutaneous tissue, while a deep infection involved fascial and muscular layers; a deeper infection is called an organ space infection.

Microorganisms involved are Gram-positive in most cases (almost 60%) of the Staphylococcus species (aureus in 37.9% and epidermidis in 22.7%). Other microorganisms involved are summarized in **Table 20.2**. The higher frequency of Staphylococci justifies the use of cefazolin for prophylaxis.[102,106]

Diagnosis is both clinical and radiological. Clinical signs are wound reddening or dehiscence, purulent drainage, local pain, and neurological signs; laboratory tests used are increase of white blood cells (WBCs), C reactive protein (CRP), procalcitonin, erythrocyte sedimentation rate, and anemia in long-term infection. For radiological diagnosis in emergency, a CT scan with contrast enhancement can be enough, however, an MRI with contrast enhancement is advisable to better identify tissues involved and the state of the bone in case of instrumented surgery. The follow-up includes wound healing, blood tests, and MRI; in detail, normalization of WBCs and CRP correspond to a clinical resolution, while the negativity of radiological imaging is delayed (up to 6 months are necessary to view significant improvement).

Table 20.2 Microorganism most frequently involved in surgical site infection[101]

Microorganism	Occurrence
Staphylococcus	50.2%
	Aureus 37.9%
	Epidermidis 22.7%
	Methicillin-susceptible 30%
	Methicillin-resistant 23.1%
Escherichia	13%
Acinetobacter	10%
Klebsiella	8.3%
Enterococcus	8.2%
Streptococcus	6.9%

The therapy for SSI is primarily represented by surgical revision with debridement of the purulent material and infected tissues (in the majority of cases, more than one surgery is necessary for the complete resolution). Implant removal in case of instrumented surgery is performed only if necessary, based on MRI imaging, because this can compromise spinal stability, and in case of late infection (> 1 month). Finally, prolonged targeted antibiotic therapy is usually necessary. The choice of antibiotic agent is guided by the culture of the material obtained during debridement or drainage procedures.

The local application of vancomycin powder seems to reduce the risk of infection but some studies contradict this conclusion. In a recent paper, Gande et al stated that its use can compromise wound healing and instrumentation fusion.[107–109]

Take-home Points

General and Neurological Complications

- VTE is a notable complication of posterior approaches to the cervical spine. Mechanical and sometimes medical prophylaxis and early mobilization are key to prevention. High suspicion is important for timely diagnosis and treatment of potentially fatal PE.

- Blindness associated with prone position has many causes. Prevention includes avoidance of pressure on the face, for example, by placing the head in a Mayfield clamp; keeping the face at or slightly above heart level if possible; limiting the duration of each operation—potentially staging very long prone operations.

- Nerve root palsies after posterior decompression usually involve C5 and mostly resolve within 3 to 6 months. Avoidance of traction of the nerve roots and excessive motion of the spinal cord may help prevent this condition, and physical therapy has been used to aid recovery. However, there is no proven prevention or treatment method.

- Unintentional durotomy has been reported in 0.5 to 3% cases; mostly small and controllable at the initial operation. Use of ultrasonic devices rather than a high-speed drill may help avoid some of the durotomies.

- Vertebral artery injury is uncommon but potentially severe. Permanent neurologic injury or death occurred in 5.5% and 4.5% of cases, respectively. Avoidance involves careful preoperative planning with review of MRI and CT, and doing a CT angiogram if unusual anatomy is suspected. Intraoperative fluoroscopy or CT can help in cases with difficult anatomy.

Wound Problems

- Posterior approaches to the cervical spine are associated with more wound healing problems compared to anterior approaches.

- Renal failure, obesity, and malnutrition are key factors associated with poor wound healing.

- Zinc deficiency and severe protein malnutrition are among the factors to watch for related to wound healing.

- Steroid use may contribute to poor wound healing.

- Surgical technique such as avoiding hardware, shorter operations, placement of a drain, or planned muscle flap closure can mitigate healing problems.

Bleeding

- Spinal epidural hematoma is a common radiological finding after posterior cervical surgery but only 0.1 to 2% of patients are symptomatic and require emergency surgery.

- It is necessary to weigh between risk of hemorrhage and thrombotic risk for the management of anticoagulant/antiplatelet drugs.

- Patients undergoing cervical spine surgery can start pharmacological prophylaxis safely 48 hours after surgery with heparin, either LMWH or UFH. The screening for VTE is reserved to symptomatic patients.

Infection

■ The overall pooled incidence of SSI in cervical spine surgery is 3.4%, and the overall rates is higher in posterior and open approach and in instrumented surgery.

■ In almost 50% of cases, microorganism involved is Staphylococcus.

■ Therapy requires surgical debridement and, if necessary, implant removal and prolonged antibiotic therapies.

References

1. Slavin J, Lewis EM, Sansur CA. Complication avoidance in spine surgery. In: Winn HR, ed. Youmans and Winn Neurological Surgery. 7th ed. Philadelphia, PA: Elsevier; 2017:2344–2347

2. Sebastian AS, Currier BL, Clarke MJ, Larson D, Huddleston PM III, Nassr A. Thromboembolic disease after cervical spine surgery: a review of 5,405 surgical procedures and matched cohort analysis. Global Spine J 2016;6(5):465–471

3. Yamada K, Suda K, Matsumoto Harmon S, et al. Rapidly progressive cervical myelopathy had a high risk of developing deep venous thrombosis: a prospective observational study in 289 cases with degenerative cervical spine disease. Spinal Cord 2019;57(1):58–64

4. Gephart MG, Zygourakis CC, Arrigo RT, Kalanithi PS, Lad SP, Boakye M. Venous thromboembolism after thoracic/thora-columbar spinal fusion. World Neurosurg 2012;78(5):545–552

5. Bono CM, Watters WC III, Heggeness MH, et al. An evidence-based clinical guideline for the use of antithrombotic therapies in spine surgery. Spine J 2009;9(12):1046–1051

6. Hirsh J, Dalen J, Guyatt G; American College of Chest Physicians. The sixth (2000) ACCP guidelines for antithrombotic therapy for prevention and treatment of thrombosis. Chest 2001; 119(1, Suppl)1S–2S

7. Lee LA, Roth S, Posner KL, et al. The American Society of Anesthesiologists Postoperative Visual Loss Registry: analysis of 93 spine surgery cases with postoperative visual loss. Anesthesiology 2006;105(4):652–659, quiz 867–868

8. Stambough JL, Dolan D, Werner R, Godfrey E. Ophthalmologic complications associated with prone positioning in spine surgery. J Am Acad Orthop Surg 2007;15(3):156–165

9. Shen Y, Drum M, Roth S. The prevalence of perioperative visual loss in the United States: a 10-year study from 1996 to 2005 of spinal, orthopedic, cardiac, and general surgery. Anesth Analg 2009;109(5):1534–1545

10. Baig MN, Lubow M, Immesoete P, Bergese SD, Hamdy EA, Mendel E. Vision loss after spine surgery: review of the literature and recommendations. Neurosurg Focus 2007; 23(5):E15

11. Uribe AA, Baig MN, Puente EG, Viloria A, Mendel E, Bergese SD. Current intraoperative devices to reduce visual loss after spine surgery. Neurosurg Focus 2012;33(2):E14

12. Myers MA, Hamilton SR, Bogosian AJ, Smith CH, Wagner TA. Visual loss as a complication of spine surgery. A review of 37 cases. Spine 1997;22(12):1325–1329

13. Patil CG, Lad EM, Lad SP, Ho C, Boakye M. Visual loss after spine surgery: a population-based study. Spine 2008;33(13):1491–1496

14. Stevens WR, Glazer PA, Kelley SD, Lietman TM, Bradford DS. Ophthalmic complications after spinal surgery. Spine 1997;22(12): 1319–1324

15. Walick KS, Kragh JE Jr, Ward JA, Crawford JJ. Changes in intraocular pressure due to surgical positioning: studying potential risk for postoperative vision loss. Spine 2007; 32(23):2591–2595

16. Epstein NE. Cervical myelopathy: laminectomy. In: Benzel EC, ed. The Cervical Spine. 5th ed. Philadelphia, PA: Lippincott Williams & Wilkins; 2012:970–979

17. Rhee KJ, Green W, Holcroft JW, Mangili JA. Oral intubation in the multiply injured patient: the risk of exacerbating spinal cord damage. Ann Emerg Med 1990;19(5):511–514

18. Muckart DJ, Bhagwanjee S, van der Merwe R. Spinal cord injury as a result of endotracheal intubation in patients with undiagnosed cervical spine fractures. Anesthesiology 1997;87(2):418–420

19. Saldua NS, Harrop JS. Iatrogenic spinal cord injuries. In: Benzel EC, ed. The Cervical Spine. 5th ed. Philadelphia, PA: Lippincott Williams & Wilkins; 2012:1321–1325

20. Frank E, Keenen TL. A technique for cervical laminoplasty using mini plates. Br J Neurosurg 1994;8(2):197–199

21. Jin SW, Kim SH, Kim BJ, et al. Modified open-door laminoplasty using hydroxyapatite spacers and miniplates. Korean J Spine 2014;11(3):188–194

22. Ono A, Yokoyama T, Numasawa T, Wada K, Toh S. Dural damage due to a loosened hydroxyapatite intraspinous spacer after spinous process-splitting laminoplasty. Report of two cases. J Neurosurg Spine 2007; 7(2):230–235

23. Kanemura A, Doita M, Iguchi T, Kasahara K, Kurosaka M, Sumi M. Delayed dural laceration by hydroxyapatite spacer causing tetraparesis following double-door laminoplasty. J Neurosurg Spine 2008;8(2): 121–128

24. Wada E, Yonenobu K. Treatment of cervical myelopathy: laminoplasty. In: Benzel EC, ed. The Cervical Spine. 5th ed. Philadelphia, PA: Lippincott Williams & Wilkins; 2012: 980–994

25. Itoh T, Tsuji H. Technical improvements and results of laminoplasty for compressive myelopathy in the cervical spine. Spine 1985;10(8):729–736

26. Zdeblick TA, Zou D, Warden KE, McCabe R, Kunz D, Vanderby R. Cervical stability after foraminotomy. A biomechanical in vitro analysis. J Bone Joint Surg Am 1992; 74(1):22–27

27. Sakaura H, Hosono N, Mukai Y, Ishii T, Yoshikawa H. C5 palsy after decompression surgery for cervical myelopathy: review of the literature. Spine 2003;28(21):2447–2451

28. Greiner-Perth R, Elsaghir H, Böhm H, El-Meshtawy M. The incidence of C5-C6 radiculopathy as a complication of extensive cervical decompression: own results and review of literature. Neurosurg Rev 2005; 28(2):137–142

29. Sakaura H, Hosono N, Mukai Y, Ishii T, Iwasaki M, Yoshikawa H. Long-term outcome of laminoplasty for cervical myelopathy due to disc herniation: a comparative study of laminoplasty and anterior spinal fusion. Spine 2005;30(7):756–759

30. Chen Y, Chen D, Wang X, Guo Y, He Z. C5 palsy after laminectomy and posterior cervical fixation for ossification of posterior longitudinal ligament. J Spinal Disord Tech 2007;20(7):533–535

31. Takemitsu M, Cheung KM, Wong YW, Cheung WY, Luk KD. C5 nerve root palsy after cervical laminoplasty and posterior fusion with instrumentation. J Spinal Disord Tech 2008;21(4):267–272

32. Imagama S, Matsuyama Y, Yukawa Y, et al; Nagoya Spine Group. C5 palsy after cervical laminoplasty: a multicentre study. J Bone Joint Surg Br 2010;92(3):393–400

33. Dafford KA, Hart RA. Postsurgical C5 nerve root palsy. In: Benzel EC, ed. The Cervical Spine. 5th ed. Philadelphia, PA: Lippincott Williams & Wilkins; 2012:1316–1320

34. Wang T, Wang H, Liu S, Ding WY. Incidence of C5 nerve root palsy after cervical surgery: A meta-analysis for last decade. Medicine (Baltimore) 2017;96(45):e8560

35. Chiba K, Toyama Y, Matsumoto M, Maruiwa H, Watanabe M, Hirabayashi K. Segmental motor paralysis after expansive open-door laminoplasty. Spine 2002;27(19): 2108–2115

36. Seichi A, Takeshita K, Kawaguchi H, Nakajima S, Akune T, Nakamura K. Postoperative expansion of intramedullary high-intensity areas on T2-weighted magnetic resonance imaging after cervical laminoplasty. Spine 2004;29(13):1478–1482, discussion 1482

37. Sakaura H, Hosono N, Mukai Y, Fujii R, Iwasaki M, Yoshikawa H. Segmental motor paralysis after cervical laminoplasty: a prospective study. Spine 2006;31(23): 2684–2688

38. Sasai K, Saito T, Akagi S, Kato I, Ohnari H, Iida H. Preventing C5 palsy after laminoplasty. Spine 2003;28(17):1972–1977

39. Komagata M, Nishiyama M, Endo K, Ikegami H, Tanaka S, Imakiire A. Prophylaxis of C5 palsy after cervical expansive laminoplasty by bilateral partial foraminotomy. Spine J 2004;4(6):650–655

40. Tanaka N, Nakanishi K, Fujiwara Y, Kamei N, Ochi M. Postoperative segmental C5 palsy after cervical laminoplasty may occur without intraoperative nerve injury: a prospective study with transcranial electric motor-evoked potentials. Spine 2006; 31(26):3013–3017

41. Nakamae T, Tanaka N, Nakanishi K, et al. Investigation of segmental motor paralysis after cervical laminoplasty using intraoperative spinal cord monitoring with transcranial electric motor-evoked potentials. J Spinal Disord Tech 2012;25(2):92–98

42. Yonenobu K, Hosono N, Iwasaki M, Asano M, Ono K. Neurologic complications of surgery for cervical compression myelopathy. Spine 1991;16(11):1277–1282

43. Huang RC, Girardi FP, Poynton AR, Cammisa FP Jr. Treatment of multilevel cervical spondylotic myeloradiculopathy with posterior decompression and fusion with lateral mass plate fixation and local bone graft. J Spinal Disord Tech 2003;16(2):123–129

44. Hannallah D, Lee J, Khan M, Donaldson WF, Kang JD. Cerebrospinal fluid leaks following cervical spine surgery. J Bone Joint Surg Am 2008;90(5):1101–1105

45. Graham JJ. Complications of cervical spine surgery. A five-year report on a survey of the membership of the Cervical Spine Research Society by the Morbidity and Mortality Committee. Spine 1989;14(10):1046–1050

46. Cammisa FP Jr, Girardi FP, Sangani PK, Parvataneni HK, Cadag S, Sandhu HS. Incidental durotomy in spine surgery. Spine 2000;25(20):2663–2667

47. Adamson TE. Microendoscopic posterior cervical laminoforaminotomy for unilateral radiculopathy: results of a new technique in 100 cases. J Neurosurg 2001; 95(1, Suppl): 51–57

48. Jagannathan J, Sherman JH, Szabo T, Shaffrey CI, Jane JA. The posterior cervical foraminotomy in the treatment of cervical disc/osteophyte disease: a single-surgeon experience with a minimum of 5 years' clinical and radiographic follow-up. J Neurosurg Spine 2009;10(4):347–356

49. Parker SL, Kretzer RM, Recinos PF, et al. Ultrasonic BoneScalpel for osteoplastic laminoplasty in the resection of intradural spinal pathology: case series and technical note. Neurosurgery 2013; 73(1, Suppl Operative):ons61–ons66

50. Eskander MS, Drew JM, Aubin ME, et al. Vertebral artery anatomy: a review of two hundred fifty magnetic resonance imaging scans. Spine 2010;35(23):2035–2040

51. Lunardini DJ, Eskander MS, Even JL, et al. Vertebral artery injuries in cervical spine surgery. Spine J 2014;14(8):1520–1525

52. Hsu WK, Kannan A, Mai HT, et al. Epidemiology and outcomes of vertebral artery injury in 16 582 cervical spine surgery patients: an AOSpine North America Multicenter Study. Global Spine J 2017; 7(1, Suppl)21S–27S

53. Winter F, Okano I, Salzmann SN, et al. A novel and reproducible classification of the vertebral artery in the subaxial cervical spine. Oper Neurosurg (Hagerstown) 2020;18(6):676–683

54. Hong JT, Park DK, Lee MJ, Kim SW, An HS. Anatomical variations of the vertebral artery segment in the lower cervical spine: analysis by three-dimensional computed tomography angiography. Spine 2008;33(22):2422–2426

55. Peng CW, Chou BT, Bendo JA, Spivak JM. Vertebral artery injury in cervical spine surgery: anatomical considerations, management, and preventive measures. Spine J 2009;9(1):70–76

56. Huang DG, Hao DJ, Fang XY, Zhang XL, He BR, Liu TJ. Ponticulus posticus. Spine J 2015;15(11):e17–e19

57. Lee CK, Tan TS, Chan C, Kwan MK. Is C1 lateral mass screw placement safe for the Chinese, Indians, and Malays? An analysis of 180 computed tomography scans. J Orthop Surg (Hong Kong) 2017;25(1):2309499017692683

58. Tambawala SS, Karjodkar FR, Sansare K, et al. Prevalence of Ponticulus posticus on lateral cephalometric radiographs, its association with cervicogenic headache and a review of literature. World Neurosurg 2017;103:566–575

59. Arslan D, Ozer MA, Govsa F, Kıtıs O. The Ponticulus posticus as risk factor for screw insertion into the first cervical lateral mass. World Neurosurg 2018;113:e579–e585

60. Tripodi D, Tieri M, Demartis P, Però G, Marzo G, D'Ercole S. Ponticulus posticus: clinical and CBCT analysis in a young Italian population. Eur J Paediatr Dent 2019;20(3):219–223

61. Kaye ID, Marascalchi BJ, Macagno AE, Lafage VA, Bendo JA, Passias PG. Predictors of morbidity and mortality among patients with cervical spondylotic myelopathy treated surgically. Eur Spine J 2015; 24(12):2910–2917

62. Greiner-Perth R, Allam Y, El-Saghir H, Röhl F, Franke J, Böhm H. Analysis of reoperations after surgical treatment of degenerative cervical spine disorders: a report on 900 cases. Cent Eur Neurosurg 2009;70(1):3–8

63. Choy W, Lam SK, Smith ZA, Dahdaleh NS. Predictors of 30-day hospital readmission after posterior cervical fusion in 3401 patients. Spine 2018;43(5):356–363

64. Martin CT, Pugely AJ, Gao Y, Mendoza-Lattes SA, Weinstein SL. The impact of renal impairment on short-term morbidity risk following lumbar spine surgeries. Spine 2015;40(12):909–916

65. Bains RS, Kardile M, Mitsunaga L, et al. Does chronic kidney disease affect the mortality rate in patients undergoing spine surgery? J Clin Neurosci 2017;43:208–213

66. Sudo H, Ito M, Abumi K, et al. Long-term follow up of surgical outcomes in patients with cervical disorders undergoing hemodialysis. J Neurosurg Spine 2006;5(4):313–319

67. Glassman SD, Alegre G, Carreon L, Dimar JR, Johnson JR. Perioperative complications of lumbar instrumentation and fusion in patients with diabetes mellitus. Spine J 2003;3(6):496–501

68. Smith DK, Bowen J, Bucher L, et al. A study of perioperative hyperglycemia in patients with diabetes having colon, spine, and joint surgery. J Perianesth Nurs 2009;24(6):362–369

69. Cross MB, Yi PH, Thomas CF, Garcia J, Della Valle CJ. Evaluation of malnutrition in orthopaedic surgery. J Am Acad Orthop Surg 2014;22(3):193–199

70. Kobayashi Y, Inose H, Ushio S, et al. Body mass index and modified glasgow prognostic score are useful predictors of surgical site infection after spinal instrumentation surgery: a consecutive series. Spine 2020;45(3):E148–E154

71. Sandstead HH, Shepard GH. The effect of zinc deficiency on the tensile strength of healing surgical incisions in the integument of the rat. Proc Soc Exp Biol Med 1968;128(3):687–689

72. Lin PH, Sermersheim M, Li H, Lee PHU, Steinberg SM, Ma J. Zinc in wound healing modulation. Nutrients 2017;10(1):E16

73. Binnebösel M, Grommes J, Koenen B, et al. Zinc deficiency impairs wound healing of colon anastomosis in rats. Int J Colorectal Dis 2010;25(2):251–257

74. Vaxman F, Olender S, Lambert A, Nisand G, Grenier JF. Can the wound healing process be improved by vitamin supplementation? Experimental study on humans. Eur Surg Res 1996;28(4):306–314

75. Koerner JD, Vives MJ, O'Connor JP, et al. Zinc has insulin-mimetic properties which enhance spinal fusion in a rat model. Spine J 2016;16(6):777–783

76. Marquez-Lara A, Nandyala SV, Sankaranarayanan S, Noureldin M, Singh K. Body mass index as a predictor of complications and mortality after lumbar spine surgery. Spine 2014;39(10):798–804

77. Pesenti S, Pannu T, Andres-Bergos J, et al; Scoliosis Research Society (SRS). What are the risk factors for surgical site infection after spinal fusion? A meta-analysis. Eur Spine J 2018;27(10):2469–2480

78. Phan K, Kothari P, Lee NJ, Virk S, Kim JS, Cho SK. Impact of obesity on outcomes in adults undergoing elective posterior cervical fusion. Spine 2017;42(4):261–266

79. Zhang GA, Zhang WP, Chen YC, Hou Y, Qu W, Ding LX. Impact of elevated body mass index on surgical outcomes for patients undergoing cervical fusion procedures: a systematic review and meta-analysis. Orthop Surg 2020;12(1):3–15

80. Blume C, Wiederhold H, Geiger M, Clusmann H, Müller CA. Lacking benefit of intraoperative high-dose dexamethasone in instrumented surgery for cervical spondylotic myelopathy. J Neurol Surg A Cent Eur Neurosurg 2018;79(2):116–122

81. Farshad M, Burgstaller JM, Held U, Steurer J, Dennler C. Do preoperative corticosteroid injections increase the risk for infections or wound healing problems after spine surgery?: a swiss prospective multicenter cohort study. Spine 2018;43(15):1089–1094

82. Keam J, Bilsky MH, Laufer I, et al. No association between excessive wound complications and preoperative high-dose, hypofractionated, image-guided radiation therapy for spine metastasis. J Neurosurg Spine 2014;20(4):411–420

83. Takemoto E, Yoo J, Blizzard SR, Shannon J, Marshall LM. Preoperative prealbumin and transferring: Relation to 30-day risk

of complication in elective spine surgical patients. Medicine (Baltimore) 2019;98(9): e14741

84. Oichi T, Oshima Y, Matsui H, Fushimi K, Tanaka S, Yasunaga H. Can elective spine surgery be performed safely among nonagenarians?: analysis of a national inpatient database in Japan. Spine 2019;44(5):E273–E281

85. Gubin AV, Prudnikova OG, Subramanyam KN, Burtsev AV, Khomchenkov MV, Mundargi AV. Role of closed drain after multi-level posterior spinal surgery in adults: a random-ised open-label superiority trial. Eur Spine J 2019;28(1):146–154

86. Franck P, Bernstein JL, Cohen LE, Härtl R, Baaj AA, Spector JA. Local muscle flaps minimize post-operative wound morbidity in patients with neoplastic disease of the spine. Clin Neurol Neurosurg 2018;171:100–105

87. Ridwan S, Grote A, Simon M. Safety and efficacy of negative pressure wound therapy for deep spinal wound infections after dural exposure, durotomy, or intradural surgery. World Neurosurg 2020;134:e624–e630

88. Zenga J, Sharon JD, Santiago P, et al. Lower trapezius flap for reconstruction of posterior scalp and neck defects after complex occipital-cervical surgeries. J Neurol Surg B Skull Base 2015;76(5):397–408

89. Mericli AF, Mirzabeigi MN, Moore JH Jr, Fox JW IV, Copit SE, Tuma GA. Reconstruction of complex posterior cervical spine wounds using the paraspinous muscle flap. Plast Reconstr Surg 2011;128(1):148–153

90. Kusin DJ, Ahn UM, Ahn NU. The influence of diabetes on surgical outcomes in cervical myelopathy. Spine 2016;41(18):1436–1440

91. Kusin DJ, Ahn UM, Ahn NU. The effect of smoking on spinal cord healing following surgical treatment of cervical myelopathy. Spine 2015;40(18):1391–1396

92. Stamates MM, Cui MX, Roitberg BZ. Clinical outcomes of cervical laminoplasty: results at two years. Neurosurgery 2017;80(6): 934–941

93. Guppy KH, Paxton EW, Harris J, Alvarez J, Bernbeck J. Does bone morphogenetic protein change the operative nonunion rates in spine fusions? Spine 2014;39(22):1831–1839

94. Glotzbecker MP, Bono CM, Wood KB, Harris MB. Postoperative spinal epidural hematoma: a systematic review. Spine 2010;35(10):E413–E420

95. Halvorsen CM, Lied B, Harr ME, et al. Surgical mortality and complications leading to reoperation in 318 consecutive posterior decompressions for cervical spondylotic myelopathy. Acta Neurol Scand 2011; 123(5):358–365

96. Goldstein CL, Bains I, Hurlbert RJ. Symptomatic spinal epidural hematoma after posterior cervical surgery: incidence and risk factors. Spine J 2015;15(6): 1179–1187

97. Kepler CK, McKenzie J, Kreitz T, Vaccaro A. Venous thromboembolism prophylaxis in spine surgery. J Am Acad Orthop Surg 2018;26(14):489–500

98. Steib A, Hadjiat F, Skibba W, Steib JP; French Spine Surgery Society. Focus on peri-operative management of anticoagulants and antiplatelet agents in spine surgery. Orthop Traumatol Surg Res 2011; 97(6, Suppl):S102–S106

99. Rokito SE, Schwartz MC, Neuwirth MG. Deep vein thrombosis after major reconstructive spinal surgery. Spine 1996;21(7):853–858, discussion 859

100. Du W, Zhao C, Wang J, Liu J, Shen B, Zheng Y. Comparison of rivaroxaban and parnaparin for preventing venous thromboembolism after lumbar spine surgery. J Orthop Surg Res 2015;10:78

101. Yao R, Zhou H, Choma TJ, Kwon BK, Street J. Surgical site infection in spine surgery: who is at risk? Global Spine J 2018; 8(4, Suppl):5S–30S

102. Zhou J, Wang R, Huo X, Xiong W, Kang L, Xue Y. Incidence of surgical site infection after spine surgery: a systematic review and meta-analysis. Spine 2020;45(3):208–216

103. Fang A, Hu SS, Endres N, Bradford DS. Risk factors for infection after spinal surgery. Spine 2005;30(12):1460–1465

104. Abdul-Jabbar A, Berven SH, Hu SS, et al. Surgical site infections in spine surgery: identification of microbiologic and surgical characteristics in 239 cases. Spine 2013; 38(22):E1425–E1431

105. Harel R, Stylianou P, Knoller N. Cervical spine surgery: approach-related complications. World Neurosurg 2016;94:1–5

106. Mok JM, Guillaume TJ, Talu U, et al. Clinical outcome of deep wound infection after instrumented posterior spinal fusion: a matched cohort analysis. Spine 2009; 34(6):578–583

107. Khan NR, Thompson CJ, DeCuypere M, et al. A meta-analysis of spinal surgical site infection and vancomycin powder. J Neurosurg Spine 2014;21(6):974–983

108. Eder C, Schenk S, Trifinopoulos J, et al. Does intrawound application of vancomycin influence bone healing in spinal surgery? Eur Spine J 2016;25(4):1021–1028

109. Gande A, Rosinski A, Cunningham T, Bhatia N, Lee YP. Selection pressures of vancomycin powder use in spine surgery: a meta-analysis. Spine J 2019;19(6):1076–1084

21 Minimally Invasive Techniques for the Treatment of Cervical Spondylotic Myelopathy and OPLL

Marcos Masini and João Flávio G. Madureira

Background

The exact pathogenesis of ossification of the posterior longitudinal ligament (OPLL) has only been partially clarified; nevertheless, there is a clear relationship between OPLL and cervical spondylosis. These diseases progress from a primary disc degeneration, followed by disc space reduction, and subsequent progress toward osteophyte formation, ligamentum flavum hypertrophy and facetal retrolisthesis. As a consequence, stenosis occurs in spinal and neural canal, and a myriad neurological symptoms and deficits appear. The formation of abnormal calcification/ossification will ultimately encroach the spinal canal, causing it to be compressed and leading to progressive myelopathy. Location of the ossification anterior to the spinal cord and posterior to single or multiple vertebral bodies makes direct surgical resection a challenging and dangerous surgical procedure (**Fig. 21.1**).

Anterior approaches for the treatment of cervical spine myelopathy can be dated back to the 40s when attempts were made to achieve decompression by offending material. In 1944, Speling and Sackville[1] were the first to achieve decompression via cervical laminectomy. This approach further evolved with Frykoholm[2] who, in the 50s, developed a minimal lateral foraminotomy, also known as keyhole. However, it did not allow for the removal of ventromedial lesions, allowing only an indirect decompression of the neural elements. Posterior access limitation led to the development of the anterior cervical surgical approaches in the 60s by Cloward,[3] Smith and Robinson.[4] The surgical treatment of myelopathy and other cervical spine degenerative diseases evolved considerably over the next decades. These traditional techniques rely on posterior, anterior and oblique approaches.

These techniques are focused on decompressing the spinal cord and rely on stabilization of the spinal segments, a procedure necessary to increase stability. As a consequence, patients suffer with mobility reduction due to consequent arthrodesis.[5]

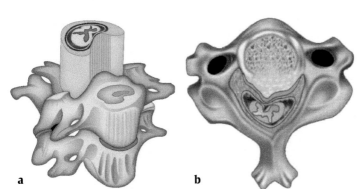

Fig. 21.1 (a, b) Scheme illustrating sagittal (left) and three-dimensional and axial (right) views of anterior spinal cord compression. Note the ossification growth which compresses and misshapes the spinal and neural canal. (These images are provided courtesy of Gustavo Cockell [designer]).

Therefore, fixation strategies are still a subject of intense clinical discussion.

The history of spine minimal decompression dates back to 1968 with Verbiest and Lesoin.[6,7] Minimally invasive approaches were first developed by Celestre[8] in 2012 and are becoming increasingly popular in recent years. These minimally invasive procedures are intended to treat anterior compressive lesions, which do not require the use of traditional techniques to achieve direct and complete decompression, maintaining vertebral functions and while preserving stability and mobility of the affected segment. Minimal decompression is preferable since it can achieve comparable outcomes with less blood loss, minimized tissue damage, and reduced recovery time and hospital stay.[9] Moreover, minimal decompression avoids spine fusion and further complications related to the grafting material, even reducing the probability of adjacent level disease. These techniques are classified as minimally invasive and motion-preserving procedures. Some of the most recent minimally invasive techniques advancements are further detailed in this chapter.

Minimally Invasive Surgical Techniques

Anterior "Uncoforaminotomy"[10]

This is a very localized procedure. The exposed field involves the lateral portion of the superior vertebral body, including the corresponding *processus uncinatus* (PU) of the inferior vertebral body and the lateral third of the intervertebral disc. Using a high-speed drill and a 1.8 mm spherical bur, proceed to cut the external side of the PU, matching a semioval orifice of 2 to 3 mm wide and 8 to 10 mm deep. Drilling is performed, reaching the posterior cortical laminae or directly to the dura of the corresponding nerve root. Using a 2 mm spherical diamond drill, proceed to resect the thinned posterior cortical layer and the posterior part of the lateral wall of the PU, carefully drilling through it. Through this procedure, posterolateral osteophytes as well as the external and foraminal part of the PU were removed and so the underlying root is decompressed under microscopic view. One can also perform an anterior canal decompression by enlarging the oblique view in the spinal canal (**Fig. 21.2**).

Indications

Patients are indicated to this approach based on the following criteria:

- Unilateral cervical radiculopathy refractory to medical therapy after 6 weeks of optimal treatment.
- The oblique extension to midline in cases that associate a refractory to medical treatment of myelopathy with central compression and compatible image diagnosis. It is a minimally invasive procedure, simple to perform, preserve motion and stability of the spine, preserve most of the intervertebral discs, and minimal aggression to the bone structure.[11]

It is not indicated to patients with osteoporosis. There is a need of surgical microscope and high-speed drill as the only condition required to perform this procedure, which makes it an effective and inexpensive technique.

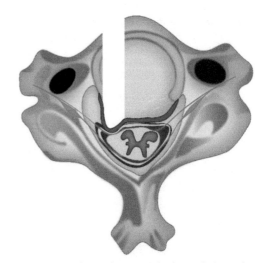

Fig. 21.2 Schematic coronal view of the spine showing the anterior "uncoforaminotomy" surgical approach.

Anterior Cervical Transcorporeal– "Tunnel Approach"[12]

This is a minimal invasive procedure aimed to resect small and localized osteophytes or calcifications, resulting in cervical myelopathy. The advance to the cervical spine can be done by the conventional approach (Smith and Robinson), anterior minimally invasive approach, or tubular or partial or full endoscopic by anterior single or multiple disc space decompression. The hole is performed in the middle of the vertebral body and pointed to the localized osteophyte or calcification, avoiding the medial wall of the transverse foramen and attempting to preserve the lower endplate and disc space heights. The main goals and advantages of this technique are direct anterior decompression, preservation of disc height, motion preservation, avoidance of complications related to anterior fusion surgery, prevention of exposure and injury to the vertebral artery and cervical sympathetic chain, and no need for postoperative immobilization **(Fig. 21.3)**.

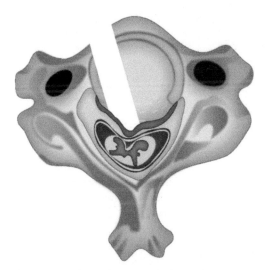

Fig. 21.3 Schematic coronal view of the spine showing the anterior cervical transcorporeal, "tunnel approach". Note how the hole is performed in the middle of the vertebral body and pointed to the localized osteophyte or calcification.

Indications

Patients are indicated for surgery based on the following criteria:
- Unilateral compression of spinal cord and roots not responding to conservative treatment.
- Imaging studies corresponding to clinical features.

It is not indicated in patients with, dominant axial neck pain, cervical instability, cervical infection or tumor, and high cervical levels (C3-C4 or above).

Multiple Midline or Oblique "Corpectomy (ies)"[13–15]

The classical approach first described by Cloward and Smith Robinson in 1958[3,4] requires the addition of surgical microscope and microinstruments. The localization of the area of decompression is done with radioscopy or/and neuronavigation. As dealing with a spinal cord lesion prevention, one should use preoperative corticosteroids and intraoperative monitoring. Using the "fish mouth" approach, the resection of the degenerated disc and osteophytes can be accomplished with precision and direct protection of spinal cord and roots. With microscopic approach, the ossified ligament can be cut and resected. One can perform a multilevel decompression without destabilization of the spine.[16,17] Notably, in these cases, the surgeon must prevent blood loss using bone wax on a cancellous bone. As the disc prolapses and osteophytes are not symmetrical, a variety of resections can be made accordingly **(Figs. 21.4 and 21.5)**.

Indications

Patients are indicated for surgery based on the following criteria:
- Failure of conservative treatment.
- Persistent and intractable pain.
- (Progressive) myelopathy, with or without radiculopathy, and if kyphosis is present.

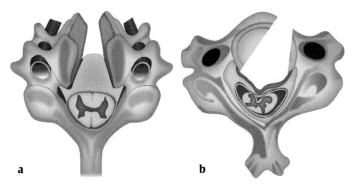

Fig. 21.4 (a, b) Schematic coronal views of the spine showing midline and oblique corporectomies (left and right, respectively).

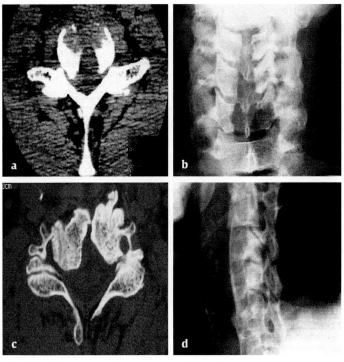

Fig. 21.5 Upper row, images taken by **(a)** CT left, axial view and **(b)** X-ray, right, anterior/posterior view, immediately after a midline multilevel corpectomy. Lower row, images taken by **(c)** CT, left axial view and **(d)** X-ray, right lateral view, 3 years after midline multilevel corpectomy.

The main advantages of this technique are as follows: the positioning is easy and less risky; direct and quick dissection of the anatomic planes; allows direct approach to the vertebral bodies and discs; allows decompression of the spinal cord and roots; less damage to the ligaments; remodeling of the canal; wide area for decompression and fusion; controlled blood loss; short time surgery; inclined approaches can be accomplished; less postoperative pain; and reduced time to return to social activities. Importantly, there is a need to leave the bone opening exposed. The opening can be filled with bone powder and bone growth factors, which have been shown to increase bone formation locally. Over time, the bone grows through this media and closes the opening while respecting the neural anatomy.

Discussion

Corpectomy technique and its variations preserve over half of the vertebral body and maintain intact nature of two of three columns without compromising spinal stability. Therefore, bone grafts or instrumentation for arthrodesis are not necessary.[18] To perform the anterior central corpectomy, we will not manipulate the sympathetic chain, and approaches above C3 will not retract the accessory nerve. The vertebral artery is not exposed and consequently protected by the bilateral part (piece) of the vertebral body.

The first pitfall is the use of the irrigation/suction device, with the drilling tip protected from dural heating or lesion. The second pitfall is the exposition of the image study accessible during all the surgical procedure. When there is a tight adherence between dura mater and calcified ligament, the decompression may be accomplished by only widening the vertebral canal and drilling the posterior part of the vertebral body.

Authors suggest pre- and postoperative evaluation by the Japanese Orthopedic Association (JOA) score. Note that inclusion of some modifications, as suggested by Salvatore[13], can increase global recovery to 95%. The aim is to stop progression of myelopathy, and recovering is related to the rehabilitation and physiotherapy program.

Conclusion

An ideal procedure should be objective, easy to perform, highly effective, safe and, if possible, not expensive.

Patients with anterior compression of the spinal cord are frequently old (60 years of age or more). Due to aging, many present degenerative compromises of the cervical vertebral bodies and discs, which can cause a reduction of mobility and consequent stabilization (fusion) of the spine. Anterior and lateral osteophytes are to blame for this stabilization. The design of the surgical approach should ensure preservation of the physiological fusion.

In this chapter, the authors attempted to systematize surgical techniques from unilateral to bilateral and multilevel approaches to intentionally explain the variety of constructions the surgeon can use for minimal invasive technique without instrumentation. Their experience with elderly patients confirms that each surgery is different from previous cases and technical choices should be carefully accessed on a case-by-case scenario, with decisions and modifications being potentially made during the procedure. Some of these approaches should be applied by an experienced surgeon, knowing deeply the clinical neurological deficit immediately prior to the intubation and appropriate imaging available at the surgical theater. Therefore, electrophysiologic monitoring and neuronavigation by image assessment (CT-MRI) should be used along with surgery.

Although multilevel corpectomy remains a rather demanding technique with a substantial learning curve, authors believe it is a valid alternative for the management of multisegmental cervical spondylosis. A variety of cervical anterior corpectomy resections can be performed once the vertebral osteophytes and ossifications of the anterior longitudinal ligaments are asymmetrical. The surgeon will decompress using a variety of asymmetric ways. Minimal invasive techniques will help to customize each approach to each patient's needs. Of course, there are limits to this technique as for all the others, and the surgeon must identify the right moment to abort it and use the most adequate and secure way to treat each patient. The incidence of early and late postoperative complications is lower. Bone grafting and heavy instrumentation are not necessary. It is adequate for elderly patients with diabetes, obesity, hypertension, and other associated comorbidities, which will not allow for time consuming and complicated procedures. It allows early patient mobilization with no postoperative immobilization. Optimal results rely on scrupulous selection of patients and adequate designing of the decompression without destabilization of the spine.

References

1. Spelling RG, Sackville WB. Lateral rupture of the cervical Intervertebral disc. A common cause of shoulder and arm pain. Surg Gynecol Obstet 1944;798:350–358

2. Frykholm R, Sackavillle WB. Root compression resulting from disc degeneration and root sleeve fibrosis. Acta Chir Scand 1951;160:1–158

3. Cloward RB. The anterior approach for removal of ruptured cervical disks. J Neurosurg 1958;15(6):602–617

4. Smith GW, Robinson RA. The treatment of certain cervical-spine disorders by anterior removal of the intervertebral disc and interbody fusion. J Bone Joint Surg Am 1958;40-A(3):607–624

5. Hakuba A. Trans-unco-discal approach. A combined anterior and lateral approach to cervical discs. J Neurosurg 1976;45(3): 284–291

6. Verbiest H. Chapter 23. The management of cervical spondylosis. Clin Neurosurg 1973;20:262–294

7. Lesoin F, Biondi A, Jomin M. Foraminal cervical herniated disc treated by anterior discoforaminotomy. Neurosurgery 1987; 21(3):334–338

8. Celestre PC, Pazmiño PR, Mikhael MM, et al. Minimally invasive approaches to the cervical spine. Orthop Clin North Am 2012;43(1):137–147, x

9. Choi G, Lee SH, Bhanot A, Chae YS, Jung B, Lee S. Modified transcorporeal anterior cervical microforaminotomy for cervical radiculopathy: a technical note and early results. Eur Spine J 2007;16(9):1387–1393

10. Baabor M, Piedimonte F, Vergara C, et al. Microsurgical anterior cervical foraminotomy (uncoforaminotomy) for the treatment of compressive radiculopathy. Spine Research 2017;3(2):11

11. Lee SH, Lee JH, Choi WC, Jung B, Mehta R. Anterior minimally invasive approaches for the cervical spine. Orthop Clin North Am 2007;38(3):327–337, abstract v

12. Choi G, Arbatti NJ, Modi HN, et al. Transcorporeal tunnel approach for unilateral cervical radiculopathy: a 2-year follow-up review and results. Minim Invasive Neurosurg 2010;53(3):127–131

13. Salvatore C, Orphee M, Damien B, Alisha R, Pavel P, Bernard G. Oblique corpectomy to manage cervical myeloradiculopathy. Neurol Res Int 2011;2011:734232

14. Masini M. Cervical spondylotic myelopathy treated with partial central corpectomy without grafting or plating. Paper presented at: Book of Abstracts of the World Spine I; 2000; Berlin, Germany

15. Masini M. Role of corpectomy in the surgical management of cervical disc herniation. In: Ramani PS, Motoi S, Zileli M, Dohrmann GJ, eds. Surgical Management of Cervical Disc Herniation (WFNS Spine Committee), 2012, pages 134/139, Jaypee Publishers, India. 2012

16. Bruneau M, Cornelius JF, George B. Multilevel oblique corpectomies: surgical indications and technique. Neurosurgery 2007; 61(3, Suppl):106–112, discussion 112

17. Rocchi G, Caroli E, Salvati M, Delfini R. Multilevel oblique corpectomy without fusion: our experience in 48 patients. Spine 2005;30(17):1963–1969

18. Chen CS, Cheng CK, Liu CL, Lo WH. Stress analysis of the disc adjacent to interbody fusion in lumbar spine. Med Eng Phys 2001; 23(7):483–491

22 Technical Challenges and Tips in Minimally Invasive Posterior Decompression in Cervical Spondylotic Myelopathy

José Antonio Soriano Sánchez and José Alberto Israel Romero Rangel

Background

Cervical spondylotic myelopathy (CSM) is the leading cause of myelopathy in patients older than 55 years.[1] Surgical approaches include anterior or posterior fusion as well as laminectomy and laminoplasty.[2] In complex cases, the choice to treat by an anterior or posterior approach is ambiguous.[3] We agree with other authors that anterior decompression and reconstruction is a safe and appropriate treatment in the setting of single or two-level disease, as more than two-level corpectomy is associated with a very high instrumentation-failure rate. Besides, in complex cases with a multilevel disease, the posterior approach is better suited, avoiding any fistula risk due to anterior dural calcification.[3-5] Evidence-based medicine (EBM) highlights the role of fixation (whether anterior or posterior), providing faster recovery and improved neurological functions.[6] Authors do reserve fixation for high-instability cases, as most of the patients with ossification of the posterior longitudinal ligament have a "natural" self-provided anterior fusion.

EBM favors posterior surgical approach when there exists predominant posterior pathology, patients with more than two-level disease along with preserved lordosis, presence of ossified posterior longitudinal ligament (OPLL), multilevel CSM with short segment of instability and kyphosis, and multilevel CSM with apical kyphosis along with overall lordosis.[7,8]

Decompressing the cervical spine requires thoughtful knowledge, skillful hands, and a proper mental construct of the steps required to afford a suitable decompression.

To be considered a minimally invasive spine surgery (MISS), it must include respecting the midline raphe, avoiding the usual postoperative pain, while preserving the muscles, ligaments, and the stability of the spine. In this chapter, the authors will provide a step-by-step technique with tips and tricks to obtain adequate MISS posterior decompression.

Step 1: Position and Planning

Improper surgical positioning in spinal procedures leads to a variety of complications, including vision loss, nerve palsies, thromboembolic complications, pressure sores, lower extremity compartment syndrome, and shoulder dislocation.[9-12] Myelopathic patients requiring surgery have substantial neurological deficits; any minor postoperative complication will have a significant clinical impact, ultimately affecting their quality of life or make them seek the surgeon's liability.[13] Prone positioning exposes the patient to a variety of intraoperative complications that can affect the outcome or halt a medical procedure, for example, surgical bleeding because of abdominal compression;[14,15] besides, it is mandatory for the treatment of CSM.

Tip: Authors encourage spine surgeons to expend the needed time to reach optimal surgical positions; a wrong position can drive a 1-hour surgery into a longer surgery because of decreased vision, need to transfuse, or difficulties to afford a full decompression because of excessive bleeding.

Trick: Authors recommend concord positioning with the head in military position to decrease bleeding risk: Concord positioning requires the patient to be prone and straight forward with slight semi-fowler and knees, legs should be below the heart and the head above. Military positioning of the head requires to be neutral (looking straight forward from the chest) on the sagittal and axial axis. This position helps to increase the venous drainage of the head while avoiding excessive venous pressure from the abdominal compartment (**Fig. 22.1**). To proceed uneventfully, authors recommend to set up the surgical room; surgeons should be by the side of patient's predominant symptoms, first assistant and nurse in front of him and second assistants to the feet of the patient, neurophysiology stations should be aside of anesthesiologist, C-arm should be just in front of the patients head, with microscope to the side of the surgeon's position (**Fig. 22.2**).

Finally, as part of the planning process, the authors recommend total intravenous anesthesia (TIVA) without neuromuscular blocking to avoid interfering with neuromonitoring.

Step 2: Surgical Approach and Progressive Muscle-Splitting Dissection

Approach-related complications are rare but relevant, such as postoperative hematoma or vascular injuries.[16] Soft-tissue damage can also lead to muscle atrophy, loss of lordosis, pain, and lower functional scores in the postoperative period.[17,18]

Tip: Authors suggest spine surgeons handle the soft tissues properly while finding the anatomic corridor to the posterior cervical spine.

Trick: The incision 2 cm wide is made immediately beside the spinous processes. Because of the cervical lordosis, the entrance could serve to achieve up to three contiguous levels tilting the tube in a craniocaudal way. Use of microscope starting with the skin incision offers a better view of soft-tissue structures. Authors encourage surgeons to dissect the muscle bundles, following the direction of their fibers in each progressive plane; it offers the opportunity to make meticulous hemostasis during the approach, maintaining deep dry planes and favoring a perfect vision. To complete this task, the authors employ two thin esophagus retractors and bipolar forceps (**Fig. 22.3**).

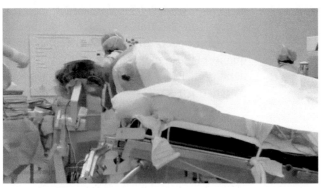

Fig. 22.1 Patient positioning: The patient clamped on head-holder and concord positioning lateral view.

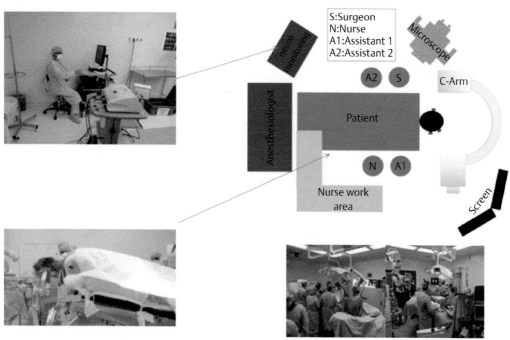

Fig. 22.2   Patient positioning: Schematic and live room setup.

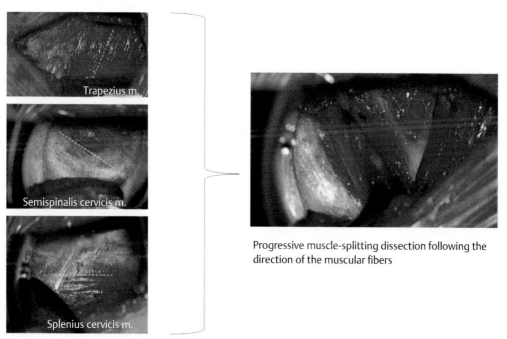

Progressive muscle-splitting dissection following the direction of the muscular fibers

Fig. 22.3   Approach. Soft-tissue dissection. Use of microscope since skin incision is recommended to better handle soft tissue, permitting a progressive muscle-splitting dissection to reduce unnecessary trauma by muscle splitting.

Step 3: Placement of Tubular Retractor

Posterior cervical muscles of the neck are directly attached to the spinous process; they serve as a power source for cervical motion and mobilizing neck. These muscles are removed from the spinous process in conventional procedures, resulting in persistent neck pain, shoulder stiffness, restricted range of motion, and spinal malalignment. Minimally invasive approaches serve to preserve the extension mechanism of the spine by carefully entering transmuscular working channels.[19] The tubular retractor system has many advantages over other conventional MISS techniques. It offers direct visualization of the operative field, anatomical familiarity with spine surgeons, and minimizes tissue trauma. In posterior cervical approaches, it has several advantages. It reduces postoperative pain, but more importantly, it preserves the ligamentous attachments of the neck muscle to the laminae and spinous process. Several posterior muscle groups, particularly the semispinalis cervicis and multifidus muscle, function as dynamic stabilizers of the neck.[20] In the past, the recommendation was to introduce a K-wire and then dilate crossing in a blind-fashion all muscular planes with imminent risk to chop the spinal cord.

Tip: The use of tubular retractors to minimize soft-tissue trauma, in order to prevent postoperative axial pain and decrease the amount of muscle removal required to visualize specific structures **(Fig. 22.4)**.

Trick: Authors prefer to avoid the use of K-wires. Instead, they recommend a progressive splitting-muscle dissection, using esophagus retractors, docking the last tube (working channel), and taking advantage of that corridor, thereby avoiding muscle entering the surgical field below the working tube.

Step 4: Soft-tissue Removal– Exposure of Bony Anatomy

It is of paramount importance to dissect soft tissue underlying tube border, and remove any redundant muscle, as minimal disinsertion helps identify bony landmarks and precise entry point to the surgical target.[21]

Tip: Use specific landmarks to guide bone resection; the upper and lower laminar borders are the respective craniocaudal limits of resection, while the laminar–facet cleft and the underlying pedicle in the opposite side are the lateral references.

Trick: Identifying the limit among the two laminae and facet joints (laminar–facet junction) is the essential anatomic landmark. Tube placement should be over the interlaminar space, focusing two-thirds of the superior and one-third of the inferior laminae, among the one-quarter medial part of the facet joint and spinous process–laminae junction, parallel to the intervertebral disc **(Fig. 22.5)**.[2]

Step 5: Ipsilateral Laminotomy

Conventionally, high-speed drilling is used to perform laminectomy. These devices have simplified spinal surgery in recent years;[22] however, they produce unwanted frictional heat during the bone resection.[23] The use of ultrasonic devices minimizes heat-related damage risk to neurological structures.[22]

Tip: Special instruments to protect neurological structures should be preferred. Ultrasonic

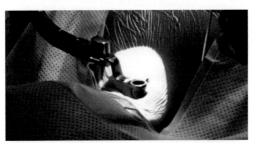

Fig. 22.4 Placement of tubular retractor. Authors prefer to avoid the use of K-wires. Instead, they recommend a progressive splitting-muscle dissection using esophagus retractors and then docking the last tube (working channel), taking advantage of that corridor avoiding muscle entering the surgical field below the working tube.

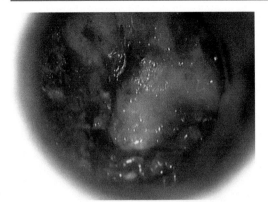

Fig. 22.5 Soft-tissue removal/exposure of bony anatomy. Identifying the limit between the two laminae and facet joints (laminar–facet junction) is the essential anatomic landmark. Tube placement should be over the interlaminar space focusing two-thirds of the superior and one-third of the inferior laminae, among the one-quarter medial part of the facet joint and spinous process-laminae junction, parallel to the intervertebral disc.

devices for bone removal help reduce iatrogenic complications by respecting soft-tissue structures and reducing heat to neurological structures.

Trick: Tilting the bed to the contralateral side and tilting the tube to the midline is vital to achieving a good vision of the spinous process base and an excellent parallel direction to the contralateral laminae while maintaining the entrance of the working channel perpendicular to the floor, in order to promote a healthy and ergonomic position between the surgeon, the surgical field and the microscope, making the surgical procedure comfortable. For conventional bone drilling, authors use a 3-mm fluted match-head drill bit (side-cutting burr with a blunt tip). The blunt tip of the drill rests on the ligamentum flavum (LF) as the side-cutting burr removes the bone.[2] While using ultrasonic devices, a frontal hook with a frontal-cut claw or microclaw is preferred, as it cuts in front and protects the dural sack below (**Fig. 22.6**).

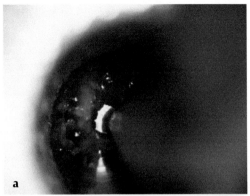

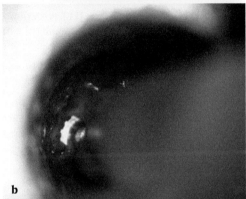

Fig. 22.6 Ipsilateral laminotomy: (**a**) A frontal-cut claw is used on an ultrasonic device to resect bone in the interlaminar space. (**b**) Bone removal is done straight forward until the insertion of ligamentum flavum (LF) is visualized; it is recommended to keep moving the claw to avoid overheating neurological structures.

Step 6: Ligamentum Flavum (LF) Resection

Once drilling has been completed, and the ipsilateral cranial-caudal and lateral limits of the LF are disinserted with blunt dissection, a rongeur is used to remove it from the surgical field.[2]

Tips: To disinsert the LF with safety, a ball-tip probe should be used to detach it at the exact point of insertion in each of its limits, applying controlled force with slight lateral movements.

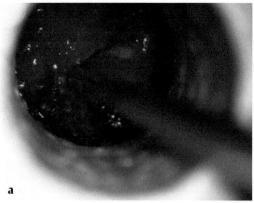
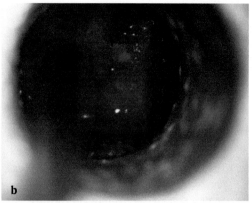

a   b

Fig. 22.7 **Ligamentum flavum (LF) resection**: **(a)** A ball-tip hook is used to disinsert LF from its craniocaudal and lateral attachments, and **(b)** a rongeur is used to remove LF in one piece (complete LF or ipsilateral half LF, depending on surgeon's preference).

Trick: LF protects the underlying dura; therefore, it should be resected after completing laminotomy. Caution should be taken not to violate the laminar–facet junction, as going too laterally will increase the risk of instability; the lateral insertion of the LF is just below the laminar–facet cleft. Ipsilateral LF resection is recommended to early decompress neurological structures; authors have clinically observed that this helps to improve neurophysiological potentials early too; otherwise, full LF resection can be completed after over the top decompression in the contralateral side (**Fig. 22.7**).

Step 7: Contralateral Decompression: Over the Top Drilling

Cervical decompression by a tubular approach requires a unilateral approach with over the top decompression in the contralateral side[2] (**Fig. 22.8**).

Tip: To accurately find and drill the contralateral limits of LF insertion, decrease surgical time and increase the chances to fulfill a complete decompression of the spinal cord and foramen.

Trick: Verify clinical, radiological, and neurophysiological correlation, as patients might

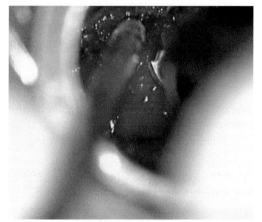

Fig. 22.8 **Contralateral decompression**: Over the top drilling. Medial wanding is performed to reach the contralateral side; then, over-the-top decompression is done by drilling over ligamentum flavum (LF) on the contralateral side (if complete LF is to be removed in one-piece, over-the-top decompression should be carried out first to protect the underlying dura).

have asymmetric findings.[24,25] Expert neurophysiological monitoring is mandatory, as unilateral symptoms are usually alleviated by unilateral decompression,[26] saving time, reducing soft-tissue damage and minimizing surgical risks, while obtaining significant clinical improvement. Neurophysiological studies are of paramount importance in preoperative decision-making.

Step 8: Inspect Decompression

The tubular retractor is "wanded" in all directions to assure complete resection of the LF (**Fig. 22.9**).

Tip: The contralateral decompression should extend to the medial wall of the contralateral pedicle.

Trick: Disc visualization is blocked to the surgeon's sight by neurological structures in posterior approaches. Traditionally, authors remove any compressing disc by blunt hooks; however, on the contralateral side, it can be very challenging, especially in the OPLL cases. Authors use the frontal-cutting attachment of ultrasonic devices to remove ossified disc just if they were resecting tumors; it offers precision and protects the nerve root.

Step 9: Hemostasis and Retractor Removal

Strict hemostasis using bipolar electrocautery and/or hemostatic agents is obtained. It is imperative to achieve hemostasis, as a postoperative hematoma in this region can result in devastating neurologic injury[2]

Tip: Surgeons must keep in mind different methods to attain hemostasis, controlling blood pressure (slight hypotension) and temperature.[27]

Trick: A proper surgical approach with muscle dissection will decrease the need for hemostatic agents before finishing the procedure (**Fig. 22.10**). If venous bleeding continues after a proper technique, authors recommend the use of tranexamic acid, as recent reviews in the field support an evidence level I in spinal surgery.[27]

Step 10: Closure

The muscle fascias are then reapproximated, followed by the deep dermal layer and skin. They inject local anesthetic for postoperative pain control[2] (avoiding any profound anesthetic leakage to prevent high cervical nerve conduction block).

Tip: Blunt muscle-fibers dissection will decrease muscle damage and the need for bipolar hemostasis, as stated before. Cerebrospinal fluid (CSF) leakage requires strict watertight closure of fascia layers (**Fig. 22.11**).

Trick: A practical and simple maneuver to treat CSF fistula from small dural defects is

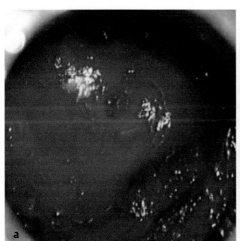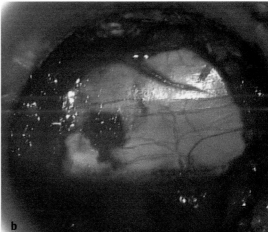

Fig. 22.9 Inspect decompression: (**a**) Complete decompression should be verified; any constricting band or ligamentum flavum (LF) remnant should be removed, (**b**) tube wanding can help assure that dural sac is clear of any compressing structure.

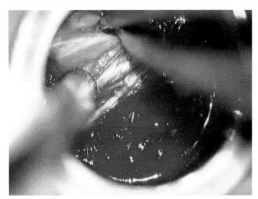

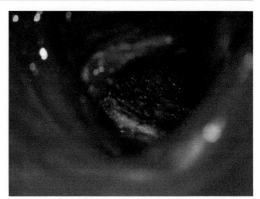

Fig. 22.10 Hemostasis and retractor removal: Proper muscle dissection will reduce the need for bipolar cauterization.

Fig. 22.11 Closure: Muscle-fibers dissection at the beginning of the surgical procedure will ease closure by clear visualization of muscle layers, permitting a watertight muscle fascia closure.

to change its pressure gradients. In the cervical spine, this goal is met by placing the patient as close to a 90° position or inverse Trendelenburg position.[28] Authors do it by starting ambulation as early as possible just after surgery (in the absence of dural puncture symptoms, such as headache). They have managed their patients with this protocol and have never needed a second surgery to solve fistula. For more prominent dural defects, authors use separate stitches, with fatty pads, if needed, and watertight fascial closure, just as in tumor resection cases.[29]

Indications

Indications of this surgical technique are below:

- Moderate-to-severe spondylotic myelopathy, three or more levels of multisegment disease, preserved cervical lordosis, posterior ligament hypertrophy, and ossification as major source of pathology[30]
- Neutral alignment with absent instability by anterior intervertebral fusion or from OPLL.
- Elderly patients.[30]
- Young patients with early onset of symptoms (< 4 months).[8]

Advantages

The most common surgical procedure for CSM is posterior decompression;[30] no major learning curve required. The improvement in Japanese Orthopaedic Association (JOA) score has been estimated to be more than 50%.[30]

Disadvantages

Complications such as postoperative kyphosis may develop. It is an indirect decompression for OPLL and nerve root damage, especially those with the former.[8]

Outcomes

Factors associated with the best outcome from posterior approaches are younger patients (< 57%), early symptom onset (< 4 months), and high preoperative JOA score (> 10).[8]

Authors previously described their surgical outcomes with this technique in a case series.[2] Fifteen patients underwent one- to three-level surgery. The mean age was 73 years; mean operative time was 125 minutes, mean blood loss was 57 mL, a mean hospital stay was 36 hours, with no complications found in 16 months follow-up. Mean improvements were as followed: visual analog scale (VAS) scores from 6.4 to 2.4, neck disability index (NDI) from 46.4 to 7.0, and modified Japanese Orthopaedic Association Score (mJOA) from 11.3 to 14.5.[2]

Complications

The most frequent complication is kyphosis, reported in up to 20% of the cases in the laminectomy series.[31] Nevertheless, laminectomy implies removal of the spinous processes, interspinous and supraspinous ligaments, laminae, and LF and loss of the capsules of the facet joints that comprise the posterior stabilizers.[30] In the present surgical technique, authors perform a limited laminotomy (either unilateral or bilateral) with LF resection and preservation of paraspinal muscle complexes and ligaments of the posterior tension band. Other reported complications include wound infection and CSF leakage,[32] the last one calculated between 0.3 and 13% and up to 18% in revision surgery.[33] Authors in their series have demonstrated a 0% complication rate with this technique (including kyphosis, infection or CSF leakage).[2]

Conclusion

In conclusion, authors consider the best way to prevent a complication is to implement quality-control protocols for hospitals and their surgical teams, focusing on technical (surgical) and nontechnical (effective communication and efficient team work) skills, as they help them increase patient safety.[34]

Illustrative Case

A 60-year-old male presenting after 2 years of repeated falls with gait instability, bilateral upper and lower limb weakness, severe disability with spondylotic myelopathy C3–C6. His Oswestry disability Index (ODI) was 86 points, NDI was 74%, and mJOA was 9 points. The patient underwent a posterior decompression with significant improvement at two years follow-up, with NDI of 8%, recovering bilateral upper and lower leg weakness, and improved disability by way of ODI of 30 and mJOA 12 points. Preoperative and postoperative images are shown in **Fig. 22.12**.

Take-home Points

- Posterior decompression is the most frequently performed procedure to solve CSM.

- Minimally invasive posterior decompression is best suited for elderly patients, and young patients with early onset symptoms (<4 months), and high JOA Scores (>10 points) with multilevel disease.

- Cervical lordosis or neutral alignment with anterior fusion (either intervertebral osteophytes or by OPLL) are key points to avoid kyphotic complications.

- The present technique comprises a limited laminotomy (either unilateral or bilateral) with LF resection and preservation of paraspinal muscles and posterior tension band, with complication rates demonstrated to be as low as 0% once mastered.

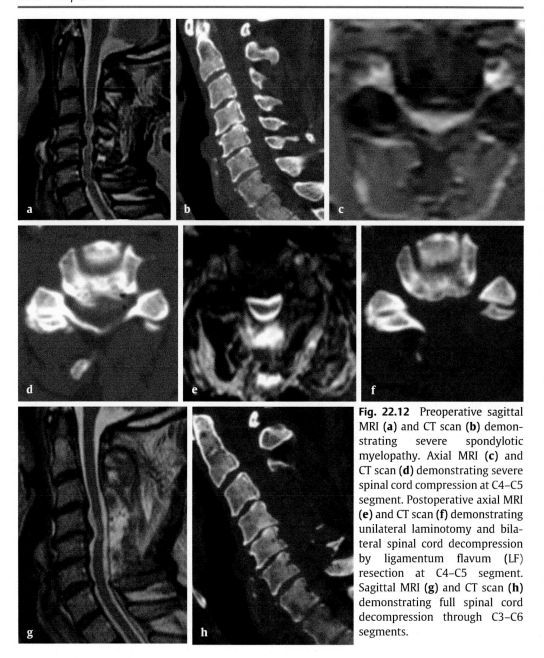

Fig. 22.12 Preoperative sagittal MRI (**a**) and CT scan (**b**) demonstrating severe spondylotic myelopathy. Axial MRI (**c**) and CT scan (**d**) demonstrating severe spinal cord compression at C4–C5 segment. Postoperative axial MRI (**e**) and CT scan (**f**) demonstrating unilateral laminotomy and bilateral spinal cord decompression by ligamentum flavum (LF) resection at C4–C5 segment. Sagittal MRI (**g**) and CT scan (**h**) demonstrating full spinal cord decompression through C3–C6 segments.

References

1. Lawrence BD, Jacobs WB, Norvell DC, Hermsmeyer JT, Chapman JR, Brodke DS. Anterior versus posterior approach for treatment of cervical spondylotic myelopathy: a systematic review. Spine 2013; 38(22, Suppl 1):S173–S182

2. Hernandez RN, Wipplinger C, Navarro-Ramirez R, et al. Ten-step minimally invasive cervical decompression via unilateral tubular laminotomy: technical note and early clinical experience. Oper Neurosurg (Hagerstown) 2020;18(3):284–294

3. Kommu R, Sahu BP, Purohit AK. Surgical outcome in patients with cervical ossified

posterior longitudinal ligament: A single institutional experience. Asian J Neurosurg 2014;9(4):196–202

4. Liu X, Zhu B, Liu X, Liu Z, Dang G. Circumferential decompression via the posterior approach for the surgical treatment of multilevel thoracic ossification of the posterior longitudinal ligaments: a single institution comparative study. Chin Med J (Engl) 2014;127(19):3371–3377

5. Epstein NE. What you need to know about ossification of the posterior longitudinal ligament to optimize cervical spine surgery: A review. Surg Neurol Int 2014;5(Suppl 3): S93–S118

6. Mehdi SK, Alentado VJ, Lee BS, Mroz TE, Benzel EC, Steinmetz MP. Comparison of clinical outcomes in decompression and fusion versus decompression only in patients with ossification of the posterior longitudinal ligament: a meta-analysis. Neurosurg Focus 2016;40(6):E9

7. Wilson JR, Tetreault LA, Kim J, et al. State of the art in degenerative cervical myelopathy: an update on current clinical evidence. Neurosurgery 2017;80(3S):S33–S45

8. Jain, Ak, Rustagi T, Prasad G, Deore T, and Bhojraj SY. 2017. "Does Segmental Kyphosis Affect Surgical Outcome after a Posterior Decompressive Laminectomy in Multisegmental Cervical Spondylotic Myelopathy? Asian Spine J 11(1):24–30

9. Shriver MF, Zeer V, Alentado VJ, Mroz TE, Benzel EC, Steinmetz MP. Lumbar spine surgery positioning complications: a systematic review. Neurosurg Focus 2015; 39(4):E16

10. Kamel I, Barnette R. Positioning patients for spine surgery: avoiding uncommon position-related complications. World J Orthop 2014;5(4):425–443

11. Biscevic M, Sehic A, Biscevic S, et al. Kyphosis—A risk factor for positioning brachial plexopathy during spinal surgeries. Acta Orthop Traumatol Turc 2019;53(3):199–202

12. Yoshihara H, Pivec R, Naam A. Positioning-related neuromonitoring change during anterior cervical discectomy and fusion. World Neurosurg 2018;117:238–241

13. Kutteruf R, Wells D, Stephens L, Posner KL, Lee LA, Domino KB. Injury and liability associated with spine surgery. J Neurosurg Anesthesiol 2018;30(2):156–162

14. Pearce DJ. The role of posture in laminectomy. Proc R Soc Med 1957;50(2):109–112

15. Phillips WA, Hensinger RN. Control of blood loss during scoliosis surgery. Clin Orthop Relat Res 1988; (229):88–93

16. Mayer HM, Siepe C, Korge A. Der mikrochirurgische anteriore Zugang zur Halswirbelsäule beim zervikalen Bandscheibenersatz. Oper Orthop Traumatol 2010;22(5-6):454–467

17. Ashana AO, Ajiboye RM, Sheppard WL, Sharma A, Kay AB, Holly LT. Cervical paraspinal muscle atrophy rates following laminoplasty and laminectomy with fusion for cervical spondylotic myelopathy. World Neurosurg 2017;107:445–450

18. Fortin M, Wilk N, Dobrescu O, Martel P, Santaguida C, Weber MH. Relationship between cervical muscle morphology evaluated by MRI, cervical muscle strength and functional outcomes in patients with degenerative cervical myelopathy. Musculoskelet Sci Pract 2018;38:1–7

19. Shiraishi T, Kato M, Yato Y, et al. New techniques for exposure of posterior cervical spine through intermuscular planes and their surgical application. Spine 2012;37(5): E286–E296

20. Kim YB, Hyun SJ. Clinical applications of the tubular retractor on spinal disorders. J Korean Neurosurg Soc 2007;42(4):245–250

21. Bodon G, Patonay L, Baksa G, Olerud C. Applied anatomy of a minimally invasive muscle-splitting approach to posterior C1-C2 fusion: an anatomical feasibility study. Surg Radiol Anat 2014;36(10):1063–1069

22. Tarazi N, Munigangaiah S, Jadaan M, McCabe JP. Comparison of thermal spread with the use of an ultrasonic osteotomy device: Sonopet ultrasonic aspirator versus misonix bonescalpel in spinal surgery. J Craniovertebr Junction Spine [Internet] 2018;9(1):68–72

23. Yu Z, He D, Xiong J, et al. Extensor muscle-preserving laminectomy in treating multilevel cervical spondylotic myelopathy compared with laminoplasty. Ann Transl Med 2019;7(18):472–472

24. Ginsberg L. Myelopathy: chameleons and mimics. Pract Neurol 2017;17(1):6–12

25. Toledano M, Bartleson JD. Cervical spondylotic myelopathy. Neurol Clin 2013;31(1): 287–305

26. Jho HD. Spinal cord decompression via microsurgical anterior foraminotomy for spondylotic cervical myelopathy. Minim Invasive Neurosurg 1997;40(4):124–129

27. Mikhail C, Pennington Z, Arnold PM, et al. Minimizing blood loss in spine surgery. Global Spine J 2020; 10(1, Suppl):71S–83S

28. Oertel JM, Burkhardt BW. Full endoscopic treatment of dural tears in lumbar spine surgery. Eur Spine J 2017;26(10):2496–2503

29. Soriano Sánchez JA, Soto García ME, Soriano Solís S, et al. Microsurgical resection of intraspinal benign tumors using non-expansile tubular access. World Neurosurg 2020;133:e97–e104

30. Bajamal AH, Kim SH, Arifianto MR, et al; World Federation of Neurosurgical Societies (WFNS) Spine Committee. Posterior surgical techniques for cervical spondylotic myelopathy: WFNS Spine Committee Recommendations. Neurospine 2019;16(3): 421–434

31. Kaptain GJ, Simmons NE, Replogle RE, Pobereskin L. Incidence and outcome of kyphotic deformity following laminectomy for cervical spondylotic myelopathy. J Neurosurg 2000; 93(2, Suppl)199–204

32. Cheung JPY, Luk KDK. Complications of anterior and posterior cervical spine surgery. Asian Spine J 2016;10(2):385–400

33. Epstein NE, Hollingsworth R. Anterior cervical micro-dural repair of cerebrospinal fluid fistula after surgery for ossification of the posterior longitudinal ligament. Technical note. Surg Neurol 1999;52(5):511–514

34. Soriano Sánchez JA, Soriano Solís S, Romero Rangel JAI. Role of the checklist in neurosurgery, a realistic perspective to "the need for surgical safety checklists in neurosurgery now and in the future—a systematic review". World Neurosurg 2020; 134:121–122

23 Endoscopic Decompression for Cervical Spondylosis

Enrique Osorio-Fonseca, Jorge Felipe Ramírez-León, José Gabriel Rugeles-Ortíz, Nicolás Prada-Ramírez, Carolina Ramírez-Martínez, and Gabriel Oswaldo Alonso-Cuéllar

Introduction

Cervical spondylosis is a degenerative pathology that affect vertebral bodies, intervertebral discs (IVD), facets and associated ligaments, causing a direct compression of neurological and vascular surrounding structures. These anatomical changes cause cervical stenosis with the subsequent cervical spondylotic radiculopathy (CSR), and in advanced cases can precipitate neurological damages and cervical spondylotic myelopathy (CSM).[1] Certainly, CSR and CSM are the most common types of cervical spondylosis[2,3] and both pathologies require surgical intervention, nevertheless CSM can potentially produce a long-term disability and major neurological impairments.[1] For this reason, the most important thing is to establish an effective treatment with the aim to avoid irreversible spinal cord damage and before CSM occurs. Currently, the most widely used surgical treatment for neurological decompression in cervical spondylosis is the open conventional technique, either posterior or anterior approach, with or without fusion.[4,5] Open surgical options have a proven track record for more than 30 years as a safe and effective means to treat cervical spondylosis, although this procedure can lead to anatomical biomechanical changes, pseudarthrosis, and complications like dysphagia, dysphonia, adjacent segment disease and even death.[6] In contrast, endoscopic cervical approach has advantages such as clear view, minimal trauma, local anesthesia, outpatient procedure, and less complications. Taking account that cervical spondylosis is a common pathology in patients over 56 years, many of them with comorbidities, it is mandatory to develop less invasive alternatives with a minor possibility of complications.

In this chapter, authors report their experience with anterior endoscopic cervical decompression procedure for CSR. The authors have used endoscopic methods for the treatment of cervical spondylosis for the last 22 years.

Background

CSR is a clinical condition resulting from compression of cervical nerve roots.[7,8] Compression is caused by a narrowing of the window for the exiting nerve roots, which is also called cervical lateral stenosis. Stenosis is the main phenomena resulting from this degenerative process. Foraminal stenosis can be caused by herniated disc, presence of osteophytes (degeneration or microfractures of adjacent bony structures), or combination of both resulting from a degenerative disease like spondylosis. In the early stages, cervical degenerative disease may be asymptomatic,[9] but when CSR develops, symptoms are broad and vary from pain and sensory deficit up to diminished reflexes or its combinations.[8] When radiating pain occurs, its distribution corresponds to the dermatome of the affected level.[10] Diagnosis is based on a detailed physical examination, history, onset and type of pain, and corresponding diagnostic information including radiography (AP, lateral, flexion and extension views), MRI and CT scans. Approximately 25% of patients with degenerative processes of the cervical spine may require surgery once persistent symptoms are nonresponsive to conservative care such as the use of analgesics, physiotherapy, soft collar, epidural steroid injections, and selective nerve blocks.[7] Therefore, nonoperative therapeutic measures should be tried first. Typically, a minimum of 6 weeks of nonoperative treatment is thought to be appropriate before considering surgery.[11] Surgery is generally considered when nonoperative measures for the patient's intense, unrelenting pain, or progressive neurological deficit have failed.[10] Surgical options for CSR can generally be divided into two groups: open or conventional surgical procedures and minimally invasive spine surgery (MISS) including endoscopic approaches.[12–14]

Conventional procedure was reported by Robinson and Smith in 1955 and is a technique for cervical discectomy and fusion. Since then, anterior cervical discectomy and fusion (ACDF) has remained the principal surgery for cervical spondylosis and now is widely accepted as gold standard surgical treatment for cervical radiculopathy.[4,12] Although many studies have proven the effectivity of open procedures, there are still many controversies about the use of these alternatives, many of them for the need for fusion after the procedure and the rate of complications reported like adjacent segment.[10,12,15] With the intent of minimizing morbidity associated with conventional open procedures, MISS procedures have been recently developed for spinal stenosis, including at cervical segment.

Nowadays, with the technological advances, there are several cervical MISS options, with important advantages over the open surgery among decreased approach-related problems including blood loss, postoperative pain, and muscle atrophy.[5] Some of the most effective MISS alternatives for cervical decompression are endoscopic procedures, including anterior and posterior approach.[16] The author's experience is based on the anterior approach, using a blunt technique.

Anterior Endoscopic Cervical Approach for Cervical Spondylosis

Anterior endoscopic cervical decompression (AECD) is the removal of degenerated tissue, compressing nerve structures in the foraminal area under an endoscope view from an anterior percutaneous approach. The surgical principle is the same as in open decompression and aims to expand the foraminal window, and remove the hypertrophic tissue and osteophytes to achieve decompression of neural structures.[17] One of its advantages is that it can be performed in one or several levels without the need for fusion.[10]

Equipment and Instrumentation

Cervical spine endoscopic surgery requires special high-technology devices for its implementation. Among the key devices, we have the following: video-endoscopic tower, C-arm, source of heat energy (radiofrequency [RF]) and cervical discoscope with their respective instrumental set-like forceps and chisels (**Fig. 23.1**). The tower used by the authors in the cervical decompression includes equipment such as the following: monitor, video processor, light source and camera, shaver console and irrigation pump, devices available in a variety of brands. With the aim to do a thermal therapy, a bipolar radiofrequency console (Surgimax, Elliquence LLC, NYC) and a probe are used (Trigger Flex Elliquence LLC). The RF devices allow coagulation, annuloplasty and nucleoplasty with a probe which passes through the working channel of the endoscope and reaches the intradiscal space. The instrumental complementary are a set of spinal needles, dilators, cannula, trephines, burrs, and punch clamps (**Fig. 23.1**).

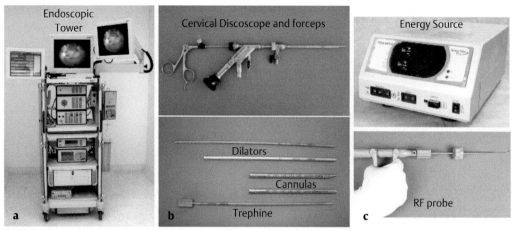

Fig. 23.1 Equipment and instrument set for anterior endoscopic cervical decompression (AECD). **(a)** Endoscopic Tower (Richard Wolf, Germany), **(b)** Cervical discoscope set (Richard Wolf, Germany), and **(c)** Radiofrequency thermal energy set (Elliquence LLC NYC).

Surgical Technique

The patient is placed on supine position with cervical extension. With the aim to get cervical lordosis, a pillow under the shoulders is placed; thus, there is no necessity to use any type of mechanical hyperextension system **(Fig. 23.2)**. Anatomical landmarks correspond to the intersection of the level affected and medial edge of the sternocleidomastoid muscle **(Fig. 23.3)**. Intervertebral level and point of entry of the blunt-ended cannula is secured using biplanar fluoroscopy.

Once this point is identified, the patient's head is slightly tilted toward contralateral side of the approach. In order to displace the esophagus and trachea medially and the neurovascular bundle laterally, the surgeon's finger firmly presses on the space between the muscle and the trachea (tracheoesophageal groove). Under an abundant local anesthetic infiltration, a 4-mm skin incision is made. Then, a cannula and a dilator are inserted, turning gently both until the anterior edge of the annulus **(Fig. 23.3)**. When the dilator blunt tip is just in front of the disc, one can withdraw the dilator, and through the cannula, the needle is advanced up to the posterior third of the disc. At this point, it is

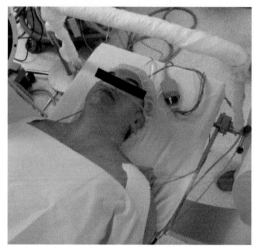

Fig. 23.2 Patient position during anterior endoscopic cervical decompression (AECD).

very important to reach a blunt technique, in order to avoid an undesirable puncture of a vascular structure[5] **(Fig. 23.3)**. Cannula and dilator are part of MiniDiscFx system for cervical nonendoscopic thermodiscoplasty (Elliquence LLC, NYC).

Once the needle is inserted into the disc, if the surgeon chooses to do it, discography and discogenic tests are performed. The purpose of the discogenic test is to verify that the disc

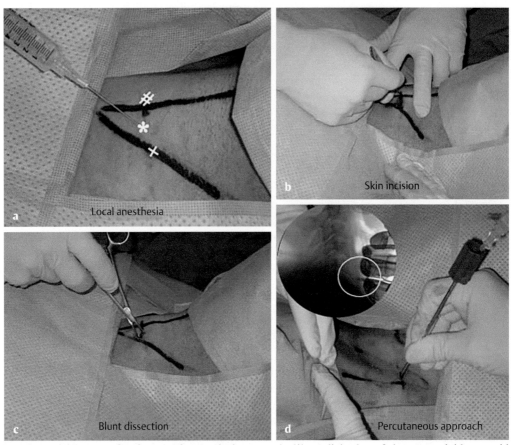

Fig. 23.3 **(a)** Entry point for anterior cervical approach. (*) medial edge of the sternocleidomastoid muscle; (+) intersection of the level affected; (#) entry point and entrance with blunt-tipped cannula within the intervertebral disc. **(b–d)** The blunt-tipped cannula is softly advanced up to the annulus anterior edge with circular movements and under fluoroscopic view.

is positive (> 5 points in visual analog scale [VAS]) and the symptoms are consistent with familiar concordant pain, taking advantage of the fact that the patient is awake. Also, to demonstrate the anatomical outlines of the disc, it is useful to use methylene blue to view internal disruptive dye patterns and leakage of dye, suggesting the location of annular tears as well as extruded disc material and their relationship to the posterior longitudinal ligament and the uncovertebral joint complex **(Fig. 23.4)**.

With a safe entry point, one can pull out the nonendoscopic set and replace it with the endoscopic set. The first step involves changing the cannula for the endoscopic dilator.

Using a guide wire over the needle, authors secure their approach **(Fig. 23.4)**. Once the position of the guide wire is confirmed, the needle is removed, and the set of dilators and cannulas for the endoscope are placed over the annulus of the disc **(Fig. 23.5)**. Then, the dilator is replaced with trephine and advanced with a rotating hand motion until the annulotomy is accomplished. Then, trephine is replaced by the discoscope. When endoscope is positioned, it is frequently necessary to achieve a better visualization and improve dissection through the anterior cervical prevertebral fascia with the use of a bipolar radiofrequency probe. The latter also helps with coagulation of small vessels,

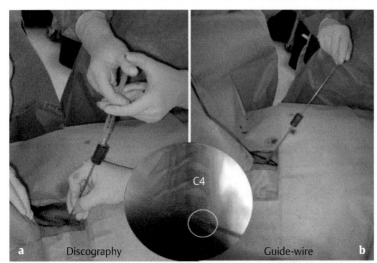

Fig. 23.4 (a) Discography and discogenic test and **(b)** placement of guide wire into the disc.

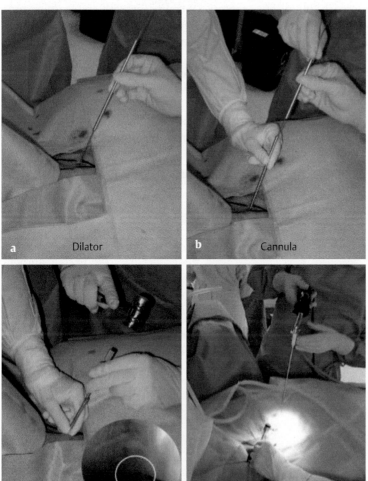

Fig. 23.5 (a–d) Step-by-step changing of nonendoscopic set with the endoscopic set.

thus improving the endoscopic differentiation of anatomical structures. Through the working channel of the endoscope, grasping forceps are inserted to perform a mechanic discectomy; also, authors complemented decompression with RF and thermal discectomy (**Fig. 23.6**). Finally, osteophytes located in the foraminal window are endoscopically removed using a shaver. Sometimes, due to the size of the osteophytes compressing the neural structures, it is necessary to use a chisel (**Fig. 23.7**). Complete decompression is then verified by directly visualizing the released cervical nerve root (**Fig. 23.7**).

Learning Curve

Although with this new approach, injury of vital structures are extremely uncommon, it is very important to consider the presence of relevant anatomic structures in the neck anterior zone. The surgeon must be mindful of the applied surgical anatomy in the anterior cervical area. An important factor to achieve a successful technic is appropriate and sufficient training. The learning curve

of the procedure is steep, and the outcomes are directly related to the skills of the surgeon. The authors recommend beginning performing 20 to 30 cases of MISS nonendoscopic and endoscopic techniques on lumbar area; thereafter, performing 10 to 15 cases of nonendoscopic cervical technics such as cervical thermodiscoplasty, and performing endoscopic techniques for nonextruded hernias under the supervision of an experienced surgeon. Finally, with total confidence about the technics and with the complete set of instruments, the surgeon must be able to perform a cervical endoscopic foraminotomy. Also, authors strongly suggest making more cadaver laboratories and workshops, and visiting fellowships on spine and training centers. Of course, as with any learning process, it is important to have adequate patience and perseverance.[18] Throughout their experience, they have realized about the importance of properly choosing patients, making constant training processes and cadaveric specimens, and advancing the selection and use of improved technologies. These should be considered and integrated into surgical

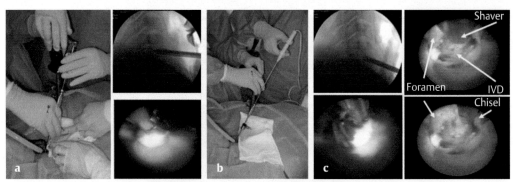

Fig. 23.6 (**a–c**) Endoscopic decompression with forceps, radiofrequency, shaver, and chisel.

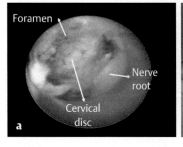

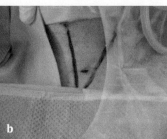

Fig. 23.7 (**a**) Free nerve root and (**b**) wound incision after surgery.

residency and fellowship spine training programs, as it is a timely fit with the ongoing demand of patients and payers alike for less complicated, cost-effective, and reliable solutions to treat cervical radiculopathy.[19]

It is also important to have the necessary and sufficient equipment for performing the technique; although it is a minimally invasive technique, it remains a highly complex surgery. Of course, one of the most important aspects that directly affect the success of surgery is the human resources, so there must be a surgical team which is trained, updated and, possibly, constant. Authors' team of orthopedists and neurosurgeons have started in 1993.

Clinical Outcomes

Endoscopic technique through an anterior approach for cervical radiculopathy was introduced in Latin America by the authors in October 1997. Until 2020, a total of 232 procedures on 169 patients (1 to 3 levels per patient) were performed. The main indication for the procedure was degenerative disc disease and disc hernia among 94.39% (219/232). Specifically, for the treatment of lateral stenosis, a total of 13 (4.9%) procedures have been performed until August 2019.

MacNab criteria, VAS, and neck disability index (NDI) were used to evaluate clinical outcomes. At 12 months follow-up with MacNab criteria, 90% of patients were rated to have had excellent and good outcomes; fair and poor outcomes were reported by 7% and 3% of patients, respectively. In Vernon and Moir's NDI (a cervical modification of Oswestry low back pain index), the authors obtained excellent and good improvement of their neck and arm pain in 66% of patients; poor improvement of symptoms was reported by 34% of patients. Finally, the VAS score (1 no pain to 10 worst pain possible) on average was reported; preoperatively 8 and postoperatively 2. In this cervical stenosis series, no intraoperative or postoperative relevant complications or reoperations associated with the procedure occurred.

Clinical Case

A 33-year-old male patient presented to us with a 2 years history of radiated right arm pain. He is an elite high-performance weightlifter, and 1 year before, he participated in the 2008 Beijing Olympics, suffering an adverse result in the form of an intense wrist-arm pain. After that, he returned to Colombia and was diagnosed a C6–C7 cervical hernia (**Fig. 23.8**). His doctors proposed him an AECD, but he reiterated his strong wish to

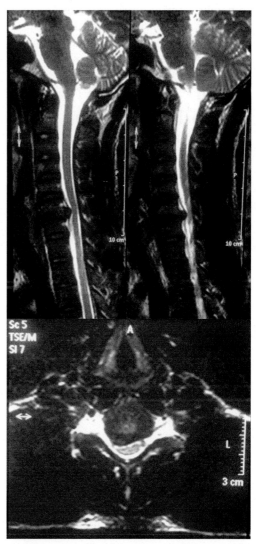

Fig. 23.8 T2 sequence of cervical MRI revealed the presence of IDH at C6–C7 level.

return to competing on London Olympic Games in 2012. The authors' team proposed an anterior endoscopic spine surgery. Under local anesthesia and sedation, they performed a full-endoscopic discectomy in C6–C7 IVD. The patient was discharged on the same day. MRI performed at 4-week postsurgery showed a complete disc decompression; then, he started his normal training. He began participating in professional competitions at 10 months postsurgery. At 40 months from surgery, he participated in London Olympic Games 2012 and won the silver medal; also he obtained the Olympic record in "clean & jerk" in his category: 62 kg. At 48 months follow-up, MRI showed a relief of arm pain and a complete decompression (**Fig. 23.9**).

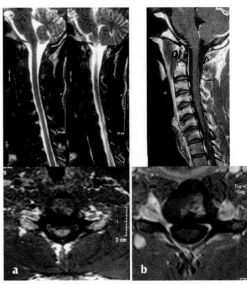

Fig. 23.9 Postoperative MRI showing complete decompression of cervical disc herniation at 1 month (**a**) and at 48 months (**b**).

Anterior Endoscopic Cervical Approach for OPLL and CSM

Ossification of the posterior longitudinal ligament (OPLL) has been described as a common disease in East Asian countries.[20] Here, in Latin America, at least in the authors' experience, they do not have any cases. For cases of severe CSM, the use of AECD is contraindicated. Nevertheless, recently some authors described the feasibility of the use of an anterior endoscopic approach for OPLL and CSM using anterior full-endoscopic percutaneous transcorporeal procedure.[6,21] The approach has been successfully used in a case report of OPLL,[6] and in a study with 2 years follow-up for single segment CSM.[21] It Is clear that there is a need to implement high level of evidence studies.

Conclusion

When one speaks about degenerative spine pathologies, one of the most important factors to be taken into account is the longevity and its global impact. More than ever before, human beings are living longer. Nevertheless, our bodies have a limited capacity, and therefore degenerative diseases begin to appear among the elderly. Older patients with comorbidities are looking for a better quality of life and pain relief treatments. Spine surgeons must be capable to offer more safe, effective and advanced procedures with less associated comorbidities and complications.

Clinical outcomes obtained by the anterior endoscopic cervical technique in the treatment of cervical spondylosis are similar to open conventional techniques in terms of improvement and symptom resolution. When compared with literature, endoscopic anterior approach outcomes are not significantly different from those reported with open or mini-open techniques. With regard to the low complication rate and other advantages of MISS (in terms of decreased length of stay, blood loss, postoperative pain, narcotic utilization, as well as shorter operative times), it is clear that anterior endoscopic cervical foraminotomy is an attractive alternative to open and other MISS techniques.[5,10]

Take-home Points

- Longevity phenomena leads to patients becoming older every day; thus, the age-related degenerative diseases are becoming increasingly common.

- Many of those patients have comorbidities and their surgical management is an important challenge. So, it is necessary to establish safer treatments.

- Current literature suggests that results obtained with different versions of anterior cervical discectomy and foraminotomy techniques are similar to those achieved by anterior endoscopic approaches. Nevertheless, inherent benefits of MISS technics could be a decision factor for the surgeons.

- Anterior cervical endoscopic approach can be a safe alternative for the management of stenosis related with cervical spondylosis.

References

1. McCormick JR, Sama AJ, Schiller NC, Butler AJ, Donnally CJ III. Cervical spondylotic myelopathy: a guide to diagnosis and management. J Am Board Fam Med 2020; 33(2):303–313

2. Li C, Tang X, Chen S, Meng Y, Zhang W. Clinical application of large channel endoscopic decompression in posterior cervical spine disorders. BMC Musculoskelet Disord 2019;20(1):548

3. Yamaguchi S, Mitsuhara T, Abiko M, Takeda M, Kurisu K. Epidemiology and overview of the clinical spectrum of degenerative cervical myelopathy. Neurosurg Clin N Am 2018;29(1):1–12

4. Pingel A, Kandziora F. Anterior decompression and fusion for cervical neuroforaminal stenosis. Eur Spine J 2013;22(3):671–672

5. Ruetten S, Komp M, Merk H, Godolias G. A new full-endoscopic technique for cervical posterior foraminotomy in the treatment of lateral disc herniations using 6.9-mm endoscopes: prospective 2-year results of 87 patients. Minim Invasive Neurosurg 2007; 50(4):219–226

6. Kong W, Xin Z, Du Q, Cao G, Liao W. Anterior percutaneous full-endoscopic transcorporeal decompression of the spinal cord for single-segment cervical spondylotic myelopathy: The technical interpretation and 2 years of clinical follow-up. J Orthop Surg Res 2019; 14(1):461

7. Woods BI, Hilibrand AS. Cervical radiculopathy: epidemiology, etiology, diagnosis, and treatment. J Spinal Disord Tech 2015; 28(5):E251–E259

8. Iyer S, Kim HJ. Cervical radiculopathy. Curr Rev Musculoskelet Med 2016;9(3):272–280

9. Roh JS, Teng AL, Yoo JU, Davis J, Furey C, Bohlman HH. Degenerative disorders of the lumbar and cervical spine. Orthop Clin North Am 2005;36(3):255–262

10. Ramírez León JF, Rugeles Ortíz JG, Martínez CR, Alonso Cuéllar GO, Lewandrowski KU. Surgical treatment of cervical radiculopathy using an anterior cervical endoscopic decompression. J Spine Surg 2020;6 (Suppl 1):S179–S185

11. Childress MA, Becker BA. Nonoperative management of cervical radiculopathy. Am Fam Physician 2016;93(9):746–754

12. Ruetten S, Komp M, Merk H, Godolias G. Full-endoscopic anterior decompression versus conventional anterior decompression and fusion in cervical disc herniations. Int Orthop 2009;33(6):1677–1682

13. Clark JG, Abdullah KG, Steinmetz MP, Benzel EC, Mroz TE. Minimally invasive versus open cervical foraminotomy: a systematic review. Global Spine J 2011;1(1):9–14

14. Ramírez León JF, Rugeles Ortiz JG, Ramírez Martínez C, Osorio Fonseca E, Prada N, Alonso Cuéllar GO. Anterior percutaneous cervical discectomy. Two-year follow-up of a blunt technique procedure. Coluna/Columna 2017;16(4):261–264

15. Ahn Y, Lee SH, Shin SW. Percutaneous endoscopic cervical discectomy: clinical outcome and radiographic changes. Photomed Laser Surg 2005;23(4):362–368

16. Yang JS, Chu L, Chen L, Chen F, Ke ZY, Deng ZL. Anterior or posterior approach of full-endoscopic cervical discectomy for cervical intervertebral disc herniation? A comparative cohort study. Spine 2014;39(21):1743–1750

17. Saringer WF, Reddy B, Nöbauer-Huhmann I, et al. Endoscopic anterior cervical foraminotomy for unilateral radiculopathy: anatomical morphometric analysis and preliminary clinical experience. J Neurosurg 2003;98(2, Suppl):171–180

18. Ramírez León JF, Alonso Cuéllar GO, Rugeles Ortiz JG, Ramírez Martínez C. Multispecialty and multilanguage training in spine surgery: a Latin-American experience. Educ Med 2016; 17:61–66

19. Ramírez León JF. The motivators to endoscopic spine surgery implementation in Latin America. J Spine Surg 2020;6(Suppl 1): S45–S48

20. Stapleton CJ, Pham MH, Attenello FJ, Hsieh PC. Ossification of the posterior longitudinal ligament: genetics and pathophysiology. Neurosurg Focus 2011;30(3):E6

21. Kong W, Ao J, Cao G, Xia T, Liu L, Liao W. Local spinal cord decompression through a full endoscopic percutaneous transcorporeal approach for cervicothoracic ossification of the posterior longitudinal ligament at the T1-T2 level. World Neurosurg 2018; 112:287–293

24 Outcome Measures for Patients with Cervical Spondylotic Myelopathy and OPLL

Eko Agus Subagio, Abdul Hafid Bajamal, Muhammad Faris, and Khrisna Rangga Permana

Introduction

Controversy over which surgery is best for cervical spondylotic myelopathy (CSM) and ossification of posterior longitudinal ligament (OPLL) continues. In determining the benefits of surgery for CSM and OPLL, and various factors that affect outcomes, it is very important to have an objective and reproducible way to measure the patient's disability before and after surgery.[1]

Because CSM and OPLL have similar myelopathic symptoms, they will be discussed together. The authors tried to choose an outcome measure that is often used. Outcome measure instruments have various pressure points such as assessment of function, pain due to physical disability, patient satisfaction, and general health. Hence, the selection of outcome measure instruments should be adjusted according to the corresponding objectives. It is important to assess outcome by comparing patient's condition before and after intervention, or comparing one intervention with others. Favorable outcomes can be used as a measure of the effectiveness and efficiency of an intervention.[2]

Background

We already know the various surgical options for this condition include anterior cervical discectomy and fusion, anterior corpectomy, posterior foraminotomy, laminectomy, laminectomy and fusion, and laminoplasty.

In the assessment of outcome measures of surgical procedures such as decompression of CSM or OPLL, one should avoid subjective assessment by physician's or patient's impressions. Experience has shown the possibility of a mismatch between the expected results of the doctor and the functional results reported by the patient such as pain and activities in daily life.[3,4]

The increasing prevalence of CSM and OPLL, the advancement of new surgical techniques, advances in instrumentation, and the economic impact of treatment require careful evaluation of the results of surgery. The following chapter will present the most widely used posttreatment outcome measures for CSM and OPLL in the literature.[5]

Outcome Measures

Various measurement methods are used by surgeons to measure the progress of the disease, determine the selection of surgical procedures, and find out the results of the surgical procedure.[1] In addition to data of age, sex, and comorbid conditions, clinical picture measurements are needed, which are mostly related to functional measurements. The radiological picture is not included in this paper because it requires a broader explanation.

Many functional outcome measures are used in the literature, but one should ideally choose the one which measures well at each stage of the disease.[3]

Long-distance assessments using telephone, video calls, or other means are important things to consider. There is no single measurement which is perfect, as evaluation may use a combination of several measurements to provide complementary results.

Nurick's grade, short form-36 (SF-36) health survey, myelopathy disability index (MDI), modified Japanese Orthopaedic Association (mJOA) scale, neck disability index (NDI), and the 30-m walking test, are methods that are widely used in CSM and OPLL.[2] We will discuss each one at a time.

Nurick's Grade

Nurick's[6] grade is a functional measurement that measures the degree of disability and the ability to walk. The higher the gradation, the greater the disability rate. Nurick's grade has good reliability, according to Singh and Crockard. Its simplicity, ease of use, and provision of quick ambulatory status compared to other scorings are the advantages of this measurement.[2,7] It also provides quick ambulatory status compared to other scorings. However, it cannot provide complete assessment, so it still needs other scores to assess another domain of functionality. This measurement is also less sensitive in detecting postoperative improvement in CSM patients.[8]

Modified Japanese Orthopaedic Association Scale (mJOA)

The JOA scale is a functional measurement which was developed in 1975, and then modified several times, so that it is patient-oriented. One of those scales was modified by Benzel et al which uses a scale from 0 to 18.[9]

This modified version is the most acceptable version, especially in its psychometric properties, and has a good and moderate correlation with Nurick's grade in preintervention and postintervention period.[8,10,11] This score can be used as supplementary with another score. Sometimes, a disagreement may appear if mJOA scores are compared

to another score.[8] After conducting studies in the mild or moderate CSM group, there was a convergent construct validity of the mJOA with MRI and diffusion tensor imaging (DTI).[11,12]

Short Form-36 (SF-36) Health Survey

The SF-36 survey instrument[13] provides a measurement of functional quality of life. This scale records the patient's health status with regard to the following: mental health, physical functioning, bodily pain, physical role limitations, general health, vitality, social functioning, and emotional role limitations. The lower the score, the greater the handicap. After comparing with other scores, it is found that the SF-36 has proven to be reliable and responsive.[2,14,15]

SF-36 has great validity as an outcome tool after major elective surgery, even though the sensitivity of instruments for detecting small changes in health status remains uncertain.[16] SF-36 has the advantage of assessing outcome after major elective surgery; also, it is simple and easy to administer.[8] SF-36 is culturally sensitive, which means it is easily adapted and translated into different languages across the globe. SF-36 shows adequate data quality, concurrent and discriminant validity, and reliability among populations with different languages in its cross-cultural adaptation and psychometric evaluation.[17]

Neck Disability Index (NDI)

NDI is a modification of the Oswestry low back pain index which consists of a 10-item questionnaire. It measures how everyday activities such as reading, driving, working, and sleeping, are affected by neck pain. The higher the value, the more severe the condition. NDI has been validated in patients undergoing neck surgery. In a recent study, NDI and JOA have also been validated in patients with cervical myelopathy or radiculopathy with strong repeat tests.[2,18]

NDI has a good correlation with other scores. It has good sensitivity, convergent validity, and is associated with scores before and after the intervention. However, the sensitivity of measuring emotional states still requires further research.[19]

The most commonly used measures to quantify CSM are JOA scale and Nurick's grade, but they are not adequate for mild disease. The shortcoming in Nurick's grade is that it relies too much on mobility and employment of the patient.[2] SF-36 and NDI are used to evaluate improvement after surgery as the most commonly used self-report measure for neck pain.[20]

Myelopathy Disability Index (MDI)

This scale specifically describes the strength and quality of hand and foot movements in everyday life with the help of 10 items. The higher the handicap, the higher the score. It has proven validity, reliability, and responsiveness in studies. MDI was reported to have high sensitivity to detect postsurgical outcome.[1,2,7]

MDI is capable of providing prognostic information and can serve as the basis for future studies comparing surgical outcomes between different surgical groups and treatment options. MDI provides responsiveness in specific measures following surgery. However, MDI does not evaluate emotional state and quality of life.[21]

The 30-m Walking Test (30MWT)

This is a quantitative and objective test that was developed in 1999. This test assesses the ability of a person to stand alone from a sitting position and then walk 15 meters to measure the ability and speed of walking, turning, and walking backward as fast as possible. Measurements are based on the time taken and the number of steps indicated. Good convergent validity was found with SF-36v2 PCS, mJOA, and Nurick's scale.[2] Gait analysis has also been proven to be a valid and reliable outcome measurement tool in patients

undergoing surgery for CSM.[22,23] The 30MWT does not have high overall responsiveness, but it is significantly improved in severe myelopathy evaluation. Language is not a barrier for this measure. It provides additional gait evaluation, even though it cannot replace Nurick's grade and mJOA Score.[24]

Conclusion

Spine care management involves complex multidimensional variables, which will certainly have an impact on many aspects including financing, so we need a tool that can measure the outcome of an intervention. Various outcome parameters for myelopathy due to cervical stenosis are available. It takes careful selection of outcomes measurement, including validity, reliability, simplicity, and ease of use. No single existing scale is ideal; further development needs to be carried out continuously, especially aimed at unresolved clinical problems.

Take-home Points

- No single existing scale is ideal. It is recommended to use a combination of functional measures with quantitative measures to evaluate the development of the patient both before surgery and as a postsurgical follow-up. From the available functional outcome measures in the literature, Nurick's scale, JOA, SF-36 scale, NDI, and MDI, have been shown to be valid and reliable in assessing patients undergoing intervention for CSM and OPLL. Further development of outcome measures needs to be carried out continuously.

References

1. Casey ATH, Bland JM, Crockard HA. Development of a functional scoring system for rheumatoid arthritis patients with cervical myelopathy. Ann Rheum Dis 1996; 55(12):901–906
2. Zileli M, Maheshwari S, Kale SS, Garg K, Menon SK, Parthiban J. Outcome measures

and variables affecting prognosis of cervical spondylotic myelopathy: WFNS Spine Committee Recommendations. Neurospine 2019;16(3):435–447

3. Singh A, Tetreault L, Casey A, Laing R, Statham P, Fehlings MG. A summary of assessment tools for patients suffering from cervical spondylotic myelopathy: a systematic review on validity, reliability and responsiveness. Eur Spine J 2015;24(Suppl 2):209–228

4. Singh A, Gnanalingham KK, Casey AT, Crockard A. Use of quantitative assessment scales in cervical spondylotic myelopathy—survey of clinician's attitudes. Acta Neurochir (Wien) 2005;147(12):1235–1238, discussion 1238

5. Holly LT, Matz PG, Anderson PA, et al; Joint Section on Disorders of the Spine and Peripheral Nerves of the American Association of Neurological Surgeons and Congress of Neurological Surgeons. Functional outcomes assessment for cervical degenerative disease. J Neurosurg Spine 2009;11(2):238–244

6. Nurick S. The pathogenesis of the spinal cord disorder associated with cervical spondylosis. Brain 1972;95(1):87–100

7. Singh A, Crockard HA. Comparison of seven different scales used to quantify severity of cervical spondylotic myelopathy and post-operative improvement. J Outcome Meas 2001-2002;5(1):798–818

8. Revanappa KK, Rajshekhar V. Comparison of Nurick grading system and modified Japanese Orthopaedic Association scoring system in evaluation of patients with cervical spondylotic myelopathy. Eur Spine J 2011;20(9):1545–1551

9. Benzel EC, Lancon J, Kesterson L, Hadden T. Cervical laminectomy and dentate ligament section for cervical spondylotic myelopathy. J Spinal Disord 1991;4(3):286–295

10. Kopjar B, Tetreault L, Kalsi-Ryan S, Fehlings M. Psychometric properties of the modified Japanese Orthopaedic Association scale in patients with cervical spondylotic myelopathy. Spine 2015;40(1):E23–E28

11. Furlan JC, Kalsi-Ryan S, Kailaya-Vasan A, Massicotte EM, Fehlings MG. Functional and clinical outcomes following surgical treatment in patients with cervical spondylotic myelopathy: a prospective study of 81 cases. J Neurosurg Spine 2011; 14(3):348–355

12. Ellingson BM, Salamon N, Grinstead JW, Holly LT. Diffusion tensor imaging predicts functional impairment in mild-to-moderate cervical spondylotic myelopathy. Spine J 2014;14(11):2589–2597

13. Ware JE Jr, Sherbourne CD. The MOS 36-item short-form health survey (SF-36). I. Conceptual framework and item selection. Med Care 1992;30(6):473–483

14. King JT Jr, Roberts MS. Validity and reliability of the short form-36 in cervical spondylotic myelopathy. J Neurosurg 2002; 97(2, Suppl): 180–185

15. Guilfoyle MR, Seeley H, Laing RJ. The Short Form 36 health survey in spine disease—validation against condition-specific measures. Br J Neurosurg 2009; 23(4):401–405

16. Mangione CM, Goldman L, Orav EJ, et al. Health-related quality of life after elective surgery: measurement of longitudinal changes. J Gen Intern Med 1997;12(11): 686–697

17. Mbada CE, Adeogun GA, Ogunlana MO, et al. Translation, cross-cultural adaptation and psychometric evaluation of yoruba version of the short-form 36 health survey. Health Qual Life Outcomes 2015;13:141

18. Gupte G, Peters CM, Buchowski JM, Zebala LP. Reliability of the Neck Disability Index and Japanese Orthopedic Association questionnaires in adult cervical radiculopathy and myelopathy patients when administered by telephone or via online format. Spine J 2019;19(7):1154–1161

19. Howell ER. The association between neck pain, the Neck Disability Index and cervical ranges of motion: a narrative review. J Can Chiropr Assoc 2011;55(3):211–221

20. Kalsi-Ryan S, Singh A, Massicotte EM, et al. Ancillary outcome measures for assessment of individuals with cervical spondylotic myelopathy. Spine 2013; 38(22, Suppl 1): S111–S122

21. Tamimi AF, Juweid M. Epidemiology and outcome of glioblastoma. In: De Vleeschouwer S, ed. Glioblastoma. Brisbane: Codon Publications; 2017

22. Singh A, Crockard HA. Quantitative assessment of cervical spondylotic myelopathy

by a simple walking test. Lancet 1999; 354(9176):370–373

23. Kuhtz-Buschbeck JP, Jöhnk K, Mäder S, Stolze H, Mehdorn M. Analysis of gait in cervical myelopathy. Gait Posture 1999;9(3): 184–189

24. Bohm PE, Fehlings MG, Kopjar B, et al. Psychometric properties of the 30-m walking test in patients with degenerative cervical myelopathy: results from two prospective multicenter cohort studies. Spine J 2017;17(2):211–217

25 Enhanced Recovery after Surgery (ERAS) Spine Care Pathways for Cervical Spondylotic Myelopathy and OPLL

Scott C. Robertson

Introduction

Enhanced recovery after surgery (ERAS) proposes a multimodal, evidence-based approach to perioperative care. Numerous specialties have implemented ERAS programs across the globe, providing a foundation for spine surgeons to begin the process themselves. ERAS pathways have been shown to help reduce complications, hospital length of stay (LOS), 30-day readmission rates, pain scores, and ultimately surgical costs while improving patient satisfaction scores and outcomes in multiple surgical subspecialties.[1-6] Over the last few years, a significant number of papers have been addressing ERAS pathways for spinal surgery.[7-19] The majority have addressed the lumbar spine.[9,20-26] The number of cervical ERAS pathways have been limited.[27,28] There are currently several spine programs that have begun the implementation process, incorporating principles and interventions to various spine surgical procedures. Although differences in implementation across programs exist, there are a few common elements that promote a successful enhanced recovery approach.[11,16,23,25,29-32] This chapter will describe a framework for the development and implementation of ERAS pathway for patients undergoing cervical surgery for spondylotic myelopathy and ossified posterior longitudinal ligament (OPLL).

ERAS Pathway for Cervical Spondylotic Myelopathy and OPLL

The spine ERAS pathway provides a guide for the patient's journey. ERAS pathways are generally divided into three phases: preoperative, perioperative, and postoperative. Within these phases, they can be further divided into prehospital, preoperative, intraoperative, postoperative and postdischarge phases (**Table 25.1**).

Prehospital and Preoperative Phase

The prehospital/ preoperative phase is to maximize the physical and functional status of the patient prior to surgical intervention as well as to engage and educate the patient about surgical expectations. The timeline for this portion of the ERAS is variable for each patient and can range from days to weeks.

Patient Education

Once the patient has elected to proceed with surgery, the educational process begins. The surgical procedure and expectations are reviewed with the patient. Surgical risk, benefits, and alternatives are explained as part of a typical informed consent. Several preoperative educational topics covered are reiterated

Table 25.1 Cervical ERAS phases

Prehospital phase	Preoperative phase	Intraoperative phase	Postoperative phase	Postdischarge phase
Medical clearance	Limited fasting light meal up to 6 hrs	Opioid sparing/ multimodal anesthesia	Early mobilization	Minimal Restriction of ADL
Patient optimization			Early diet	
Patient education	Carbohydrate beverage up to 2 hrs preop	Surgical safety checklist	Discontinue IVF	Phone follow-up
Expectation setting			Discontinue drains and foley	Scheduled follow-up visit
Nutritional instructions	Initiation of multimodal analgesia	Minimal invasive surgical techniques	Bowel regimen	Home health/PT
Pain management plan	Chlorhexidine skin cleaning	Nausea/vomiting prophylaxis	Multimodal analgesia	Reduction of multimodal analgesia
Cervical assessment testing	Preemptive anti-nausea medication	Avoid catheters and drains	Early PT/OT evaluation	Resource for questions, either written, hotline, digital app.
		Normothermia	Discharge planning	
	Review procedure with patient/ family	Normovolemia	Patient education on wound care, activity, and medications	Outcome assessment
Prehabilitation		Local analgesia		
Orthotic fitting		Limited muscle relaxant		
Preop surgical checklist	Antibiotics	Vancomycin powder in wound	Schedule follow-up	
RAPT	DVT prophylaxis			
Postop medications review				

Abbreviations: ADL, activities of daily living; ERAS; enhanced recovery after surgery; OT, occupational therapy; PT, physical therapy; RAPT, risk assessment and prediction tool.

during the perioperative and postoperative phases to reinforce the information. Group preoperative clinics to cover the educational topics can help save time in a busy clinic. Patients scheduled for similar surgeries will meet with the surgeon, nurse, and other members of the team, including anesthesia providers and physical therapist (PT).

The pathways include information about necessary appointments and consultations prior to surgery, postoperative expectations and disposition, preadmission testing, perioperative eating and drinking, surgical site care, postoperative medications, physical restrictions, orthotic care, postoperative discharge needs, and appointments.

A detailed clinical assessment should always be interpreted in conjunction with supplemental assessment tools, including imaging, electrodiagnostic tools, and standardized disease-specific assessment tools. Some useful cervical assessment tools include the myelopathy disability index, Japanese Orthopaedic Association (JOA) score, Short Form-36 (SF-36), and neck disability index (NDI) to help discussions on outcome expectations after surgery and determine postoperative rehabilitation planning.[33–36]

Medical Clearance and Optimization

Preoperative preparation should include smoking cessation and alcohol reduction. Smoking is a well-established risk factor for nonunion in spinal fusions. Smoking cessation can decrease risk of infection, perioperative respiratory problems, and wound complications. Weight loss in obese patients is encouraged. Holding antiplatelet and anticoagulation medications are needed prior to surgery. Obstructive sleep apnea (OSA) management is important in cervical surgery.

Nutrition is a modifiable risk factor which can be optimized. Checking albumin is important, since hypoalbuminemia is a predictor of complications. In addition, low prealbumin, retinol-binding protein and transferrin levels are associated with increased infection risk.[37] Diabetes is also associated with poor postoperative outcomes affecting wound healing and increased infections. Tight glycemic control prior to spinal surgery is recommended. Other things to consider are calcium and vitamin D supplements in osteopenic patients and erythropoietin treatment in anemic patients prior to surgery.

Surgical site wound care, including preoperative cleaning with antimicrobial solution (chlorohexidine gluconate), reduces bacterial skin flora and helps reduce wound infections.

Pain Management Plan

Screen for chronic opioid users who are analgesic-tolerant and drug-dependent. Chronic opioid users undergoing spinal surgery have been found to have worse outcomes compared to those who do not use opioids preoperatively. Opioid tolerant patients experience greater acute pain and slower resolution of pain despite therapeutic doses.[38,39] Pain is common and expected after surgery. Developing realistic expectations and a treatment plan is important. Inform patients of the possibility of dysphagia, incisional pain, cervical muscle tension, and persistent neurogenic pain. Postoperative prescriptions are placed for patients to pick up before surgery and have available when they get home. This prevents any delays in their medication regimen and assures the medications are available prior to the surgery.

Prehabilitation

Preoperative physical therapy or rehabilitation, also known as prehabilitation, is practiced, accelerating the recovery process. Therapy prehabilitation is designed to build up muscle activity, promote the importance of physical activity, and provide equipment to improve independence where required. Cervical range of motion (ROM) exercises and strengthening may improve postoperative functional recovery. The patients begin early mobilization and exercising right after surgery; thus, preventing any delays waiting for physical therapy referrals. A postoperative plan for gradual increase in activity is reviewed and limitations are provided to the patient.

Cervical Collar Care and Instructions

When cervical collars are used, fitting and care instructions are performed preoperatively. This allows for proper fitting while the patient is not in pain and can concentrate on the instructions. Patients are instructed to bring the devices to surgery, in order to prevent delays in postoperative mobilization of the patient. The nursing team and therapist should all be aware of proper fitting and use of cervical collars.

Preoperative Surgical Checklist

Communication with the operating room team in advance to assure equipment and supplies are available for the procedure is essential. A basic checklist, which can be modified to individual surgical techniques, is provided (**Box 25.1**). Items among the checklist include surgical table, fixation frames, and equipment; imaging including fluoroscopy, O-arm, and neuronavigation, if needed; scheduling of neuromonitoring and other ancillary services; and contacting instrument companies for implants to be available. For surgical revision, obtain old operative reports and equipment for revision if needed. Any special medications from pharmacy or the

---

> **Box 25.1 Preoperative checklist for enhanced recovery after surgery (ERAS)**
>
> - OR equipment.
> - Surgical implants and vendors.
> - Ancillary services nerve monitoring, blood bank, pharmacy.
> - Surgical supplies and medications.
> - Radiology needs—fluoroscopy, O-arm, neuronavigation.
> - Outside records and operative reports, if indicated.

blood bank should be conveyed. This pre-planning will reduce surgical time and reduce omissions in the intraoperative pathway.

Discharge Planning

The risk assessment and prediction tool (RAPT) can determine if patient will be returning home or will require discharge to a secondary facility.[40] The expected hospital stay and discharge process is reviewed with the family. In addition, postoperative wound care, medications, and activities are reviewed, and follow-up appointments discussed. These discussions prior to surgery will facilitate the patient and family's expectations postoperatively and prevent readmissions.

Perioperative Phase

The perioperative phase focuses on the time of admission, the intraoperative period, and the immediate postoperative period. Having standardized perioperative protocols for elective surgery has been shown to reduce LOS and complications.[41] Preoperatively, meet with the patient and family to review the surgical procedure and sign consent. Also, providing family with an estimate of surgical and recovery time will help reduce the anxiety while waiting.

Immediately prior to surgery, communication with OR team members to confirm all equipment, medications, instruments, and supplies are available is essential. In addition, surgeons should review the anesthesia plan,

emphasizing a multimodal analgesia regimen with providers. Confirm all ancillary services including nursing, surgical technicians, radiology, pharmacy, and blood banks are prepared. Perioperative antibiotics, sequential compression devices (SCD), and prevention of hypothermia are a standard part of all surgeries.

Nutrition

Prolonged fasting is avoided, because it has been proven to exert negative effects on the metabolism and musculature. The use of carbohydrate supplements has been found to be safe, reducing the physiologic stress that fasting has on the body. Limited fasting of light meal up to 6 hours preoperatively are the new guidelines, with a carbohydrate beverage up to 2 hours preoperative.[42]

Analgesia

A multimodal analgesia regimen is used to help reduce postoperative pain and reduce opioid usage. Preemptive analgesia aims to prevent postoperative pain through a multimodal approach. Medications include regional anesthesia, nonsteroidal anti-inflammatory drugs (NSAIDs), opioids, anticonvulsants, and acetaminophen. Initially, acetaminophen and gabapentin were administered preoperatively. General anesthesia with endotracheal intubation to secure the airway with total intravenous anesthesia (TIVA) is used intraoperatively with propofol, ketamine, ketorolac, lidocaine, antiemetics, opioids, and permissible inhalation agents.

Some specific recommendations include gabapentin 600 mg immediately preoperative, scopolamine patches for nausea for those with history of postoperative nausea, and IV acetaminophen 975 mg every 6 hours for 24 hours. Dexamethasone 6 to 10 mg IV is routinely used even in diabetic patients. Standard use of local anesthetics such as bupivacaine or extended release (exparel) bupivacaine can be used at the time of closure of the wound. In posterior cervical approach cases, an additional deep layer injection along the facet joints and muscle layer will help reduce pain. Muscle relaxants like valium and cyclobenzaprine, ketamine and ketorolac are also used as adjuncts for pain reduction. Judicious use of intravenous fluids (IVF) should be used to prevent fluid overload. In the immediate postoperative recovery, nursing should continue with multimodal pain management and limit opioid usage to reduce nausea, sedation, and prevent early mobilization of patient.

Surgery

Cervical spondylotic myelopathy (CSM) and OPLL may be treated with either an anterior or posterior approach. There are advantages and disadvantages to both approaches. In addition, newer minimally invasive techniques have been developed utilizing both approaches. The surgical approach selected will be determined, based on the pathology and surgeon preference. In either case, a standardized surgical approach should be used, which all team members are familiar with. The detailed surgical steps are beyond the scope of this chapter. Patients are positioned and padded appropriately to reduce secondary injuries and cautery pads applied. Individual items can be added or deleted to basic pathways, depending on the surgical approach selected. Minimally invasive approaches can improve outcomes, and reduce hospital stay and narcotics usage. A surgical safety checklist is recommended to help standardize the procedure and reduce complications and errors (**Box 25.2**). All attempts to reduce surgical time, blood loss, and tissue trauma will improve outcomes. Injection of wound with local anesthetic prior to wound closure is useful in managing postoperative pain and earlier patient mobilization. Application of vancomycin powder to reduce infections has been recommended. If excessive blood loss is expected, tranexamic acid has been reported to reduce blood loss during surgery. Skin closure with medical glues provide a waterproof barrier, which can facilitate wound healing, reduce infections, and make wound care easier.

Neurologic status should be assessed in the operating room or immediately upon arrival to the postoperative care unit. Communication with the family to update them on completion of the surgery, patient disposition, and time in recovery is conveyed. Many hospitals have implemented electronic notifications through monitors, pagers, or smartphones, which can facilitate this. The importance of early mobilization, multimodal pain management, and resumption of activities of daily living (ADLs) is reiterated to the patient and family members.

Postoperative Phase

Nutrition

Early dietary intake encouraged and chewing gum has been found to reduce postoperative ileus and increase intestinal motility.[43–46]

Box 25.2 Surgical safety checklist for enhanced recovery after surgery (ERAS)

- Confirm patient and procedure.
- Confirm patient preoperative imaging.
- Preop antibiotics given and antibiotic irrigation used intraoperatively.
- Neuromonitoring assessment.
- Confirmation of surgical levels.
- Surgical decompression/stabilization.
- Secure hemostasis and minimize drain placement.
- Vancomycin powder application.
- Local anesthetic.
- Time-out to confirm all indicated procedures completed and sponge counts are correct.
- Final postoperative imaging and wound closure.

Regular use of stool softeners is ordered. Dysphagia from cervical surgery can be a problem, so speech pathology referral and appropriate dietary recommendations should be followed to reduce aspiration risk. Fluid overload should be avoided. IVFs should be stopped once taking oral liquids or 4 hours after surgery.

Respiratory Management

Early incentive spirometry is started in the postoperative area. Spirometry is recommended every hour when awake to reduce atelectasis. Patients are encouraged to continue regular spirometry for 3 days postoperatively. Early mobilization including walking up to chair for meals will improve respiratory status. Identify any patients with sleep apnea or additional respiratory needs. Breathing treatments should be provided as needed. Close observation of the neck is essential to identify any wound swelling which could compromise the airway. Hematomas, particularly in anterior cervical approaches, can be life-threatening complications, which need to be addressed emergently.

Wound Care

Wounds need to be checked and redressed daily. If medical glue is used on the wound ointments, soap should be avoided, which can cause early breakdown of the glue. Wound should be kept clean and dry. A standardized wound care protocol should be established for inpatients. These same wound care and bathing instructions should be reviewed and provided in a written form for discharge home. Specific care instructions for wound care and bathing should be provided to post-acute care facilities, including rehabilitation and skilled nursing facilities. Cervical collar care and usage should also be provided.

Mobility

Postoperative fear of movement is strongly associated with pain, disability, and physical recovery. Addressing the fear of movement and expectations after surgery will help prepare the patient for early mobilization in the perioperative and postoperative phases. Early mobilization has significant benefits in the postoperative recovery.[47] A mobility plan with input from nursing and physical therapy should be developed to have better compliance. Postoperative mobility is encouraged 2 hours after surgery including walking in halls, to the bathroom, and up to chair for meals. Early discontinuation of all drains, IVF and SCDs will allow for easier mobilization of the patients. Ambulatory assist devices/walkers should be provided early in the postsurgical phase and assessment of home needs reevaluated.

Analgesia

Traditional postoperative patient controlled analgesic pumps using opioids is discouraged. Multimodal analgesic will continue until discharge. Explain to patients that pain is normal and review treatments are available to reduce pain. Regularly scheduled doses of acetaminophen, anti-inflammatories, gabapentin, and muscle relaxants can manage most pain. Opioids should be used sparingly for breakthrough pain. It is important for the nursing staff and patients to differentiate types of pain (incisional, muscle, nerve) they are experiencing, so the appropriate medications for treatment can be used. Cryotherapy in the form of ice packs or cooling devices can be used to help reduce neck pain and swelling. Early paracervical and periscapular muscle ROM is encouraged to reduce muscle tension. Additional dexamethasone can be used 2 to 3 days postoperatively to reduce pain and swelling. Continuing a scheduled multimodal analgesic plan for the first week postoperatively can keep most pain under control. Postoperative access to medical providers for issues pertaining to pain or other questions is essential to reduce complications and prevent readmissions.

Physical Therapy (PT)/Occupational Therapy (OT)

Many patients with cervical myelopathy and hand weakness benefit from additional therapy services. PT and OT referrals are initiated on day of surgery. Home needs including walkers, elevated toilet seats, grabbers, and accessibility needs are determined and provided prior to discharge; case management evaluation for support services and discharge planning initiated. When the disposition of patients require inpatient rehabilitation services or skilled nursing facility, postoperative care instructions should be shared with them. These facilities should continue the ERAS pathway with an emphasis on early mobilization, wound care, and multimodal analgesic to reduce pain. Scheduled surgical follow-ups should be kept.

Discharge Planning

Education including collar instructions, wound care, medications, activity level, and follow-up appointments are reviewed. In addition, numbers to contact for questions and postoperative appointments provided. These educational sessions can be held in a group setting for several patients when time and resources are limited. This information can be provided in a booklet the patient receives or through websites or smartphone applications.

Postdischarge Phase

Patients will continue with home health if indicated. Physical therapy regimen either at home or as an outpatient is usually recommended for 4 to 6 weeks. Longer treatment may be needed for patients with significant cervical disease or cord injury. Each patient should be contacted the next day after discharge by phone and then seen in the office for a 2-week wound check. Close monitoring of symptoms or changes in health should be conveyed to the surgeon's office and assistance sought if needed. Dedicated nursing hotline for questions should be established at the hospital or surgeon's office. Patients are encouraged to resume daily activities with minimal restrictions. Outcome assessment can be determined using the same preoperative cervical assessment tools used.

Smartphones can be used to send photos of the wound for evaluation. Some mobile applications can track data, including visual analogue scale (VAS) and vital signs, and provide alerts to patients and physicians.[30] The educational discharge information may also be provided in an electronic format they can retrieve from their phone or computer. The use of e-health is very promising, allowing for personalized 24-hour monitoring, and does not force postoperative problems onto the general practitioner or external emergency services.

Discussion

The traditional approach to surgical spine care emphasized the surgery and did not address some of the pre- and postoperative issues. No standardized pathways existed, which allowed for inconsistent care. Traditional approaches called for overnight fasting and minimal perioperative analgesic management. Spine patients were given controlled analgesia using IV morphine and hydromorphone and oral narcotics. No intraoperative checklists were used to avoid complications and errors of omissions during surgery. Foley catheters and IVFs were continued for days, significantly limiting mobility and increasing infection risk. Ambulation was limited, including mobility out of bed, with meals consumed in bed, resulting in deep venous thrombosis (DVT) and pneumonia. Incentive spirometry and sleep apnea machines were not routinely used. Recent studies have showed all these issues have resulted in more complications, LOS, readmissions and costs. Arnold et al[48] found the complications with the largest effect on LOS in anterior cervical discectomy and fusion (ACDF) surgery was pulmonary, urinary, and cardiac complications. Many of these could have been avoided with earlier intervention and prevention protocols.

Immobility was often encouraged with no set physical therapy instructions or direction for the nursing staff. Patients requiring additional inpatient rehabilitation services were not often identified until a few days postoperatively, leading to delays in referrals and extended LOS. Opioid-related adverse drug events have been shown to occur in over 13% of patients undergoing surgery.[49] These adverse events lead to 55% longer LOS, 47% higher cost of care, 36% increased risk of 30-day readmission, and 3.4 times higher risk of inpatient mortality.

The use of spinal ERAS pathways has been shown to improve pain scores and patient satisfaction surveys, while reducing complications, hospital LOS, 30-day readmissions and hospital cost.[9,50,51] Soffin et al[28] investigated ERAS for ACDF ($n = 25$) and cervical disc arthroplasty ($n = 8$). Compliance was 85.6%, with patients receiving 18 of 19 ERAS elements. LOS was 416 minutes on average and minimal complications were reported, with no patient requiring readmission in 90 days.

Decreased length of index hospital stay, complications, and readmissions show the economic benefit of ERAS regimens.[52–54] Another benefit of ERAS for spine surgery is related to total cost savings, which accompany streamlined and less invasive methods. Wang et al[26,55] reported savings of $3442 or 15.2% per procedure with the application of ERAS methods, including endoscopic decompression versus traditional TLIF, the anesthetic technique, and liposomal bupivacaine in an acute care setting. In addition, Staartjes et al[16] showed a reduction in nursing cost of 46.8% associated with ERAS protocol reduction in LOS. Operation time after the ERAS protocol was also decreased, showing further means of potential cost-saving. Mathieson et al[39] reported that patients undergoing spine surgery who received an ERAS preoperative regimen of NSAIDs, acetaminophen, and gabapentin with incorporation of intraoperative IV ondansetron and ketamine and a postoperative NSAID course reported greater and earlier mobilization, less opioid use, and decreased nausea and sedation early postoperatively. In addition, LOS was reduced by 2 days for the ERAS intervention group compared with the pre-ERAS cohort.

Minimally invasive surgical techniques represent a logical integration in the ERAS protocol, because it has been shown to improve patient satisfaction and pain scores, minimize complications, and shorten recovery time.[55–58] Moreover, additions such as liposomal bupivacaine, incorporated in Wang and Grossman's study, have been shown to provide patients with extended local analgesia after spine surgery compared with standard preparations of bupivacaine without impairing healing. Incorporation of ERAS methods in spine surgery may also increase potential for transition to outpatient procedures. Alternatively, some protocols used short-acting opioids such as sufentanil to reduce opioid load. Opioid-free anesthesia relies on nonopioid analgesic agents such as propofol, ketamine, and dexmedetomidine and local anesthetic agents to carry out analgesia and anesthesia. Opioid usage in disorders in spine surgery are also associated with higher complication rates, extended hospitalization, and higher total costs. Nonopioid drugs may achieve intraoperative anesthesia, with reduced postoperative nausea, pain, ileus, and LOS.

Variation in spine surgery and patient populations may differ sufficiently to warrant multiple ERAS protocols, depending on indication and intervention. Based on the surgical approach elected to treat CSM, care pathways may need to be customized and outcomes assessed separately. In comparative studies for treatment of multilevel cervical spondylosis and myelopathy, an anterior approach had fewer complications, lower morbidity, and better outcome assessment scores compared to posterior cervical fusions.[59,60] Establishing a modified posterior cervical ERAS pathway may help overcome the shortcomings of this approach.

The current cervical ERAS pathways require a multifaceted team approach to patient care (**Box 25.3**). For the pathways to be effective, it requires the compliance and engagement of all parties, including the patients, surgeon, anesthesia team, nursing staff, and all other providers in each

---

Box 25.3   Cervical enhanced recovery after surgery (ERAS) guidelines

Preoperative

Medical clearance and optimization.

Surgical equipment and implants.

Imaging and laboratory workup.

Patient education– review postop medications, activity, wound care, and expectations.

Perioperative

Preop preparation– antibiotics, pneumatic compression devices, preference cards.

Anesthesia planning

Preemptive analgesia and nausea/vomiting prophylaxis.

Surgical equipment and implants.

Imaging equipment and available imaging.

Pharmaceutical needs/blood bank.

Safety surgical checklist "time out."

Standardized surgical approach.

No drains or foleys; if needed, remove early postoperative day 1 (POD1).

Postoperative

Early oral intake

Early mobilization within 2–4 hours, up to chair for meals.

Incentive spirometry.

Minimize IV fluids; discontinue when taking oral (PO).

Multimodal pain management with minimal narcotic usage.

Early physical therapy (PT)/occupational therapy (OT) evaluation for discharge planning.

Patient education– review postop medications, activity and wound care.

Postoperative monitoring and follow-up in office with surgical team.

---

department of the pathway. Maximal benefits are unlikely if there is noncompliance or poor adoption of the pathways. One of the pillars of spinal ERAS is to make the patient proactive in their surgical care. Education provided before, during, and after the surgery is essential for patient compliance in their recovery process and to improve outcomes.

Implementation of spinal ERAS pathways may need to overcome certain barriers. It is always difficult to fight against conservatism and resistance to the adoption of new procedures or innovations, and ERAS is no exception. Resistance can be found at any level and concerns all stakeholders, from the administrative levels to the healthcare staff. Basic surgical routines such as use of drains and foley catheters, the use of a collar or brace, the timing of discharge, the use of opioids, activity level, transport home in a personal car and driving, and so on can vary greatly and significantly influence the LOS. Collaboration and collegial unification of procedures and protocols of care is an essential step in the development of ERAS. Optimizing the fluidity of the patient pathway is a prerequisite, as is the appropriate postoperative follow-up. The entirety of care is extended and improved even if the physical stay is shortened.

Spine surgery represents a typically invasive intervention, with a protracted recovery phase that often requires rehabilitation and intensive postoperative pain management. Given the benefits of ERAS to decrease complications and improve patient-reported physiologic and psychological states, its incorporation into spine surgery represents a natural transition. In addition, anticipated increases in annual cases of spine surgery from an aging population portends increasing volume of spine surgery. Quantitative quality measures such as patient-reported outcomes have emerged as an objective and increasingly used metric to evaluate surgical success by way of measuring postoperative pain, functional ability, and quality of life after spine surgery. Standardization of ERAS for spine surgery may benefit such patient-reported outcomes, enhance surgeon and patient decision-making, and optimize the rehabilitative course. Opportunities for improved outcomes and decreased complication rates also make spine surgery an appropriate setting for ERAS development.

Conclusion

The literature is growing showing the benefits of spinal ERAS pathways. The primary principles of these ERAS pathways include patient education, multimodal pain management, early mobilization, and surgical techniques to reduce blood loss and reduce tissue destruction. The adoption of these pathways can be easily incorporated into most surgical practices. Because of the recent introduction of ERAS to neurosurgery, a consensus has not yet been reached for evidence-based recommendations of cervical ERAS pathways. Lumbar ERAS pathways are further along in development. This chapter provides a framework for cervical ERAS pathways to build upon. In the future, we predict multiple evidence-based cervical ERAS pathways will be available.

Take-home Points

■ Utilization of Cervical ERAS pathways will help reduce surgical LOS, complications, and hospital cost, while improving patient satisfaction and outcomes.

■ Multimodal pain management helps reduce opioid consumption and the secondary complications associated with narcotics.

■ Successful execution of the cervical ERAS requires a multifaceted team approach to patient care.

References

1. Liu JY, Wick EC. Enhanced recovery after surgery and effects on quality metrics. Surg Clin North Am 2018;98(6):1119–1127
2. Ljungqvist O. Jonathan E. Rhoads lecture 2011: insulin resistance and enhanced recovery after surgery. JPEN J Parenter Enteral Nutr 2012;36(4):389–398
3. Saidian A, Nix JW. Enhanced recovery after surgery: urology. Surg Clin North Am 2018; 98(6):1265–1274
4. Smith HJ, Leath CA III, Straughn JM Jr. Enhanced recovery after surgery in surgical specialties: gynecologic oncology. Surg Clin North Am 2018;98(6):1275–1285
5. Tiernan JP, Liska D. Enhanced recovery after surgery: recent developments in colorectal surgery. Surg Clin North Am 2018; 98(6):1241–1249
6. Zhu S, Qian W, Jiang C, Ye C, Chen X. Enhanced recovery after surgery for hip and knee arthroplasty: a systematic review and meta-analysis. Postgrad Med J 2017; 93(1106):736–742
7. Ali ZS, Ma TS, Ozturk AK, et al. Pre-optimization of spinal surgery patients: Development of a neurosurgical enhanced recovery after surgery (ERAS) protocol. Clin Neurol Neurosurg 2018;164:142–153
8. Angus M, Jackson K, Smurthwaite G, et al. The implementation of enhanced recovery after surgery (ERAS) in complex spinal surgery. J Spine Surg 2019;5(1):116–123

9. Brusko GD, Kolcun JPG, Heger JA, et al. Reductions in length of stay, narcotics use, and pain following implementation of an enhanced recovery after surgery program for 1- to 3-level lumbar fusion surgery. Neurosurg Focus 2019;46(4):E4

10. Carr DA, Saigal R, Zhang F, Bransford RJ, Bellabarba C, Dagal A. Enhanced perioperative care and decreased cost and length of stay after elective major spinal surgery. Neurosurg Focus 2019;46(4):E5

11. Dietz N, Sharma M, Adams S, et al. Enhanced recovery after surgery (ERAS) for spine surgery: a systematic review. World Neurosurg 2019;130:415–426

12. Elsarrag M, Soldozy S, Patel P, et al. Enhanced recovery after spine surgery: a systematic review. Neurosurg Focus 2019;46(4):E3

13. Fleege C, Arabmotlagh M, Almajali A, Rauschmann M. [Pre- and postoperative fast-track treatment concepts in spinal surgery : patient information and patient cooperation]. Orthopade 2014;43(12):1062–1064, 1066–1069

14. Muhly WT, Sankar WN, Ryan K, et al. Rapid recovery pathway after spinal fusion for idiopathic scoliosis. Pediatrics 2016;137(4):e20151568

15. Rao RR, Hayes M, Lewis C, et al. Mapping the road to recovery: shorter stays and satisfied patients in posterior spinal fusion. J Pediatr Orthop 2017;37(8):e536–e542

16. Staartjes VE, de Wispelaere MP, Schröder ML. Improving recovery after elective degenerative spine surgery: 5-year experience with an enhanced recovery after surgery (ERAS) protocol. Neurosurg Focus 2019;46(4):E7

17. Venkata HK, van Dellen JR. A perspective on the use of an enhanced recovery program in open, non-instrumented day surgery for degenerative lumbar and cervical spinal conditions. J Neurosurg Sci 2018;62(3):245–254

18. Wainwright TW, Immins T, Middleton RG. Enhanced recovery after surgery (ERAS) and its applicability for major spine surgery. Best Pract Res Clin Anaesthesiol 2016;30(1):91–102

19. Zhang CH, Yan BS, Xu BS, et al. [Study on feasibility of enhanced recovery after surgery combined with mobile microendoscopic discectomy-transforaminal lumbar interbody fusion in the treatment of lumbar spondylolisthesis]. Zhonghua Yi Xue Za Zhi 2017;97(23):1790–1795

20. Bradywood A, Farrokhi F, Williams B, Kowalczyk M, Blackmore CC. Reduction of inpatient hospital length of stay in lumbar fusion patients with implementation of an evidence-based clinical care pathway. Spine 2017;42(3):169–176

21. Wang MY, Chang HK, Grossman J. Reduced acute care costs with the ERAS® minimally invasive transforaminal lumbar interbody fusion compared with conventional minimally invasive transforaminal lumbar interbody fusion. Neurosurgery 2018;83(4):827–834

22. Dai B, Gao P, Dong QR, et al. [Clinical study of the application of enhanced recovery after surgery in cervical spondylotic myelopathy]. Zhongguo Gu Shang 2018;31(8):740–745

23. Smith J, Probst S, Calandra C, et al. Enhanced recovery after surgery (ERAS) program for lumbar spine fusion. Perioper Med (Lond) 2019;8:4

24. Soffin EM, Wetmore DS, Beckman JD, et al. Opioid-free anesthesia within an enhanced recovery after surgery pathway for minimally invasive lumbar spine surgery: a retrospective matched cohort study. Neurosurg Focus 2019;46(4):E8

25. Soffin EM, Vaishnav AS, Wetmore DS, et al. Design and implementation of an enhanced recovery after surgery (ERAS) program for minimally invasive lumbar decompression spine surgery: initial experience. Spine 2019;44(9):E561–E570

26. Wang MY, Chang PY, Grossman J. Development of an Enhanced Recovery After Surgery (ERAS) approach for lumbar spinal fusion. J Neurosurg Spine 2017;26(4):411–418

27. Li J, Li H, Xv ZK, et al. Enhanced recovery care versus traditional care following laminoplasty: A retrospective case-cohort study. Medicine (Baltimore) 2018;97(48):e13195

28. Soffin EM, Wetmore DS, Barber LA, et al. An enhanced recovery after surgery pathway: association with rapid discharge and minimal complications after anterior cervical spine surgery. Neurosurg Focus 2019;46(4):E9

29. Chakravarthy VB, Yokoi H, Coughlin DJ, Manlapaz MR, Krishnaney AA. Development and implementation of a comprehensive

spine surgery enhanced recovery after surgery protocol: the Cleveland Clinic experience. Neurosurg Focus 2019;46(4):E11

30. Debono B, Corniola MV, Pietton R, Sabatier P, Hamel O, Tessitore E. Benefits of Enhanced Recovery After Surgery for fusion in degenerative spine surgery: impact on outcome, length of stay, and patient satisfaction. Neurosurg Focus 2019;46(4):E6

31. Grasu RM, Cata JP, Dang AQ, et al. Implementation of an Enhanced Recovery After Spine Surgery program at a large cancer center: a preliminary analysis. J Neurosurg Spine 2018;29(5):588–598

32. Nazarenko AG, Konovalov NA, Krut'ko AV, et al. [Postoperative applications of the fast track technology in patients with herniated intervertebral discs of the lumbosacral spine]. Vopr Neirokhir 2016;80(4):5–12

33. Al-Tamimi YZ, Guilfoyle M, Seeley H, Laing RJ. Measurement of long-term outcome in patients with cervical spondylotic myelopathy treated surgically. Eur Spine J 2013; 22(11):2552–2557

34. Cheung WY, Arvinte D, Wong YW, Luk KD, Cheung KM. Neurological recovery after surgical decompression in patients with cervical spondylotic myelopathy—a prospective study. Int Orthop 2008;32(2): 273–278

35. Kalsi-Ryan S, Singh A, Massicotte EM, et al. Ancillary outcome measures for assessment of individuals with cervical spondylotic myelopathy. Spine 2013; 38(22, Suppl 1): S111–S122

36. Salvi FJ, Jones JC, Weigert BJ. The assessment of cervical myelopathy. Spine J 2006; 6(6, Suppl):182S–189S

37. dos Santos Junqueira JC, Cotrim Soares E, Rodrigues Corrêa Filho H, Fenalti Hoehr N, Oliveira Magro D, Ueno M. Nutritional risk factors for postoperative complications in Brazilian elderly patients undergoing major elective surgery. Nutrition 2003; 19(4):321–326

38. Martini ML, Nistal DA, Deutsch BC, Caridi JM. Characterizing the risk and outcome profiles of lumbar fusion procedures in patients with opioid use disorders: a step toward improving enhanced recovery protocols for a unique patient population. Neurosurg Focus 2019;46(4):E12

39. Mathiesen O, Dahl B, Thomsen BA, et al. A comprehensive multimodal pain treatment reduces opioid consumption after multilevel spine surgery. Eur Spine J 2013; 22(9):2089–2096

40. Slover J, Mullaly K, Karia R, et al. The use of the Risk Assessment and Prediction Tool in surgical patients in a bundled payment program. Int J Surg 2017;38:119–122

41. Sivaganesan A, Wick JB, Chotai S, Cherkesky C, Stephens BF, Devin CJ. Perioperative protocol for elective spine surgery is associated with reduced length of stay and complications. J Am Acad Orthop Surg 2019;27(5):183–189

42. Apelbaum J, Agarkar M, Connis RT, et al. Practice Guidelines for Preoperative Fasting and the Use of Pharmacologic Agents to Reduce the Risk of Pulmonary Aspiration: Application to Healthy Patients Undergoing Elective Procedures: An Updated Report by the American Society of Anesthesiologists Task Force on Preoperative Fasting and the Use of Pharmacologic Agents to Reduce the Risk of Pulmonary Aspiration. Anesthesiology 2017;126(3):376–393

43. Charoenkwan K, Matovinovic E. Early versus delayed oral fluids and food for reducing complications after major abdominal gynaecologic surgery. Cochrane Database Syst Rev 2014; (12):CD004508

44. Fujii T, Morita H, Sutoh T, et al. Benefit of oral feeding as early as one day after elective surgery for colorectal cancer: oral feeding on first versus second postoperative day. Int Surg 2014;99(3):211–215

45. Hoshi T, Yamashita S, Tanaka M, Motokawa K, Toyooka H. Early oral intake after arthroscopic surgery under spinal anesthesia. J Anesth 1999;13(4):205–208

46. Yin X, Ye L, Zhao L, Li L, Song J. Early versus delayed postoperative oral hydration after general anesthesia: a prospective randomized trial. Int J Clin Exp Med 2014;7(10): 3491–3496

47. Epstein NE. A review article on the benefits of early mobilization following spinal surgery and other medical/surgical procedures. Surg Neurol Int 2014;5(Suppl 3):S66–S73

48. Arnold PM, Rice LR, Anderson KK, McMahon JK, Connelly LM, Norvell DC. Factors affecting hospital length of stay following anterior cervical discectomy and fusion. Evid Based Spine Care J 2011;2(3):11–18

49. Kessler ER, Shah M, Gruschkus SK, Raju A. Cost and quality implications of opioid-based postsurgical pain control using administrative claims data from a large health system: opioid-related adverse events and their impact on clinical and economic outcomes. Pharmacotherapy 2013;33(4): 383–391

50. Fletcher ND, Shourbaji N, Mitchell PM, Oswald TS, Devito DP, Bruce RW. Clinical and economic implications of early discharge following posterior spinal fusion for adolescent idiopathic scoliosis. J Child Orthop 2014;8(3):257–263

51. Gornitzky AL, Flynn JM, Muhly WT, Sankar WN. A rapid recovery pathway for adolescent idiopathic scoliosis that improves pain control and reduces time to inpatient recovery after posterior spinal fusion. Spine Deform 2016;4(4):288–295

52. Lee L, Feldman LS. Enhanced recovery after surgery: economic impact and value. Surg Clin North Am 2018;98(6):1137–1148

53. Lee L, Mata J, Ghitulescu GA, et al. Cost-effectiveness of enhanced recovery versus conventional perioperative management for colorectal surgery. Ann Surg 2015;262(6): 1026–1033

54. Sanders AE, Andras LM, Sousa T, Kissinger C, Cucchiaro G, Skaggs DL. Accelerated discharge protocol for posterior spinal fusion patients with adolescent idiopathic scoliosis decreases hospital postoperative charges 22%. Spine 2017;42(2):92–97

55. Wang MY, Chang HK, Grossman J. Reduced acute care costs with the ERAS minimally invasive transforaminal lumbar interbody fusion compared with conventional minimally invasive transforaminal lumbar interbody fusion. Neurosurgery 2018;83(4): 827–834

56. Goldstein CL, Macwan K, Sundararajan K, Rampersaud YR. Perioperative outcomes and adverse events of minimally invasive versus open posterior lumbar fusion: meta-analysis and systematic review. J Neurosurg Spine 2016;24(3):416–427

57. Lu VM, Kerezoudis P, Gilder HE, McCutcheon BA, Phan K, Bydon M. Minimally invasive surgery versus open surgery spinal fusion for spondylolisthesis: a systematic review and meta-analysis. Spine 2017;42(3):E177–E185

58. Phan K, Mobbs RJ. Minimally invasive versus open laminectomy for lumbar stenosis: a systematic review and meta-analysis. Spine 2016;41(2):E91–E100

59. Shamji MF, Cook C, Pietrobon R, Tackett S, Brown C, Isaacs RE. Impact of surgical approach on complications and resource utilization of cervical spine fusion: a nationwide perspective to the surgical treatment of diffuse cervical spondylosis. Spine J 2009; 9(1):31–38

60. Veeravagu A, Connolly ID, Lamsam L, et al. Surgical outcomes of cervical spondylotic myelopathy: an analysis of a national, administrative, longitudinal database. Neurosurg Focus 2016;40(6):E11

26 Cervical Sagittal Balance

R. David Fessler, Onur Yaman, and Richard G. Fessler

Introduction

Cervical sagittal balance is an important component of global spinal sagittal balance that has received more attention in recent years. In addition to the contribution to global sagittal balance, compensatory movements within the cervical spine are important for maintaining horizontal gaze. In the context of cervical fusion, this must be taken into account when determining the ideal alignment for permanent fixation. While numerous articles and chapters have been published regarding cervical sagittal balance parameters, there remains a great deal of debate in the field as to which are the most important for the best clinical outcomes.[1]

Cervical Sagittal Alignment Parameters

Important cervical sagittal alignment parameters are:

K-line is the line between the midpoints of the anteroposterior canal diameter at C2 and C7.

Center of gravity (COG) of the head is measured at the anterior margin of the external auditory canal. A plum line drawn vertically from this point is used to measure COG–C7 sagittal vertical axis as well as global spinal sagittal balance (**Fig. 26.1**).

Slope of line of sight is measured as the angle between a line drawn from the inferior margin of the orbit to the superior border of external auditory canal and the horizontal (**Fig. 26.2**).

McGregor's slope is measured as the angle between a line drawn from the posterior superior corner of the hard palate to the opisthion and the horizontal. It is used for measurement of the C0–2 angle (**Fig. 26.3**).

0–2 angle is measured as the angle between McGregor's line and the inferior endplate of C2 (**Fig. 26.4**).

Chin-brow vertical angle (CBVA) is measured as the angle between a line drawn from the chin to the brow and vertical. It is commonly used to determine horizontal gaze (**Fig. 26.5**).

C1 inclination is the angle between a line drawn between the center of the C1 anterior and posterior arches and horizontal (**Fig. 26.6**).

C2 slope is the angle between the inferior endplate of C2 and horizontal (**Fig. 26.6**).

C2–7 sagittal vertical axis (SVA) is measured as the horizontal distance between a plum line drawn vertically at the midpoint of the C2 vertebral body and the posterior superior corner of the C7 vertebral body (**Fig. 26.7**).

COG–C7 SVA is measured as the horizontal distance between a plum line drawn vertically from the anterior border of the external auditory canal and the posterior superior corner of the C7 vertebral body (**Fig. 26.7**).

C7 slope is the angle between the superior endplate of C7 and horizontal. This is often used as a substitute for T1 slope, which is often difficult to visualize on X-ray (**Fig. 26.6**).

T1 slope is the angle between the superior endplate of T1 and horizontal (**Fig. 26.8**).

C2–7 lordosis is the angle between the inferior endplate of C2 and the inferior endplate of C7 (**Fig. 26.9**).

Neck tilt is the angle between vertical and a line from the center of the T1 inferior endplate and the upper end of the sternum (**Fig. 26.10**).

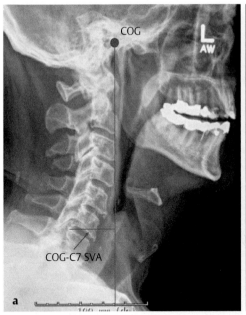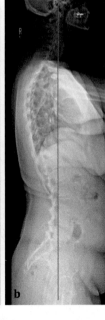

Fig. 26.1 **(a)** Center of gravity of the head (COG) and a vertical plumb line are used to calculate COG–C7 sagittal vertical axis (SVA), **(b)** Global sagittal balance aligns the COG over the femoral heads

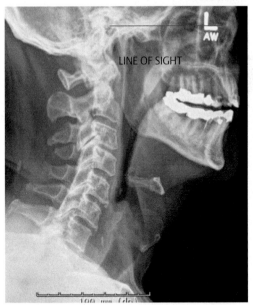

Fig. 26.2 Angle of the line of sight is measured between the line of sight (shown) and horizontal.

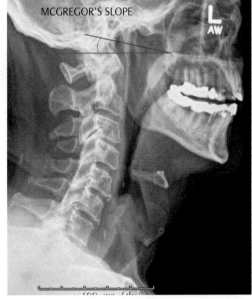

Fig. 26.3 McGregor's slope is measured between McGregor's line and horizontal line.

Thoracic inlet angle (TIA) is the angle between a line perpendicular to the superior endplate of T1 and a line from the center of the T1 inferior endplate and the superior end of the sternum **(Fig. 26.10)**. This may also be calculated as the sum of T1 slope and neck tilt (TIA = T1 slope + neck tilt), similar to the relationship of pelvic incidence (PI) to sacral slope (SS) and pelvic tilt (PT) (PI = SS + PT) **(Fig. 26.11)**.

Cervical tilt is the angle between a line perpendicular to the T1 superior endplate and a

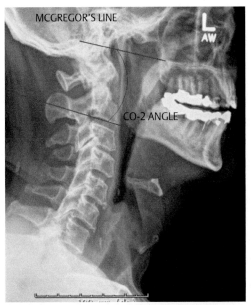

Fig. 26.4 C0–2 angle is measured between McGregor's line and the angle of the inferior endplate of C2.

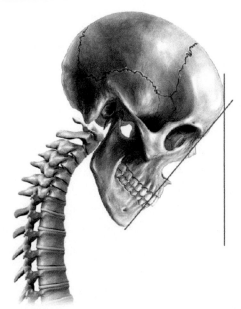

Fig. 26.5 Chin-brow vertical angle (CBVA) is measured between a line from the chin to the brow and vertical.

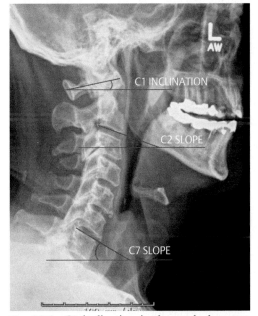

Fig. 26.6 C1 inclination is the angle between C1 and horizontal. C2 slope is the angle between the C2 inferior endplate and horizontal. C7 slope is the angle between the superior endplate of C7 and horizontal.

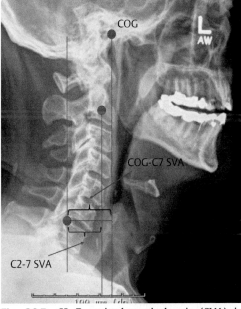

Fig. 26.7 C2–7 sagittal vertical axis (SVA) is measured as the horizontal distance between two plum lines drawn from the center of the C2 vertebral body and posterior superior corner of the C7 vertebral body.

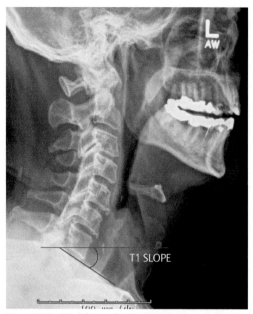

Fig. 26.8 T1 slope is the angle between the superior endplate of T1 and horizontal.

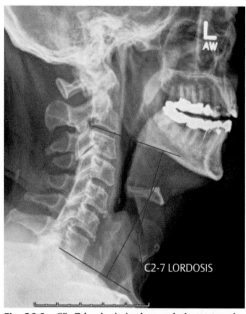

Fig. 26.9 C2–7 lordosis is the angle between the inferior endplate of C2 and the inferior endplate of C7.

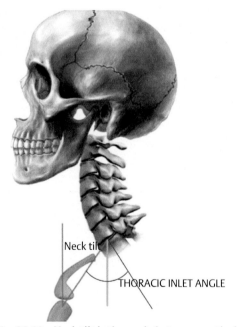

Fig. 26.10 Neck tilt is the angle between vertical and a line from the center of the superior endplate of T1 and superior end of the sternum. Thoracic inlet angle (TIA) is the angle between the line from the center of the superior endplate of T1 to the superior end of the sternum and a line drawn perpendicular to the T1 superior endplate.

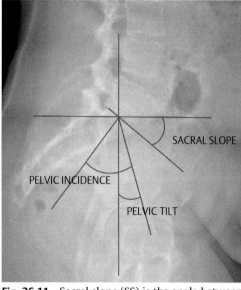

Fig. 26.11 Sacral slope (SS) is the angle between the superior endplate of the S1 and horizontal. Pelvic tilt (PT) is the angle between vertical and a line drawn from the center of the S1 superior endplate and the center of the femoral head. Pelvic incidence (PI) is the angle between a line drawn perpendicular to the S1 superior endplate and the line from the center of the S1 superior endplate to the center of the femoral head.

line from the center of the T1 superior endplate to the tip of the dens. The angle between this same line and vertical is called *cranial tilt* (**Fig. 26.12**).

Normal Sagittal Balance

The mechanical role of the cervical spine may be thought of as reconciling the alignment of the more caudal spine segments, which determine T1 slope, and the need to maintain horizontal gaze as well as maintain the COG of the head above the pelvis. As the cervical spine is the most mobile segment of the spine, it therefore has a wide range of normal

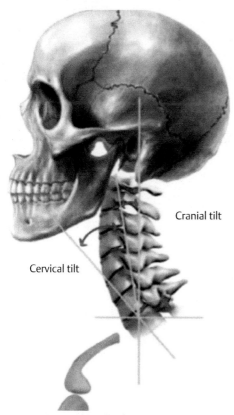

Cranial tilt

Cervical tilt

Fig. 26.12 Cranial tilt is the angle between vertical and a line drawn from the center of the T1 superior endplate to the tip of the dens. Cervical tilt is the angle between a line from the center of the T1 superior endplate to the tip of the dens and a line drawn perpendicular to the T1 superior endplate.

alignment.[2,3] In asymptomatic adults, total cervical lordosis (C1–7) is approximately – 40 degrees. The majority of this lordosis (~75–80%) comes from C1–2, while the lower cervical levels each contribute minimally to overall cervical lordosis, and O–C1 is mildly kyphotic. In fact, in a large cohort meta-analysis, Guo et al showed that only 68% of asymptomatic adults had C2–7 lordotic curvature.[4] However, subaxial lordosis varies significantly based on T1 slope, which is determined by the sagittal alignment of more caudal segments (thoracic kyphosis, lumbar lordosis, pelvic incidence, etc.).[5]

Normal C2–7 SVA should be < 4 cm, and measurements greater than this have been correlated with higher neck disability index (NDI) scores both pre- and postoperatively.[6,7] Normal C7 or T1 slope is approximately 20 degrees and should not be greater than 40 degrees.[1] T1 slope is directly correlated with cervical lordosis, as greater T1 slope requires greater cervical lordosis to maintain horizontal gaze.[1,8] T1 slope is also strongly directly correlated with C2–7 SVA.[1] By association, TIA is also directly correlated with cervical lordosis and C2–7 SVA (TIA = T1 slope + neck tilt).

In aging and elderly patients, degenerative processes lead to loss of lumbar lordosis, pelvic retroversion, increased thoracic kyphosis, and thereby an increase in T1 slope. With this increase in T1 slope, cervical lordosis and C2–7 SVA increase (**Fig. 26.13**).[9,10] If the subaxial cervical segments are unable to compensate for this increased T1 slope, then sagittal balance or horizontal gaze may be compromised. Furthermore, the degree of lordosis required for this compensation may lead to spinal cord tension and myelopathy.[11–13]

Improving Clinical Outcomes

The ability of the cervical spine to compensate for caudal deformity often makes it difficult to assess the nature of cervical spine deformity. It is therefore imperative to obtain

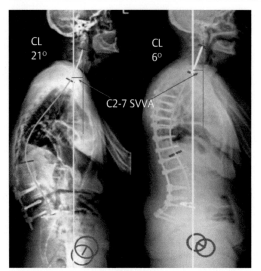

Fig. 26.13 In the aging spine, as T1 slope increases, cervical lordosis and C2–7 sagittal vertical axis (SVA) increase. Correction of thoracolumbar sagittal balance can improve T1 slope, thus decreasing cervical lordosis and C2–7 SVA.

long segment standing X-rays in patients suspected of cervical sagittal imbalance. As cervical sagittal balance is greatly dependent on T1 slope, a thoracic or lumbar procedure to address the primary sagittal deformity may improve T1 slope and resolve the cervical malalignment.[14]

When cervical reconstruction is indicated, the primary goals of the reconstruction should be to obtain a T1 or C7 slope of < 40 degrees and C2–7 SVA of less than 4 cm. Both of these parameters are associated with improved clinical outcomes. Minimal lordosis within the subaxial cervical spine is required for normal alignment as long as T1 slope is < 40 degrees. Care should be taken not to provide significant lordosis at these levels, as hyperlordosis may not only lead to spinal cord tension but may also interfere with functional downward gaze, particularly if the fusion extends to the occiput. This may lead to falls from a patient's inability to watch their feet, often in the setting of myelopathy.

Conclusion

Cervical sagittal balance is an important component of global spinal sagittal balance, and as the most mobile segment of the spine, it is responsible for reconciling the alignment of the thoracolumbar spine with the requirements of horizontal gaze and maintaining the COG of the head over the pelvis. While numerous alignment parameters exist for evaluation of the cervical spine, T1 slope and C2–7 SVA (measured on long segment lateral X-rays) are most significant for consideration during sagittal reconstruction. Much further study is needed into the complex biomechanics of the cervical spine, a greater understanding of which will lead to improved clinical outcomes.

Take-home Points

- Cervical sagittal balance is an important component of global spinal sagittal balance.

- Cervical spine acts as a compensation mechanism to maintain the horizontal gaze.

- T1 slope and C2–7 SVA are most significant measurements for consideration during sagittal reconstruction.

References

1. Ling FP, Chevillotte T, Leglise A, Thompson W, Bouthors C, Le Huec JC. Which parameters are relevant in sagittal balance analysis of the cervical spine? A literature review. Eur Spine J 2018;27(Suppl 1):8–15

2. Ames CP, Blondel B, Scheer JK, et al. Cervical radiographical alignment: comprehensive assessment techniques and potential importance in cervical myelopathy. Spine 2013; 38(22, Suppl 1):S149–S160

3. Hardacker JW, Shuford RF, Capicotto PN, Pryor PW. Radiographic standing cervical segmental alignment in adult volunteers without neck symptoms. Spine 1997;22(13): 1472–1480, discussion 1480

4. Guo GM, Li J, Diao QX, et al. Cervical lordosis in asymptomatic individuals: a meta-analysis. J Orthop Surg Res 2018;13(1):147

5. Lee SH, Son ES, Seo EM, Suk KS, Kim KT. Factors determining cervical spine sagittal balance in asymptomatic adults: correlation with spinopelvic balance and thoracic inlet alignment. Spine J 2015;15(4):705–712

6. Bao H, Varghese J, Lafage R, et al. Principal radiographic characteristics for cervical spinal deformity: a health-related quality of life analysis. Spine 2017;42(18):1375–1382

7. Iyer S, Nemani VM, Nguyen J, et al. Impact of cervical sagittal alignment parameters on neck disability. Spine 2016;41(5):371–377

8. Kim B, Yoon DH, Ha Y, et al. Relationship between T1 slope and loss of lordosis after laminoplasty in patients with cervical ossification of the posterior longitudinal ligament. Spine J 2016;16(2):219–225

9. Le Huec JC, Charosky S, Barrey C, Rigal J, Aunoble S. Sagittal imbalance cascade for simple degenerative spine and consequences: algorithm of decision for appropriate treatment. Eur Spine J 2011;20(Suppl 5):699–703

10. Tang R, Ye IB, Cheung ZB, Kim JS, Cho SK. Age-related changes in cervical sagittal alignment: a radiographic analysis. Spine 2019;44(19):E1144–E1150

11. Chavanne A, Pettigrew DB, Holtz JR, Dollin N, Kuntz C IV. Spinal cord intramedullary pressure in cervical kyphotic deformity: a cadaveric study. Spine 2011;36(20):1619–1626

12. Farley CW, Curt BA, Pettigrew DB, Holtz JR, Dollin N, Kuntz C IV. Spinal cord intramedullary pressure in thoracic kyphotic deformity: a cadaveric study. Spine 2012;37(4):E224–E230

13. Jarzem PF, Quance DR, Doyle DJ, Begin LR, Kostuik JP. Spinal cord tissue pressure during spinal cord distraction in dogs. Spine 1992;17(8, Suppl):S227–S234

14. Smith JS, Shaffrey CI, Lafage V, et al; International Spine Study Group. Spontaneous improvement of cervical alignment after correction of global sagittal balance following pedicle subtraction osteotomy. J Neurosurg Spine 2012;17(4):300–307

27 Surgery for Cervical Deformity

Toshihiro Takami and Nobuyuki Shimokawa

Introduction

Cervical deformity occurs predominantly as cervical kyphosis.[1,2] Cervical deformity may develop postoperatively or secondary to aging disc degeneration, trauma, neoplasm, infection, or inflammation. Progression of cervical deformity may lead to the aggravation of neurological function or neck pain, although cervical deformity may be relatively asymptomatic. Symptoms associated with cervical deformity include pain, neurological deficits of myelopathy, radiculopathy or both, limitation of horizontal gaze, and problems with appearance. Cervical deformity may also have significant negative impacts on health-related quality of life. Evidence from clinical studies has suggested a relationship between radiographic parameters and health-related quality of life.[3] Surgical correction may be available, but it carries a possible risk of surgery-related complications.[1,4–7] Posterior decompression surgery alone may not be good enough to improve the neurological symptoms. The primary goals of surgery for cervical deformity include neural decompression, deformity correction, and rigid osseous stabilization of the cervical spine with minimal surgery-related complications. This chapter provides a comprehensive discussion of surgery for cervical deformity.

Assessment of Cervical Deformity

Cervical deformity can be evaluated radiologically by careful imaging workup. Cervical deformity is a local structural problem, but it may be significantly affected by other parameters of global sagittal alignment.[8–14] Analysis of cervical local alignment with respect to global sagittal alignment is necessary for spine surgeons to secure the correct diagnosis and solution. The cranial gravity is positioned in the middle of the nasion-inion line, above and slightly in front of the external auditory meatus, just behind the sella turcica.[15] The axis of cranial gravity falls on and passes in front of the cervical spine. The posterior cervical elements of ligaments and paraspinal muscles are the stabilizers that maintain the cervical curvature in healthy subjects. In cases of lordotic cervical spine, the instantaneous axis of rotation of cervical spine (cervical-IAR) is positioned posteriorly in the vertebral body, but in cases of kyphotic cervical spine, cervical-IAR shifts to anterior to the vertebral body.[16–18] The cranial gravity or cervical-IAR may continue to shift anteriorly with structural fatigue of the posterior cervical element and aging disc degeneration.

Imaging parameters of cervical spine have been well discussed in the literature (**Fig. 27.1**). C2–C7 angle is defined between the horizontal line of C2 lower endplate and the horizontal line of C7 lower endplate. Thoracic inlet angle (TIA), stable morphological parameter, is defined as the angle formed by intersection of the line perpendicular to the center of T1 upper endplate and the superior point of sternum. T1 slope (TS) is defined as the angle formed between the horizontal line and the T1 upper endplate. Neck tilt (NT) is defined as the angle formed by the vertical line passing through the superior point of sternum and the line connecting the center of the T1 upper endplate with the superior point of sternum. T1 slope and TIA with respect to cervical sagittal balance may be as important as pelvic incidence (PI) with regard to lumbar lordosis (LL). It has been suggested that C2–C7 sagittal vertical axis (SVA) correlates positively with neck disability index (NDI) scores. The increase of TS results in

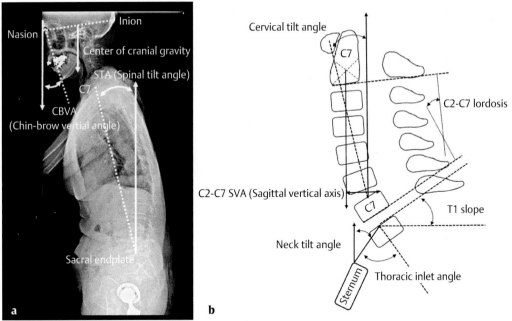

Fig. 27.1 Radiological assessment. **(a)** Relationship between cervical alignment and global spine. **(b)** Radiological parameters of cervical alignment.

C2–C7 lordosis to maintain forward gaze, finally leading to a greater degree of lordotic curvature. Similarly, the increase of TS results in the increase of C2–C7 SVA. TS can change in compensation for thoracolumbar sagittal imbalance. Such a compensatory mechanism of the cervicothoracic spine has been reported to become insufficient when the TS is > 25°. Mizutani et al retrospectively analyzed radiological parameters from patients with symptomatic primary cervical kyphosis and patients with adult thoracolumbar deformity.[19] They showed that global sagittal alignment in symptomatic patients with primary cervical kyphosis was characterized by a posterior shift in the C7 plumb line, small TS and large LL compared to patients with adult thoracolumbar deformity. Lumbar extension with C7 posterior shift would be the essence of compensatory mechanism among symptomatic patients with primary cervical kyphosis. Ames et al proposed a novel classification of cervical deformity.[20] Their classification included a deformity descriptor and five modifiers including sagittal, regional and

global spine alignments and functional condition. The modifiers included C2–C7 SVA, horizontal gaze (chin-brow vertical angle [CBVA]), TS – C2–C7 lordosis (TS – CL), degree of cervical myelopathy, and the Scoliosis Research Society (SRS)–Schwab classification for thoracolumbar deformity. Their classification helps spine surgeons to evaluate cervical deformity within the understanding of global spine alignment and clinical parameters **(Table 27.1)**.

Selection of Surgical Approach and Method

One of the goals of cervical deformity surgery is to obtain occiput–trunk harmony with global spine alignment.[21] Many different surgical options are available for correcting cervical deformity.[1,4–7] However, selection of a better or best approach that can ensure optimal outcomes after surgery is still difficult and often controversial. Cervical deformity usually results in mechanical pain, functional disability, or neurological deficits. Surgical

Table 27.1 Classification of cervical deformity as proposed by Ames et al.[20]

Deformity descriptor	
C	Primary sagittal deformity apex in cervical spine
CT	Primary sagittal deformity apex at cervicothoracic junction
T	Primary sagittal deformity apex in thoracic spine
S	Primary coronal deformity (C2–C7 Cobb angle[3] 15°)
CVJ	Primary cranio-vertebral junction deformity
Modifiers	
1. C2–C7 SVA	
0	C2-C7 SVA < 4 cm
1	C2-C7 SVA = 4–8 cm
2	C2-C7 SVA > 8 cm
2. Horizontal gaze	
0	CBVA = 1–10°
1	CBVA = -10–0° or 11–25°
2	CBVA = < – 10° or > 25°
3. TS – C2–C7 lordosis	
0	TS – CL < 15°
1	TS – CL = 15–20°
2	TS – CL > 20°
4. Myelopathy based on modified JOA score	
0	Normal
1	Mild
2	Moderate
3	Severe
5. Scoliosis Research Society–Schwab classification	
Coronal curve (> 30°)	Thoracic only, thoracolumbar/lumbar only, double curve or no coronal curve
PI – LL mismatch	0: < 10°; +: 10–20°; ++: > 20°
C7 – S1 SVA	0: < 4 cm; +: 4–9.5 cm; ++: > 9.5 cm
Pelvic tilt	0: < 20°; +: 20–30°; ++: > 30°

Abbreviations: CBVA; chin-brow vertical angle; JOA, Japanese Orthopaedic Association score; PI – LL mismatch; pelvic incidence minus lumbar lordosis mismatch; SVA, sagittal vertical axis; TS – CL; T1 slope minus cervical lordosis.

correction of cervical deformity should thus be performed in combination with neural decompression. Cervical fusion in situ without correction may not be desirable for the majority of cases of cervical deformity. Furthermore, correction of C2–C7 angle alone may not be adequate. Surgical indications and selection of surgical techniques (anterior, posterior or combined approach; osteotomy; long or short fusion) should be determined, based on optimizing the balance between patient profile, symptoms or neurological condition and imaging characteristics, including global spinal alignment as briefed below:

- Patient profile: age, social activity, and comorbidity.
- Symptoms: mechanical pain, functional or cosmetic problem.
- Neurological condition: myelopathy, radiculopathy or both.
- Imaging characteristics:
  - Flexible, stiff or rigid spine.
  - Ventral, dorsal compression, or both.
  - Local or diffuse kyphosis.
  - Ankylosed or not ankylosed.
  - Upper thoracic hyperkyphosis.

Based on the radiological assessment, a flexible structure of cervical spine **(Fig. 27.2)** may be well treated by posterior surgery alone. However, anterior and posterior combined surgery with or without osteotomy may be necessary for a relatively rigid (i.e., stiff) or rigid **(Fig. 27.3)** structure of the cervical spine.[22]

An anterior approach for the correction of cervical deformity includes anterior cervical

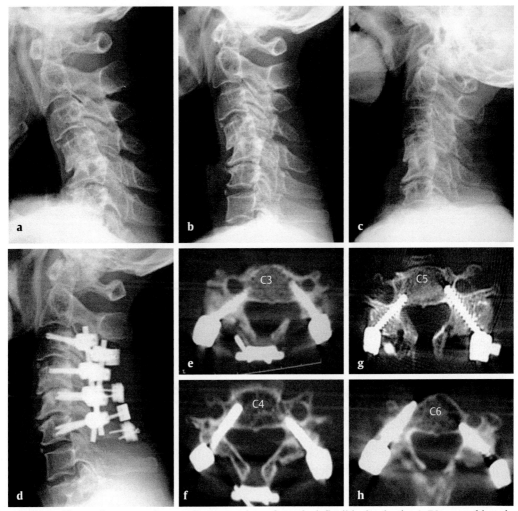

Fig. 27.2 Illustrative case of posterior correction of cervical flexible kyphosis. A 70-year-old male patient presented with severe neck pain and progressive myelopathy. (**a–c**) Preoperative cervical lateral radiographs (**a**), flexion position; (**b**), neutral position; (**c**), extension position. (**d**) Postoperative cervical lateral radiograph. (**e–h**) Postoperative axial images showing correct placement of cervical pedicle screws.

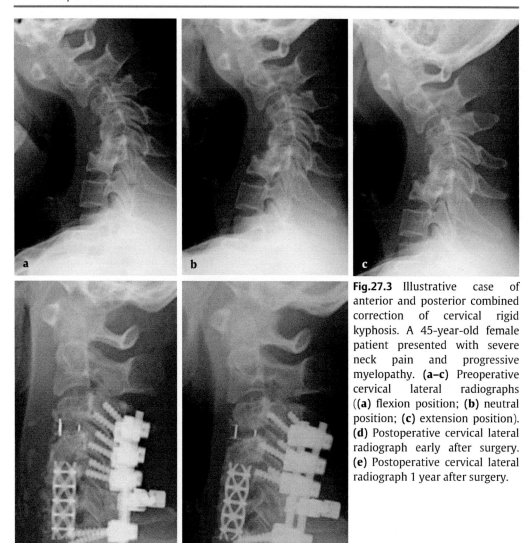

Fig.27.3 Illustrative case of anterior and posterior combined correction of cervical rigid kyphosis. A 45-year-old female patient presented with severe neck pain and progressive myelopathy. **(a–c)** Preoperative cervical lateral radiographs ((**a**) flexion position; (**b**) neutral position; (**c**) extension position). **(d)** Postoperative cervical lateral radiograph early after surgery. **(e)** Postoperative cervical lateral radiograph 1 year after surgery.

discectomy and fusion (ACDF) and anterior corpectomy and fusion (ACCF). ACDF can be applied for cases of flexible cervical kyphosis, and ACCF can be applied to treat fixed-type cervical deformity. However, multilevel ACDF or ACCF for more than three spine levels may be associated with a risk of pseudoarthrosis or instrumentation failure without posterior fusion. The surgical treatment for severe fixed cervical deformity associated with ankylosing spondylitis remains a big challenge for spine surgeons.[23–25] Tokala et al demonstrated their technique of decancellization closing wedge osteotomy of C7 accompanied by secure segmental internal fixation in eight patients.[23] Restoration of normal forward gaze was achieved in all patients. No patient suffered spinal cord injury or permanent nerve root palsy. No loss of correction or pseudoarthrosis was evident at their final follow-up. Hoh et al reported the effective technique of posterior C7–T1 osteotomy, although possible procedure-related complications including subluxation at the osteotomy level, spinal cord injury, radiculopathy, dyspha-gia, and pseudoarthrosis need to be noted.[25] Mummaneni et al demonstrated their surgical results of 30 patients with cervical kyphotic deformity who underwent combined anterior and posterior approaches.[26] Anterior proce-dures included discectomy and corpectomy/ osteotomy at one or more levels with fusion, and posterior procedures included decom-pression and/or osteotomy with lateral mass or pedicle screw fixation. They suggested that surgical management using combined ante-rior and posterior approaches can restore cervical alignment and stabilization, and it can also lead to acceptable improvements in neurological function, although surgery-related complications need to be resolved. Kim et al demonstrated surgical management of fixed cervical deformity using a technique of anterior osteotomy of the cervical spine.[27] Care should be taken during the anterior osteotomy to ensure an uncinate-to-uncinate process resection to allow for complete ante-rior release. Joaquim et al discussed the man-agement of cervical spine deformity after intradural tumor resection.[28] Assessment of the alignment and flexibility of the cervical spine is absolutely necessary to secure the surgical strategy. Although flexible deform-ity can often be treated with an anterior or posterior single approach, rigid deformity should be treated by combined anterior and posterior approaches. Tan et al demonstrated their surgical technique of anterior cervical osteotomy.[29] Anterior cervical osteotomy is effective for correcting rigid cervical deform-ity, although this technique is absolutely technically demanding. Ames et al proposed a universal nomenclature for cervical spine osteotomies.[30] They classified seven ana-tomical grades of increasing extent of bone/ soft-tissue resection and destabilization that can be applied under anterior, posterior, or combined approaches (**Table 27.2**). Grade 1 osteotomy is partial facet joint resection, grade 2 is complete facet joint/Ponte oste-otomy, grade 3 is partial or complete corpec-tomy, grade 4 is complete uncovertebral joint resection to the transverse foramen, grade 5 is opening wedge osteotomy, grade 6 is clos-ing wedge osteotomy, and grade 7 is com-plete vertebral column resection.

Clinical Outcome

The final goal of surgery for cervical deform-ity should be improvement of the patient satisfaction rate and health-related quality of life after surgery with minimum surgery-related complications. Etame et al conducted a review of the literature regarding outcomes after surgery for cervical spine deform-ity.[4] They analyzed 14 retrospective stud-ies involving a total of 399 patients. Surgical intervention included anterior, posterior, or combined approaches. The overall rate of patient satisfaction appeared high. Mortality rates ranged from 3.1% to 6.7%, and the medi-cal complication rate after surgery ranged from 3.1% to 44.4%. The overall neurological

Table 27.2 Osteotomy grade in surgery for cervical deformity as proposed by Ames et al.[29]

Grade	Definition
1	Partial facet joint resection, partial uncovertebral joint resection
2	Complete facet joint resection
3	Partial or complete corpectomy
4	Complete uncovertebral joint resection
5	Opening wedge osteotomy: complete posterior element resection
6	Closing wedge osteotomy: complete posterior element resection and pedicle resection
7	Complete vertebral column resection including complete uncovertebral joint and posterior element resection

complication rate was 13.5%. They suggested that surgery appears to be an effective option when conservative treatments finally fail, although surgery-related complications should be taken into consideration. Roguski et al examined a prospective observational study to determine whether postoperative cervical sagittal balance is an independent factor to predict the health-related quality of life outcomes after surgery for cervical spondylotic myelopathy (CSM).[31] Both pre- and postoperative C2–C7 SVA measurements were independent predictors of clinically significant improvement. Postoperative sagittal balance value correlated inversely with clinically significant improvements in health-related quality of life among patients undergoing posterior surgery, but not among those with anterior surgery. They concluded that pre- and postoperative sagittal balance measurements independently predict clinical outcomes after surgery for CSM. Smith et al examined prospective multicenter study of postoperative complication rates associated with adult cervical deformity surgery in 78 patients.[32] Enrollment required at least one of the following: cervical kyphosis > 10°, cervical scoliosis > 10°, C2–7 SVA > 4 cm, or CBVA > 25°. Surgical approaches included anterior-only (14%), posterior-only (49%), anterior-posterior (35%), and posterior-anterior-posterior (3%) approaches. Twenty-two patients (28.2%) had at least one minor complication, and 19 (24.4%) had at least one major complication. Overall, 34 patients (43.6%) had at least one complication. The most common complications included dysphagia (11.5%), deep wound infection (6.4%), new C5 motor deficit (6.4%), and respiratory failure (5.1%). One death (1.3%) occurred. Postoperative complication rates differed significantly, depending on the choice of surgical approach, at 27.3% for anterior-only, 68.4% for posterior-only, and 79.3% for anterior-posterior/posterior-anterior-posterior (p = .007). Complication rates were significantly higher with combined and posterior-only approaches compared with anterior-only approaches. Ailon conducted a prospective multicenter study with 1-year follow-up of outcomes from surgery for adult cervical deformity.[33] The impact of surgical treatment on health-related quality of life was determined. Fifty-five of the 77 patients (71%) reached 1-year follow-up. Posterior fusion was performed in 85%, and anterior fusion was performed in 53%. Three-column osteotomy was performed in 24% of patients. They demonstrated that surgical treatment resulted in the significant improvement of pain and function. Smith et al also examined a prospective multicenter study of all-cause mortality after surgery for adult cervical deformity.[34] All-cause mortality rate at a mean of 1.2 years after surgery was 9.2% (11 of the 120 patients). Causes of mortality included myocardial infarction (n = 2), pneumonia/cardiopulmonary failure (n = 2), sepsis (n = 1), obstructive sleep apnea/narcotics (n = 1), subsequently diagnosed amyotrophic lateral sclerosis (n = 1), burn injury related to home supplemental oxygen (n = 1), and unknown (n = 3). Deceased patients did not differ significantly from alive patients based on demographic, clinical, or surgical parameters assessed, except for a higher major complication rate (excluding mortality; 63.6% vs. 22.0%, p = 0.006). They suggested that causes of death were reflective of the overall high level of comorbidities. Protopsaltis et al conducted prospective multicenter assessment of radiographic outcomes after adult cervical deformity surgery.[35] A total of 71 patients were included. Factors associated with failure to correct the C2–C7 SVA included revision surgery, worse preoperative C2 pelvic tilt angle, and concurrent thoracolumbar deformity. Failure to correct the TS and cervical lordosis (CL) mismatch was associated with worse preoperative cervical kyphosis and C2 pelvic tilt angle. They also suggested that occurrence of early postoperative distal junctional kyphosis significantly affected postoperative radiographic outcomes.

Conclusion

Cervical deformity surgery is absolutely one of the biggest challenges for spine surgeons. Spine surgeons need to take preoperative evaluations into serious consideration when determining the surgical indications and selection of surgical techniques. Cervical deformity surgery may carry a high risk of surgery-related complications, leading to the aggravation of health-related quality of life after surgery. Spine surgeons need to evaluate the overall severity of the underlying conditions before surgery in every single patient, and try to consider the surgical strategy to secure safe surgery. To make cervical deformity surgery a much more reliable and convincing entity, the spine surgeons face great challenges.

Take-home Points

- Cervical deformity may develop postoperatively or secondary to aging disc degeneration, trauma, neoplasm, infection, or inflammation. Cervical deformity may also have significant negative impacts on not only activity of daily living but also health-related quality of life.

- Based on the radiological assessment, a flexible structure of cervical spine may be well treated by posterior surgery alone. However, anterior and posterior combined surgery with or without osteotomy may be necessary for a relatively rigid (i.e., stiff) or rigid structure of the cervical spine.

- Cervical deformity surgery may carry a high risk of surgery-related complications. To make cervical deformity surgery a much more reliable and convincing entity, the spine surgeons face great challenges.

References

1. Steinmetz MP, Stewart TJ, Kager CD, Benzel EC, Vaccaro AR. Cervical deformity correction. Neurosurgery 2007; 60(1, Suppl 1):S90–S97
2. Tan LA, Riew KD, Traynelis VC. Cervical spine deformity-part 1: biomechanics, radiographic parameters, and classification. Neurosurgery 2017;81(2):197–203
3. Scheer JK, Tang JA, Smith JS, et al; International Spine Study Group. Cervical spine alignment, sagittal deformity, and clinical implications: a review. J Neurosurg Spine 2013;19(2):141–159
4. Etame AB, Wang AC, Than KD, La Marca F, Park P. Outcomes after surgery for cervical spine deformity: review of the literature. Neurosurg Focus 2010;28(3):E14
5. Tan LA, Riew KD, Traynelis VC. Cervical spine deformity-part 2: management algorithm and anterior techniques. Neurosurgery 2017;81(4):561–567
6. Tan LA, Riew KD, Traynelis VC. Cervical spine deformity-part 3: posterior techniques, clinical outcome, and complications. Neurosurgery 2017;81(6):893–898
7. Dru AB, Lockney DT, Vaziri S, et al. Cervical spine deformity correction techniques. Neurospine 2019;16(3):470–482
8. Vialle R, Levassor N, Rillardon L, Templier A, Skalli W, Guigui P. Radiographic analysis of the sagittal alignment and balance of the spine in asymptomatic subjects. J Bone Joint Surg Am 2005;87(2):260–267
9. Knott PT, Mardjetko SM, Techy F. The use of the T1 sagittal angle in predicting overall sagittal balance of the spine. Spine J 2010;10(11):994–998
10. Roussouly P, Pinheiro-Franco JL. Biomechanical analysis of the spino-pelvic organization and adaptation in pathology. Eur Spine J 2011;20(Suppl 5):609–618
11. Smith JS, Shaffrey CI, Lafage V, et al; International Spine Study Group. Spontaneous improvement of cervical alignment after correction of global sagittal balance following pedicle subtraction osteotomy. J Neurosurg Spine 2012;17(4):300–307
12. Ames CP, Blondel B, Scheer JK, et al. Cervical radiographical alignment: comprehensive assessment techniques and potential importance in cervical myelopathy. Spine 2013; 38(22, Suppl 1):S149–S160
13. Kim TH, Lee SY, Kim YC, Park MS, Kim SW. T1 slope as a predictor of kyphotic alignment change after laminoplasty in patients with cervical myelopathy. Spine 2013;38(16):E992–E997
14. Yamagata T, Chataigner H, Longis PM, Takami T, Delecrin J. Posterior instrumented fusion

surgery for adult spinal deformity: Correction rate and total balance. J Craniovertebr Junction Spine 2019;10(2):100–107

15. Vital JM, Senegas J. Anatomical bases of the study of the constraints to which the cervical spine is subject in the sagittal plane. A study of the center of gravity of the head. Surg Radiol Anat 1986;8(3):169–173

16. Dimnet J, Pasquet A, Krag MH, Panjabi MM. Cervical spine motion in the sagittal plane: kinematic and geometric parameters. J Biomech 1982;15(12):959–969

17. Amevo B, Aprill C, Bogduk N. Abnormal instantaneous axes of rotation in patients with neck pain. Spine 1992;17(7):748–756

18. Anderst W, Baillargeon E, Donaldson W, Lee J, Kang J. Motion path of the instant center of rotation in the cervical spine during in vivo dynamic flexion-extension: implications for artificial disc design and evaluation of motion quality after arthrodesis. Spine 2013;38(10):E594–E601

19. Mizutani J, Verma K, Endo K, et al. Global spinal alignment in cervical kyphotic deformity: the importance of head position and thoracolumbar alignment in the compensatory mechanism. Neurosurgery 2018;82(5):686–694

20. Ames CP, Smith JS, Eastlack R, et al; International Spine Study Group. Reliability assessment of a novel cervical spine deformity classification system. J Neurosurg Spine 2015;23(6):673–683

21. Mizutani J, Strom R, Abumi K, et al. How cervical reconstruction surgery affects global spinal alignment. Neurosurgery 2019;84(4):898–907

22. Bohoun CA, Naito K, Yamagata T, Tamrakar S, Ohata K, Takami T. Safety and accuracy of spinal instrumentation surgery in a hybrid operating room with an intraoperative cone-beam computed tomography. Neurosurg Rev 2019;42(2):417–426

23. Tokala DP, Lam KS, Freeman BJ, Webb JK. C7 decancellisation closing wedge osteotomy for the correction of fixed cervico-thoracic kyphosis. Eur Spine J 2007;16(9):1471–1478

24. Khoueir P, Hoh DJ, Wang MY. Use of hinged rods for controlled osteoclastic correction of a fixed cervical kyphotic deformity in

ankylosing spondylitis. J Neurosurg Spine 2008;8(6):579–583

25. Hoh DJ, Khoueir P, Wang MY. Management of cervical deformity in ankylosing spondylitis. Neurosurg Focus 2008;24(1):E9

26. Mummaneni PV, Dhall SS, Rodts GE, Haid RW. Circumferential fusion for cervical kyphotic deformity. J Neurosurg Spine 2008; 9(6):515–521

27. Kim HJ, Piyaskulkaew C, Riew KD. Anterior cervical osteotomy for fixed cervical deformities. Spine 2014;39(21):1751–1757

28. Joaquim AF, Riew KD. Management of cervical spine deformity after intradural tumor resection. Neurosurg Focus 2015;39(2):E13

29. Tan LA, Riew KD. Anterior cervical osteotomy: operative technique. Eur Spine J 2018; 27(Suppl 1):39–47

30. Ames CP, Smith JS, Scheer JK, et al; International Spine Study Group. A standardized nomenclature for cervical spine soft-tissue release and osteotomy for deformity correction: clinical article. J Neurosurg Spine 2013;19(3):269–278

31. Roguski M, Benzel EC, Curran JN, et al. Postoperative cervical sagittal imbalance negatively affects outcomes after surgery for cervical spondylotic myelopathy. Spine 2014;39(25):2070–2077

32. Smith JS, Ramchandran S, Lafage V, et al; International Spine Study Group. Prospective multicenter assessment of early complication rates associated with adult cervical deformity surgery in 78 patients. Neurosurgery 2016;79(3):378–388

33. Ailon T, Smith JS, Shaffrey CI, et al; International Spine Study Group. Outcomes of operative treatment for adult cervical deformity: a prospective multicenter assessment with 1-year follow-up. Neurosurgery 2018;83(5):1031–1039

34. Smith JS, Shaffrey CI, Kim HJ, et al; International Spine Study Group. Prospective multicenter assessment of all-cause mortality following surgery for adult cervical deformity. Neurosurgery 2018;83(6):1277–1285

35. Protopsaltis TS, Ramchandran S, Hamilton DK, et al; International Spine Study Group (ISSG). Analysis of successful versus failed radiographic outcomes after cervical deformity surgery. Spine 2018;43(13):E773–E781

28 Recommendations for Cervical Spondylotic Myelopathy and OPLL

Mehmet Zileli and Jutty Parthiban

Introduction

The Spine Committee of the World Federation of Neurosurgical Societies (WFNS) formulated a consensus meeting on the management of cervical spondylotic myelopathy (CSM) to develop recommendations for global applicability during the Annual Conference of Neuro Spinal Surgeons Association at Nagpur, India, in September 2018. Seventeen topics were selected and presentations were done. Each topic at the end had prioritized questions and multiple answers, and consensus statements were finalized following voting from members and specialists using the Delphi method. The topics on discussion were later conjugated in five groups and the statements were published as five articles in the Neurospine Journal in 2019. The title of the articles were as follows: 1. Natural course and the value of diagnostic techniques, 2. Value of surgery and nonsurgical approaches, 3. Anterior surgical techniques, 4. Posterior surgical techniques, and 5. Outcome measures and variables affecting prognosis. The recommendations and statements published on CSM are stated below:[1–5]

Recommendations for Clinical Presentation of Cervical Spondylotic Myelopathy (CSM)

- Myelopathic signs (hyperreflexia, inverted brachioradialis reflex, Hoffmann sign, Babinski and clonus) are an integral component of clinical diagnosis of cervical myelopathy. However, they are not very sensitive and may be absent in about 20% of myelopathic patients.
- Individual myelopathic signs taken alone cannot diagnose cervical myelopathy in all patients, but at least one is present in severe myelopathy.
- Clinical diagnosis of CSM relies heavily on characteristic symptoms and signs elicited during history and physical examination, which prompt further investigation with cervical spine imaging.
- In severe myelopathic patients, after laminoplasty, major recovery in myelopathic signs occurs during the first 6 months and thereafter it plateaus.
- In patients with myelopathic signs, if there are no alternative explanations, a combination of clinical symptoms and imaging studies must form the basis of our treatment decisions. The absence of myelopathic signs does not preclude the diagnosis of CSM nor its successful surgical treatment.

Recommendations for Natural Course of CSM

- The natural course of patients with cervical stenosis and signs of myelopathy greatly vary.[1]
- Progression of the disease is possible, but prediction of those patients is not well known. Some patients may remain static for lengthy periods, and some patients with severe disability can improve without treatment.

- For patients with no symptoms but having significant stenosis (premyelopathic), risk of developing myelopathy with cervical stenosis is approximately 3% per year.

Recommendations for Value of Electrophysiology

- Electrophysiological tests to be used in CSM patients are as follows (in order of benefits): motor-evoked potential (MEP), spinal cord-evoked potential (SCEP), somatosensory-evoked potential (SEP), and electromyography (EMG).[1]
- Routine electrophysiological tests are useful in differential diagnosis of CSM from other neurological conditions. However, especially during the early course of the disease, differential diagnosis is very difficult; specific tests are necessary and mild forms of amyotrophic lateral sclerosis (ALS) and polyneuropathy may not be differentiated easily.
- Although MEP and SEP have been found as valuable tests to predict outcomes of CSM surgery, there is no evidence that they are more valuable than clinical parameters.
- Electrophysiological tests may have better outcome predictions than MR changes.
- Electrophysiological tests are not very useful in monitoring lower extremity power, and the value of monitoring during anterior cervical discectomy and fusion (ACDF) surgery is questionable.
- EMG and MEP monitoring have been found to be useful, in order to decrease C5 root palsy during CSM surgery.
- Intraoperative MEP/SEP worsening is not specific, and it does not show clinical worsening in every incidence. Intraoperative MEP/SEP changes do not necessarily prevent neurological injury and improve the outcomes.

Recommendations for Value of Canal Diameters in CT and MRI

- In spite of conflicting evidence, MRI morphometric analysis of the spine has a significant role in evaluation and prognostication of CSM, and it should be included in the preoperative workup.
- Among the many variables assessed using MRI, compression ratio (CR), maximum canal compromise (MCC) and transverse area (TA) are most importantly correlated with functional outcomes following surgery in patients with CSM. Each parameter has its own strengths and limitations; therefore, a combined assessment of MR parameters has a greater predictive yield.

Recommendations for Value of Signal Intensity Changes in MRI

- Intense spinal cord T2 hyperintensity on cervical MRI may be correlated with a worse outcome in CSM.
- Patients with lighter signal changes in T2 on cervical MRI should not be excluded from surgical treatment of CSM.
- More studies are needed to validate proposed grading systems, or to create new ones.
- T1 hyposignal should be considered as a sign of more advanced disease, with worse outcome.
- More studies are needed to assess the effect of sagittal and axial extension of T1 signal changes on outcome.

Recommendations for New Imaging Techniques for CSM

- Diffusion MRI, MR spectroscopy, and dynamic MRI (dMRI) may be a part of MR examinations for CSM protocol apart from conventional MRI. Authors suggest their usage for outcome studies. With data pooling of clinical and imaging findings, we will be able to prognosticate better and identify patients earlier before the changes and permanent damage sets in.[1]

Recommendations for Value of Surgery and Nonsurgical Approaches for CSM

- WFNS Spine Committee endorses the guidelines of Fehlings and coworkers. The new and adapted WFNS Spine Committee Recommendations after consensus are summarized below:[2]
- For patients with moderate and severe CSM, surgical intervention is recommended. We recommend using modified Japanese Orthopedic Association (mJOA) scale or its regional modifications to classify CSM as severe, moderate, or mild.
- We suggest offering surgical intervention or rehabilitation for patients with mild CSM (mJOA score 15–17). If at the beginning nonoperative management was followed, we recommend operative intervention when rapid progression of symptoms appear. Nonoperative management may be considered for slowly progressive disease.
- Nonmyelopathic patients with radiologic evidence of cord compression but without signs and symptoms of radiculopathy should not be offered a prophylactic surgery. These patients should be counselled about the potential risk of worsening, educated about the signs and symptoms of progression, and followed-up clinically regularly. An informed consent should be obtained about neurological deficits that may follow trivial injury.
- Nonmyelopathic patients with radiologic evidence of cord compression

and with clinical evidence of radiculopathy are potential candidates who may deteriorate, thus carrying high risk, and hence need to be counselled about it. These patients are recommended to undergo surgery or close observation with rehabilitation if they refuse to undergo surgery. In the event of developing myelopathic signs, they are advised to go for surgery at the earliest. An informed consent should be obtained about neurological deficits that may follow trivial injury.

- There is a consistent lack of evidence regarding the value of nonoperative treatment of cervical myelopathy in the literature. Hence, nonoperative treatment may not be the final decision in most cases.
- Predicting factors that indicate a possible deterioration during nonoperative management are as follows: circumferential cord compression in axial MRI, reduced diameter of cerebrospinal fluid (CSF) space, hypermobility of spinal segment, angular-edged deformity, instability, greater angle of vertebral slip, lower segmental lordotic angle, and presence of ossification of the posterior longitudinal ligament (OPLL).
- Important predictors of myelopathy development include the presence of symptomatic radiculopathy, prolonged MEPs and SEPs, and EMG signs of anterior horn cell lesions (low evidence).
- Duration of symptoms has a greater impact on outcomes. Substantial delay in surgical management leads to suboptimal outcome. In other words, patients are likely to achieve a better result after surgery if they have a shorter duration of symptoms (low evidence).
- As there is still clinical equipoise between surgery and conservative treatment in mild CSM, the WFNS Spine Committee strongly encourages randomized controlled trials comparing surgical versus nonsurgical

interventions in mild CSM. There is also a need to analyze the cost effectiveness, standardized methodology, and costs of long-term follow-up in mild CSM.

Recommendations for Surgical Indications for Treatment of CSM

- In patients with CSM, the indications for surgery include persistent or recurrent radiculopathy nonresponsive to conservative treatment (3 years); progressive neurological deficit; static neurological deficit with severe radicular pain when associated with confirmatory imaging (CT, MRI); and clinical-radiological correlation.[2]
- The indications of anterior surgery for patients with CSM include straightened spine or kyphotic spine with a compression level below three.

Recommendations for Comparison of Anterior Surgical Techniques for CSM

- There are many options for anterior decompression such as ACDF, anterior cervical corpectomy and fusion (ACCF), oblique corpectomy (OC), skip corpectomy, and hybrid surgery.[3]
- A corpectomy is a good option for a ventral compression of less than three vertebral segments, where a single-level disc and osteophyte excision are inadequate to decompress the cord in patients with CSM. In cases with a kyphotic deformity of the cervical spine, corpectomy can restore the normal lordotic curvature alignment.
- In cases of a multisegment disease with contiguous multisegment thecal compression, alternate segment discectomy/osteophyte removal while keeping the body of the intervening vertebra intact is biomechanically

more stable than a complete corpectomy with contiguous segment discectomy.

Recommendations for Endoscopic and Partial Corpectomy Procedures

- An oblique partial corpectomy can improve the sagittal canal diameter substantially. However, this procedure may be difficult to perform in cases with bilateral radiculopathy. If there is significant instability, OC should not be chosen.
- The incidence of the Horner's syndrome due to unilateral disruption of the sympathetic chain has decreased to less than 5% by some modifications in surgical technique.

Recommendations for CSM in Elderly

- In the elderly age groups with bony ankylosis due to osteophytes at C5–6–7, CSM may manifest at higher levels, where motion segments are preserved, especially the C3–4 level and also at lower levels such as the C7–T1 level.

Recommendations for Complications of Anterior Surgeries for CSM

- Reported complications resulting from anterior surgeries for CSM are quite variable. Approach-related complications (dysphagia, dysphonia, esophageal injury, respiratory distress, etc.) are more often than neurologic and implant-related complications. With appropriate choice of implants and meticulous surgical technique, the surgical complications should be seen only rarely.[3]

Recommendations for Success Rate of Anterior Surgeries for CSM

- Improvement after anterior surgery for CSM has been reported in 70% to 80% of patients. JOA recovery rates are around 60% to 70%.[3]
- There is no significant difference of success rates with ACDF, ACCF, and OC.
- ACDF is generally associated with less intraoperative blood loss and less operative complications than ACCF. The functional outcomes, using Odom's criteria, JOA, neck disability index (NDI), are reported to be the same.

Recommendations for Selection of Surgical Approach

- There are several factors that should be considered for selection of surgical approach in patients with CSM: sagittal curvature, locations of the compressive pathology, number of levels involved, and patient comorbidities.

Recommendations for Posterior Surgical Approaches for CSM

- Posterior surgical decompression is an effective technique in improving the neurological function of patients with CSM.[4]
- Posterior surgical techniques for CSM consist of laminectomy alone, laminectomy with fusion, and laminoplasty. These techniques are often used if there are three or more levels of anterior compressions. However, in cases with significant posterior compression at 1 or 2 levels, posterior decompressive surgeries are mandatory.
- The relative merit of different posterior decompression techniques has not been well determined. In kyphotic cases, especially if it is a flexible kyphosis, laminectomy and posterior fixation with fusion should be chosen. However, in rigid kyphosis, an anterior surgery combined with a posterior decompression should be preferred. In cases with preserved lordosis, laminoplasty is a good option. Cases with severe axial neck pain should not be a candidate for laminoplasty. However, there are always gray zone cases, such as straightened cervical spine, in which we do not know for sure which approach is better.

- Combined approach should be chosen in patients with significant ventral and dorsal osteophytic compression, which cannot be handled holistically with a single anterior or posterior surgery.
- Multiple factors must be taken into account when deciding on the appropriate operation for a particular patient. Surgeons need to tailor their preoperative discussion to alert patients about these facts.

Recommendations for Complications of Posterior Surgeries for CSM

- Complications resulting from posterior surgeries for CSM include injury to spinal cord and nerve roots, implant-related complications, C5 palsy, spring-back closure of lamina after laminoplasty, and postlaminectomy kyphosis.[4]

Recommendations for Success Rate of Posterior Surgeries for CSM

- In comparing laminectomy to laminoplasty, there is a trend toward laminoplasty being better than traditional laminectomy but relatively equivalent to newer techniques of minimally invasive skip laminectomies.

Recommendations for Future Directions about Surgical Approaches

- Current knowledge is deficient, especially considering the cost-to-benefit analysis of various surgical approaches, comparative efficacy of surgical approaches using various techniques, and long-term follow-up to determine outcomes. Therefore, continued research into outcomes of cervical spine surgery is essential.
- Since randomized controlled studies are very difficult to conduct in spine surgery, prospective registries with long-term follow-up will be important for our future decisions.

Recommendations for Outcome Measures for CSM

- There are a variety of outcome measures used for CSM. As functional measures, we recommend mJOA scale, Nurick's grade, and myelopathy disability index (MDI).[5]
- Walking tests can be used for quantitative measurements, and short form 36 (SF-36) is a good functional quality life measure.

Recommendations for Clinical Variables of Outcome

- Three clinical variables that are most commonly related with CSM are age, duration of symptoms, and severity of the myelopathy at presentation. Greater the age, the longer the duration of symptoms, and the more severe symptoms at presentation, the more adverse outcomes can be expected after surgery.[5]

- However, examination findings require more detailed study to validate their effect on the outcomes of surgery. The predictive variables which were studied and seemed to affect the outcomes in CSM are hand atrophy, leg spasticity, clonus and Babinski's sign.

Recommendations for Radiological Variables on Outcomes

- Cervical alignment parameters are correlated with general health scores and myelopathy severity. The curvature of the cervical spine has been found to be one of the most important variables.
- Cervical spine kyphosis predicts worse outcomes. Neurological improvement is significant in patients with normal cervical lordosis.
- Instability of the cervical spine is predictive for outcomes. In patients with single segmental CSM with instability, longer duration of symptoms, lower preoperative JOA score, and more preoperative physical signs, are highly predictive of a poor surgical outcome.
- Spinal cord compression ratio is a critical factor for prognosis of CSM. However, AP diameter of the spinal canal has no clinical significance.
- Spinal cord atrophy cannot predict outcomes.
- High-signal intensity on T2-weighted MR images is a negative predictor for prognosis.

Recommendations for Surgical Variables on Outcomes

- Surgery should be done from anterior or posterior if the disease is focal (one or two levels).[5]
- If the anterior compression is more than 2 levels, or if it is a diffuse narrowing, posterior decompression should better be chosen.

- The most important factor on decision-making in cases with multilevel (more than 2) CSM is cervical sagittal vertical axis.

Take-home Points

- Clinical diagnosis should be made heavily by symptoms and signs. Further investigation with imaging is then necessary.

- Prediction of progressive disease cannot be done easily with imaging or electrophysiology.

- Premyelopathic patients (no symptoms but having significant stenosis) risk of developing myelopathy is approximately 3% per year.

- Intense spinal cord T2 hyperintensity on cervical MRI is a sign of worse outcome.

- Moderate and severe CSM patients should better be operated.

- The most important factor on decision-making in multilevel cases is cervical sagittal vertical axis.

References

1. Zileli M, Borkar SA, Sinha S, et al. Cervical Spondylotic Myelopathy: Natural Course and the Value of Diagnostic Techniques -WFNS Spine Committee Recommendations. Neurospine 2019;16(3):386–402

2. Parthiban J, Alves OL, Chandrachari KP, Ramani P, Zileli M. Value of Surgery and Nonsurgical Approaches for Cervical Spondylotic Myelopathy: WFNS Spine Committee Recommendations. Neurospine 2019;16(3):403–407

3. Deora H, Kim S-H, Behari S, et al; World Federation of Neurosurgical Societies (WFNS) Spine Committee. Anterior Surgical Techniques for Cervical Spondylotic Myelopathy: WFNS Spine Committee Recommendations. Neurospine 2019;16(3):408–420

4. Bajamal AH, Kim S-H, Arifianto MR, et al; World Federation of Neurosurgical Societies (WFNS) Spine Committee. Posterior Surgical Techniques for Cervical Spondylotic Myelopathy: WFNS Spine Committee Recommendations. Neurospine 2019;16(3):421–434

5. Zileli M, Maheshwari S, Kale SS, Garg K, Menon SK, Parthiban J. Outcome Measures and Variables Affecting Prognosis of Cervical Spondylotic Myelopathy: WFNS Spine Committee Recommendations. Neurospine 2019;16(3):435–447

6. Fehlings, M. G., Kwon, B. K. and Tetreault, L. A. Guidelines for the management of degenerative cervical myelopathy and spinal cord injury: an introduction to a focus issue. Global Spine Journal, 7(3S), 2017, pp. 65–75

Index